Dietary Fiber in Human Nutrition

Dietary Fiber in Human Nutrition

Editor: Albie Copeland

FOSTER
ACADEMICS
www.fosteracademics.com

www.fosteracademics.com

FOSTER ACADEMICS

Cataloging-in-Publication Data

Dietary fiber in human nutrition / edited by Albie Copeland.
p. cm.
Includes bibliographical references and index.
ISBN 978-1-64646-565-1
1. Fiber in human nutrition. 2. Nutrition. 3. Diet therapy. I. Copeland, Albie.
QP144.F52 D54 2023
612.3--dc23

Foster Academics,
118-35 Queens Blvd., Suite 400,
Forest Hills, NY 11375, USA

ISBN 978-1-64646-565-1 (Hardback)

Contents

Preface

Every book is initially just a concept; it takes months of research and hard work to give it the final shape in which the readers receive it. In its early stages, this book also went through rigorous reviewing. The notable contributions made by experts from across the globe were first molded into patterned chapters and then arranged in a sensibly sequential manner to bring out the best results.

Fiber is made up of the indigestible parts or compounds of plants that remain unchanged when they pass through the stomach and intestines in the human digestive system. There are two types of fiber, namely, soluble fiber and insoluble fiber. Wholegrain cereals, fruits, and vegetables are considered as a good source of dietary fiber. It is crucial for keeping the gut healthy and reducing the risk of chronic health conditions. There are several benefits of a high-fiber diet. It normalizes the bowel movements by softening and increasing the weight and size of the stool. Soluble fibers present in beans, oats and flaxseeds can help reduce cholesterol levels. In diabetic patients, soluble fiber can slow the absorption of sugar and help in the regulation of blood sugar levels. Consumption of dietary fiber is beneficial in gastrointestinal disorders such as colorectal ulcer, hiatal hernias, gastroesophageal reflux disease, diverticular disease, and hemorrhoids. This book unravels the recent studies related to dietary fiber and its nutritional importance for human health. It will prove to be immensely beneficial to medical students and researchers engaged in this area of study.

It has been my immense pleasure to be a part of this project and to contribute my years of learning in such a meaningful form. I would like to take this opportunity to thank all the people who have been associated with the completion of this book at any step.

Editor

1

Role of Dietary Nutrients in the Modulation of Gut Microbiota

Qi Yang [1,2,†], Qi Liang [2,3,†], Biju Balakrishnan [2], Damien P Belobrajdic [4], Qian-Jin Feng [3] and Wei Zhang [2,*]

1 Center for Marine Drugs, State Key Laboratory of Oncogene and Related Genes, Department of Pharmacy, Renji Hospital, School of Medicine, Shanghai Jiao Tong University, Shanghai 200127, China; qi.yang@flinders.edu.au

2 Centre for Marine Biopro ducts Development, College of Medicine and Public Health, Flinders University, Adelaide, South Australia 5042, Australia; qi.liang@flinders.edu.au (Q.L.); biju.balakrishnan@flinders.edu.au (B.B.)

3 Shanxi University of Chinese Medicine, Tai Yuan 030619, China; fqj728119@aliyun.com

4 CSIRO Health and Biosecurity, Adelaide South Australia 5000, Australia; damien.belobrajdic@csiro.au

* Correspondence: wei.zhang@flinders.edu.au

† These authors have equal contribution and should be considered as co-first authors.

Abstract: Understanding how dietary nutrients modulate the gut microbiome is of great interest for the development of food products and eating patterns for combatting the global burden of non-communicable diseases. In this narrative review we assess scientific studies published from 2005 to 2019 that evaluated the effect of micro- and macro-nutrients on the composition of the gut microbiome using in vitro and in vivo models, and human clinical trials. The clinical evidence for micronutrients is less clear and generally lacking. However, preclinical evidence suggests that red wine- and tea-derived polyphenols and vitamin D can modulate potentially beneficial bacteria. Current research shows consistent clinical evidence that dietary fibers, including arabinoxylans, galacto-oligosaccharides, inulin, and oligofructose, promote a range of beneficial bacteria and suppress potentially detrimental species. The preclinical evidence suggests that both the quantity and type of fat modulate both beneficial and potentially detrimental microbes, as well as the Firmicutes/Bacteroides ratio in the gut. Clinical and preclinical studies suggest that the type and amount of proteins in the diet has substantial and differential effects on the gut microbiota. Further clinical investigation of the effect of micronutrients and macronutrients on the microbiome and metabolome is warranted, along with understanding how this influences host health.

Keywords: micronutrient; macronutrient; gut; microbiome; nutrition; health; diet; review

---

1. Introduction

Over the past two decades a plethora of studies have identified broad-spanning associated links between the gut microbiota and systemic health and disease risk [1–3]. Earlier, it was estimated that the human body harbors about 10^{14}–10^{15} microbial cells [4–6], which is thought to outnumber host cells in the human body by a ratio of at least 10:1 [7]. This was refuted recently, with an estimate that the ratio is much closer to 1:1 [6]. Importantly, the human microbiome is far more diverse than that of human cells, which adds to the complexity in trying to understand how the microbes and their metabolites effect health and modulate the development of disease [8]. This challenged the researchers to explore the roles of the human microbiota and their potential applications in managing human health and disease conditions.

The large intestine is the predominant location where microbes are present in the human gut and our understanding of the composition, interaction, and functions of these gut microbes [9] continues to develop as a result of advancement in major initiatives that have categorized the microbiome [1,10–13]. The human gut microbiome is highly dynamic during the various stages of human development and has been implicated in a variety of health and disease conditions. There are many factors that contribute to shaping the gut microbial colonization, growth, composition, and diversity. The major factors that impact microbial colonization and diversity include age [14], genetics [15–17], mode of delivery at birth [18,19], method of feeding in infants [20,21], medications (e.g., antibiotics), [22,23] geographical location [24], and the diet [25]. Metagenomics studies in a Dutch population have shown associations between gut microbiota and 126 exogenous factors, 31 intrinsic factors, 12 diseases, 19 drug groups, 4 smoking categories, and 60 dietary factors [26]. The responses of the gut microbiota to sensitive factors are considered to be a valuable tool to exploit and develop new strategies to promote human health. Among these influential factors, dietary factors, including micro- and macro-nutrients, are the most influential in shaping and modulating the human gut microbiota [27].

Interactions between the intestinal microbiota and the host are crucial to understand the role of the microbiota in biological processes, and how they contribute to health and the development of disease. Microbial diversity measures the distribution of different species on the community, the level of which is reduced during gut dysbiosis, and a richness of species indicates a "healthy gut" [28–30]. Lower bacterial diversity was reported in people suffering from inflammatory bowel disease, Type 2 diabetes (T2DM), and Coeliac disease. Recent studies have identified the dominance of some groups of gut microbes that are associated with a good health outcome [28–30], and these microbes are presented in this review as "potential beneficial microbes", that include major species from the genera *Bifidobacterium, Lactobacillus, Akkermansia, Fecalibacterium, Eubacterium, Roseburia, Ruminococcus,* and *Blautia.* Studies have also reported the abundance of specific bacteria that could potentially contribute to the development or progression of major non-communicable diseases and these microbes are presented in this review as "potential detrimental microbes", that include some species from the genera *Clostridium, Enterobacter, Enterococcus, Bacteoidetes,* and *Ruminococcus* [31–33]. Both human and animal studies report that an increase in the Firmicutes to Bacteroidetes ratio (F/B ratio) is associated with obese/lean phenotypes and may modulate energy balance [34,35].

The aim of this narrative review was to assess scientific studies that evaluated the effect of micro- and macro-nutrients on the composition of the gut microbiome using in vitro and in vivo models, and human clinical trials. Scientific studies published between 2005 and 2019 in the databases of PubMed, Scopus, and Web of Science were identified using specific search terms (Supplementary Table S1). Publications that did not specifically quantify changes in gut microbiota were excluded, resulting in a total of 213 articles that were selected for preparing this review. The major findings relating to the microbiome, including the shifts in potentially beneficial and detrimental gut microbiota, the F/B ratio, and microbial diversity, are discussed in this review. The studies reviewed included in vitro and in vivo models and human clinical trials (in that order whenever available) and were separated based on micro- and macro-nutrients.

2. Role of Dietary Micronutrients in Modulating Gut Microbiota

2.1. Polyphenols

Polyphenols, such as flavonoids, phenolic acids, stilbenes, and lignans [36] from fruits, vegetables, cereals, tea, coffee, and wine [37], have attracted research interest due to their potential anti-oxidative, anti-inflammatory, and anti-carcinogenic effects [38]. In vitro studies suggest that polyphenols could modulate human gut microbiota by inhibiting potential pathogenic organisms (such as *Helicobacter pylori, Staphylococcus* sp.) and favoring the growth of potential beneficial members, including *Lactobacillus* and *Bifidobacteria* [39,40]. Animal and clinical trials show that polyphenols can modulate gut microbes, microbial diversity, and the ratio of Firmicutes to Bacteroidetes (F/B) [41–44]. These and other studies have suggested that the prebiotic-like activities of polyphenols are the major reason behind the health benefits imparted by polyphenols in humans [45]. Herein, we discuss in vitro, animal, and clinical trial data that evaluated the effect of polyphenols on gut microbes, microbial diversity, and F/B ratio, and the major findings are summarized in Table 1.

In vitro studies have shown that flavonoids such as anthocyanins, phenolic acids (epicatechins, *p*-coumaric acid, and *o*-coumaric acid), and other polyphenols like quercetin, rutin, chlorogenic acid, and caffeic acid could increase the abundance of beneficial gut microbiota, such as *Bifidobacterium* and *Lactobacillus,* and decrease the number of potential pathogenic bacterial colonization in the human gut [39,40,46,47]. Catechins have also been shown to stimulate the growth of the *Clostridium coccoides-Eubacterium rectale* group, *Bifidobacterium* sp., and *Escherichia coli* and inhibit the growth of a potential pathogenic organism (*Clostridium hystolyticum* group) [48]. Fermentation of polyphenols increases the abundance of beneficial microbiota such as *Bifidobacteria* and reduces the F/B ratio by promoting the growth of specific members of the phylum *Bacteroidetes* [49]. It was proposed that the bio-transformed polyphenols promoted the production of short chain fatty acids (SCFAs), which are well recognized as playing an important role in gut and metabolic health [50]. By utilizing agar plate assays, Naringenin, a flavone present in citrus fruits, modulated the growth and genetic regulation of gut commensal bacteria [51]. Ethyl acetate/water polyphenol extract of Yunnan Chinese tea was reported to inhibit the growth of unfavorable bacteria species (*Clostridium* and *Bacteroides*) in vitro [52].

Preclinical studies have shown consistent evidence that a range of different polyphenols improve various measures of health by modulating gut microbiota. In animals fed a High-Fat Diet (HFD) or control background diets, polyphenols including grape [53], pomegranate peel [54], red wine [55], and green tea [56] have been shown to increase the abundance of fecal *Bifidobacteria* and *Lactobacilli*. Axling et al. (2012) [56] also found that green tea powder along with *Lactobacillus plantarum* could significantly increase bacterial diversity and increase the abundance of *Lactobacillus* and *Akkermansia* in the colon of mice [56]. The fecal microbiome of rats fed with blackberry anthocyanin rich extracts were found to have increased abundance of *Psudoflavonifractor* when compared to the standard control diet, whereas in the presence of an HFD, *Akkermansia* numbers were restored to the levels seen in a low-fat diet [57]. The anthocyanin extracts also increased the abundance of *Oscillobacter* in rats fed a control diet or HFD [57]. Phloridzin administration was found to increase the abundance, thereby restoring the beneficial species, of *Akkermansia* in a diabetic mouse model [58]. This microbial modulation and associated SCFA production are thought to reduce the lipopolysaccharide (LPS) content in Phloidzin-treated mice, and the authors suggested this as a potential mechanism behind the improvement seen in diabetic mice after the administration of Phloridzin. Grape polyphenols have been shown to increase *Bifidobacterium* numbers in rats of control group [59] and *Lactobacillus* numbers in broiler chickens [60]. A reduction in F/B ratio was demonstrated by feeding polyphenols to an HFD-induced rat model [41–44]. In a colitis mouse model, when animals were fed high levels of curcumin (standard rodent diet containing 0.2% w/w of nanoparticle curcumin), there was an increase in butyrate-producing bacteria, viz. *Clostridium* sp. cluster IV and XIVa, that activated T regulatory cells-mediated suppression of colitis in this model [61]. Genistein supplemented corn oil diet in germ-free humanized mice that received fecal transplant from breast cancer patients increased the abundance of beneficial gut microbiome in their gut [62]. The bacterial species that were increased after genistein feed in these mice included *Eubacterium dolichum*, *Lactococcus lactis*, *Akkermansia municiphila*, *Ruminococcus torques*, and *Clostridium hathewayi,* and the bacterial species that were significantly lower than that of control group included *Bacteroides eggerthii* and *Bacteroides ovatus* [62]. Based on their observation in this study the authors further hypothesized that this epigenetic regulation might have played a role in genistein-fed mice to reduce their tumor size and latency [62].

A small number of clinical trials have reported changes in the composition of the microbiome following the consumption of polyphenol-rich foods, that include cocoa, red wine, green tea, and vegetable/fruit. Cocoa-derived polyphenols (494 mg/day) when consumed for four weeks were shown to significantly increase the fecal abundance of *Bifidobacterium* and *Lactobacillus* compared to a low polyphenol diet (23 mg/day) [63]. This prebiotic-like effect was further confirmed by conducting in vitro fermentation analysis on fecal samples from the same study's participants [63]. In another study, polyphenols from red wine increased the number of *Bifidobacteria* and *Lactobacilli* in the feces of obese individuals, which correlated with an improvement in metabolic syndrome markers, including blood pressure, plasma glucose level, and plasma lipid profile [64]. In addition, red wine polyphenols increased the number of butyrate-producing microbes *Fecalibacterium prausnitzii* and *Roseburia* [64] in feces. Moreover, in a similar study, the modulation of beneficial microbiota such as *Bifidobacterium* sp. *Eubacterium rectale, Bacteroides uniformis, Prevotella* sp., *Blautia coccoides*, and *Eggerthella lenta* was also reported for participants consuming red wine polyphenols [65]. The consumption of a vegetable/fruit juice-based diet on three consecutive days could reduce the F/B ratio of healthy adults [66]. Green tea consumption increased the proportion of the *Bifidobacterium* sp. along with bacterial metabolite production [67]. In a study involving an adult population (n = 1044), it was reported that Diadzin intake could increase the equol-producing bacteria, such as *Asaccharobacter celatus* and *Slackia isoflavoniconvertens*, in the gut [68]. Findings from a study of Mayta-apaza et al. [69] suggested that the background diet and individual's microbiome may be a key determinant of the gut microbial metabolism of polyphenols. This study indicated that only when individuals had low Bacteroides numbers was polyphenol supplementation effective in increasing *Bifidobacterium* numbers. Alternatively, individuals with high numbers of Bacteroides, indicative of a low carbohydrates and fiber diet, western-style eating pattern, had a lower ability to metabolize polyphenols, thereby reducing the bioavailability and potential health benefits of polyphenols. Tart cherry juice consumption significantly changed the microbiome, and interestingly, it increased *Bacteroides, Parabacteroides*, and *Alistipes* in individuals with high levels of *Bacteroides* at baseline, and the opposite was observed for those with a low level of *Bacteroides* [70]. Pomegranate extract could increase beneficial microbiota *Akkermansia, Lactobacillus*, and *Prevotella* [71]. A study by Most et al. suggested that men and women may metabolize polyphenols differently. In that study, the supplementation of either epigallocatechin-3-gallate and resveratrol modulated gut microbiota in overweight men, with an increase in F/B ratio, but a similar association was not observed in overweight women [72]. Although studies have shown an influence of gender and body mass index on intestinal microbiota [73], the mechanisms for this difference in gender response in metabolizing polyphenols is not well understood.

It is evident that the beneficial health effects of polyphenols could be partly due to their ability to modulate gut microbiota. Major groups of polyphenols assayed in both in vitro and preclinical studies have shown their ability to modulate the gut microbiota to a beneficial pool characterized by the abundance of *Bifidobacterium, Lactobacillus, Akkermansia*, and *Fecalibacterium* sp. The beneficial mechanisms observed in those studies were mainly attributed to the production of SCFAs and other bacterial metabolites that contributed towards positive changes in gut health and reducing the inflammatory process, thereby improving systemic disease status. Although there are only limited clinical trials that have specifically evaluated the health effects of polyphenols, the results are highly promising, and the microbial modulation observed in these studies mimics that of preclinical studies. Based on these observations it is highly recommended to conduct more studies to explore the actions of specific polyphenols in modulating human gut microbiota, and thereby their effects on improving/preventing metabolic diseases and cancer.

2.2. Vitamins

Vitamins are organic compounds that are essential in very small amounts for supporting normal physiological function. They often serve a variety of roles in the body—one of the most important being their roles as cofactors for enzymes. The diet is the primary source of vitamins, as our bodies cannot synthesize them to meet our daily needs, but certain vitamins, notably vitamin K, and B group vitamins, are synthesized by gut microbiota [74]. When vitamins are deficient, chronic health conditions can be created or exacerbated, and it is common for people to consume individual or multiple vitamin supplements, which can provide very high doses of specific vitamins. Subsequently, minimal absorption of these vitamins in the upper gut can modulate the abundance and diversity of the gut microbiota. The role of dietary vitamins in the modulation of gut microbiota using both animal models and clinical trials are summarized in Table 2.

Vitamin A, a fat soluble vitamin, has been indicated as an adjuvant therapy for infectious diseases [75–78], and has a potential adjunct therapeutic effect on children with autism spectrum of disorders (ASD) [79], possibly by altering gut microbiota. The diversity of gut microbiota and key phylotypes differed significantly in children with persistent diarrhea, whose vitamin A levels differed considerably [80]. A decrease in butyrate-producing bacteria (*Escherichia coli* and *Clostridium butyricum*) and an increase in opportunistic pathogens (*Enterococcus*) might have partially caused the reduced diversity in the vitamin A deficiency group [80]. Vitamin A supplementation in the form of retinoic acid in a murine model could inhibit Murine Norovirus replication [75,76]. In this study, the researchers demonstrated that the administration of retinoic acid (physiologically active metabolite of vitamin A) significantly increased the abundance of *Lactobacillus* sp. during a norovirus infection. In an in vitro model, *Lactobacillus* showed antiviral activity against norovirus, and based on these data, the authors hypothesized that the abundance of *Lactobacillus* in the gut was partially responsible for norovirus inhibition [75,76]. It was also shown that retinoic acid administration increased the abundance of *Allobaculum*, *Aggregatibacter*, *Bifidobacterium*, *Dialister*, and *Enhydrobacter* [75,76]. Epidemiological studies have shown that the rate and clinical symptoms of norovirus infection decrease significantly with sufficient vitamin A supplementation [77]. In addition, vitamin A supplementation was reported to reduce both mortality and morbidity associated with infectious gastrointestinal diseases [78]. In a pilot study, vitamin A administration significantly increased both Bacteroidetes and Bacteroidales populations and reduced F/B ratios in children with ASD [79]. It was suggested that the supplementation of vitamin A to children with ASD improved the condition, possibly by restoring the Bacteroidetes/Bacteroidales population in their gut. Moreover, better vitamin A status in infancy may influence health, both in infancy and later in life, by promoting the establishment of a healthy microbiota. Huda et al. (2019) [81] reported that the supplementation of infants in early (6–15 week) or late (2 year) infancy with 50,000 IU vitamin A could increase the abundance of *Bifidobacterium* and *Akkermansia* in their feces, but did not affect the abundance of Proteobacteria.

The B-group vitamins are a collection of eight water-soluble vitamins essential for various metabolic processes. Even though B-group vitamins are found in many foods (e.g., animal-based foods, leafy green vegetables, beans, and peas), they are easily reduced, particularly by alcohol and cooking. Some B vitamins have been shown to promote bacterial colonization, modulate bacterial virulence, and take part in pathogen interactions with the host through modification of the host defense [82]. For example, supplementation of vitamin B12 was found to enhance the colonization of *Bacteroides thetaiotaomicron* in the gut of an experimental gnotobiotic mice model [83]. Moreover, vitamin B12 is also essential for some enteropathogens to utilize ethanolamine, which enhances *Salmonella typhimurium* growth and its virulence gene expression, as demonstrated in in vitro and in vivo models [84,85]. At the same time, all Fusobacteria and over 90% of Bacteroidetes were predicted to be the producers of B12 by biosynthesis [86]. Similarly, vitamin B6 could be produced by gut microbiota, Bacteroidetes [86], and is mainly utilized as a co-factor for many biological reactions associated with host immune response. B6 deficiency could induce atrophy of lymphoid organs, marked reduction in lymphocyte numbers, and impaired antibody responses and IL-2 production in a clinical study [82,87]. Animal experimentation and human clinical trials further demonstrated that vitamin B6 promotes the growth of *Bacteroides*, which was mediated either by modulating the host immune system or by interfering with the growth or expression of virulence factors of *Salmonella typhimurium* [87]. On the other hand, gut dysbiosis in a murine model could reduce the luminal vitamin B6 level and lead to colonization in the gut by enteropathogenic strains of *Salmonella* sp. [88]. From these preliminary studies it should be cautioned that vitamin B3 and B6 supplementation could lead to an abundance of deleterious/potentially pathogenic species in the gut, and hence could lead to unwanted side effects.

Vitamin C is the most important water-soluble antioxidant in the human body. In contrast to other water-soluble vitamins, vitamin C cannot be synthesized de novo in humans and has to be obtained from dietary sources (fruits and vegetables) via intestinal absorption [89]. The redox state could strongly modulate the gut microbiota. It was found that vitamin C intake was positively correlated with Firmicutes and its lower taxa (i.e., *Clostridium*) and negatively associated with Bacteroidetes in an assessment of a small group of free-living adults with stable cystic fibrosis [90]. Wilson et al. (2018) [91] investigated the effect of consuming two SunGold kiwifruit per day over 12 weeks on vitamin C status and fecal microbiota composition in people with prediabetes. Analysis showed an increase in the relative abundance of uncultivated members of the bacterial family Coriobacteriaceae; however, these changes were small and were not clinically significant. An animal study conducted on early-weaned piglets confirmed the antioxidant capacity of vitamin C in scavenging free radicals and restoring the gut microbiota microenvironment, increasing *Lactobacillus* and *Bifidobacterium* counts, and decreasing *E. coli* counts in the gut environment [92].

Clinical trials involving vitamin D supplementation have shown positive health outcomes to help people maintain health and prevent chronic diseases, and subsequent changes in the microbiota may be a significant mechanism [93,94]. As a fat-soluble vitamin, vitamin D is thought to participate in the process of neurotransmitter synthesis and calcium balance, protecting nerve cells by its antioxidant effects [95]. In a cohort study involving 56,366 American women aged 50 to 79 years it was shown that high levels of Vitamin D intake can significantly reduce the risk of depression [96]. Mounting evidence suggests that the alteration of gut microbiota by vitamin D could be the reason behind this. A randomized control trial [97] showed that weekly supplementation of vitamin D, (50,000 ergocalciferol IU) over 12 months increased the fecal levels of SCFA and abundance of SCFA-producing genera, such as *Ruminococcus*, *Fecalibacterium*, and *Dialister*. Vitamin D3 supplementation was also reported to have a positive impact on the gut microbiota in cystic fibrosis patients by increasing the beneficial bacteria of the genus *Lactococcus* and decreasing the abundance of *Veillonella* at genus level and *Erysipelotrichaceae* at the family level, of which many members were found to be potential pathogens [98]. Vitamin D administration could prevent or even treat various malignant tumors [99,100] and gastrointestinal inflammatory diseases [101,102]. For example, supplementation with vitamin D3 significantly decreased the relative abundance of gamma-proteobacteria and increased bacterial richness in humans [103]. In this study, vitamin D3 modulated the gut microbiome of the upper GI tract, which could explain its positive influence on gastrointestinal diseases, such as inflammatory bowel disease or bacterial infections. Vitamin D has immunomodulatory properties and hence could potentially affect the microbial colonization of the intestinal tract [104–106]. In a study of Garg et al. (2018) [107], the effect of vitamin D replacement in vitamin D-deficient patients with and without ulcerative colitis (UC) was investigated on inflammation and fecal microbiota. Vitamin D supplementation (one dose of 40,000 IU once weekly for eight weeks) was found to be associated with reduced intestinal inflammation in patients with active UC, with a concomitant increase in Enterobacteriaceae but no change in overall fecal microbial diversity. In addition, vitamin D also showed a specific influence on the bacterial communities in Crohn's disease (CD), but not in healthy controls [108]. In this study, the microbiota of the members of the genera *Alistipes, Barnesiella,* unclassified Porphyromonadaceae (both Actinobacteria), *Roseburia, Anaerotruncus, Subdoligranulum* and an unclassified Ruminococcaceae (all Firmicutes) were increased significantly after administration of vitamin D for one week in CD patients. This clearly suggests that the administration of vitamin D may have a positive effect on CD by modulating the intestinal bacterial composition and also by increasing the abundance of potential beneficial bacterial strains. Furthermore, maternal administration of vitamin D during pregnancy had a negative linear association with *Bifidobacterium* sp. and a positive association with the *Bacteroides fragilis* group in infants, suggesting that the prenatal vitamin D administration had an effect on bacterial diversity in the infants [109]. Reduced abundance of *Clostridium difficile* was associated with vitamin D supplementation of breast-fed infants whose mothers were more likely to adhere to a lifestyle with regards to dietary habits as vegetarians, or organic/macrobiotic diets. These data suggest that pre/postnatal vitamin D exposure influences the abundance of several key bacterial taxa within the infant microbiota, thereby leading to the development of health beneficial/detrimental microbiota in infant gut [109]. Luthold et al. (2017) [110] examined the association between vitamin D intake and circulating levels of 25(OH)D with gut microbiota composition, inflammatory markers, and biochemical profile in healthy individuals. *Prevotella* was more abundant, while *Haemophilus* and *Veillonella* were less abundant in the subset with the highest vitamin D intake ($\geq$ 10 μg/day). In addition, abundances of *Coprococcus* and *Bifdobacterium* were statistically inversely correlated with 25(OH)D, while vitamin D deficiency could significantly affect the fecal microbiota of healthy adults, as well as play an important role during the progression of hypertension. For example, healthy individuals who received less than 50 nmol/L 25(OH)D had a lower abundance of genus *Coprococcus* and higher abundance of genus *Ruminococcus* compared to those who received more than 75 nmol/L 25(OH)D [111]. The study of Zuo et al. (2019) [112] reported that vitamin D3 was positively correlated with health beneficial bacterial genera, including *Subdoligranulum, Ruminiclostridium, Intestinimonas, Pseudoflavonifractor, Paenibacillus,* and *Marvinbryantia*, which were thought to have antihypertensive function.

Vitamin E, well recognized for its antioxidant effects, is commonly found in a range of food products, including wheat germ oil, extra virgin olive oil, hazelnuts, peanuts, fish, oysters, eggs, and butter. It has been shown to protect against mucosal tissue damage in chemical-induced colitis models [113,114]. It has also been demonstrated that natural antioxidants may regulate the gut microbiota composition by scavenging excessive free radicals and supporting the cellular and humoral immune responses [115]. Recent findings in a mice model of ileal pouchitis, an antioxidant diet, enriched in vitamins E, selenium, and retinoic acid, may reshape the gut microbial community toward an anti-inflammatory profile, mitigating mucosal inflammation. This capacity appears to be mediated by an increase in the relative percentage of Bacteroidetes and a decrease in Firmicutes at the phylum level, with an overall increase in alpha-diversity (Shannon diversity index) [116]. Another mice model study compared the gut microbiota composition between groups with low vitamin E (0.06 mg/20 g of the body weight) and high vitamin E (0.18 mg/20 g) [117]. A reduced ratio of Firmicutes to Bacteroidetes was found in high-level consumption of vitamin E compared to control and low-level consumption. This evidence was confirmed by a human study conducted in pregnant women in the second trimester, which showed that a higher intake of vitamin E was associated with a decrease in Proteobacteria and Firmicutes and an increase in Bacteroidetes [118]. Moreover, a recent study conducted on iron-deficient infants and toddlers showed an increase of the relative abundance of the genus *Roseburia* (phylum Firmicutes), a butyrate producer, in the group supplemented with iron and vitamin E compared to that in the only iron-supplemented group [119].

It is evident from the above discussion that there is a high level of interactions between the vitamins and gut microbiota in that some vitamins are produced by the gut microbiota and others are responsible for modulating beneficial/detrimental species based on the concentration within the microenvironment. Both preclinical and clinical trials have shown the ability of vitamin A in modulating health-beneficial microbes of the genera *Bifidobacterium, Lactobacillus,* and *Akkermansia*. The F/B restorative function of vitamin A in ASD patients is very interesting and this demands further studies for its use in combinational therapy for patients suffering from ASD. Interestingly, some B complex vitamins are produced by gut commensals and some of these vitamins participate in enhancing the virulence/colonization of potential pathogenic microbes. Vitamin C, D, and E supplementation could modulate health-beneficial microbiota, especially beneficial species from the genera *Bifidobacterium* and *Lactobacillus*. Vitamin D and E also modulate health-beneficial microbes of the genera *Roseburia*. Moreover, vitamin D and E may also reduce F/B ratio. Taken together, these studies suggest that the supplementation of vitamins could modulate gut microbiota. However, the modulation depends on the vitamin level in the host, and hence further clinical trials are warranted to prevent any adverse reaction by "over supplementation" of vitamins.

2.3. Minerals and Trace Elements

Minerals and trace elements are essential micronutrients for human metabolism and perform active interaction with the gut microbiome [120,121]. Both nutritional deficiency and an excess of minerals and trace elements are responsible for various diseases in humans. The role of trace element excess or deficiency in modulating gut microbiota is an emerging field and the major findings from the published articles are summarized in Table 2.

Epidemiological data suggest that high calcium intake is associated with a lower prevalence of obesity [122]. It is suggested that a high intake of calcium leads to changes in the gut microbiota, which are associated with a lean phenotype [122,123]. In a healthy human intervention study, dietary intake of 1000 mg calcium per day for eight weeks resulted in a higher *Clostridium* XVIII in the fecal samples of men [124]. As this bacteria species is an unculturable bacteria it has not been classified as beneficial or detrimental, but calcium in combination with phosphorous (500 mg Ca and 1000 mg p) could lead to an abundance of butyrate producers in the feces. In an 18-month high-fat fed mouse study, calcium supplementation (5.25 g/kg of calcium) increased the microbial diversity and the number of *Ruminococcaceae* and *Akkermansia* in the fecal microbiome of these animals [125]. A multigenerational study was conducted to evaluate how an imbalance in maternal calcium promotes body weight gain in their offspring [107]. Excess dietary calcium (12 g/kg) in the maternal diet was associated with a decrease in *Verrucomicrobia* in the offspring's gut, and insufficient calcium in the maternal diet (2.5 g/kg) was associated with increased F/B ratio in the offspring [126]. In a nutritional intervention of shorter duration (54 days), high calcium supplementation (12 g/kg) modulated gut microbiota in a prebiotic manner by increasing the number of *Bifidobacterium* sp., and increasing *Bacteroides/Prevotella* ratio in the cecal sample of an HFD mouse model. The number of *Bifidobacterium* sp. in this study was negatively correlated with the plasma LPS level, indicating the reduction in LPS producers in the gut microbial pool [127].

Magnesium deficiency is associated with an increased incidence of chronic disease [128], but the evidence for the role of the microbiome in this association is not clear. It was reported previously that four days of magnesium deficiency could reduce the bifidobacterial content in mouse cecum, but with prolonged magnesium deficiency (three weeks) there was an increase in the intestinal content of bifidobacteria and lactobacilli [129]. In contrast, it was reported that six weeks of magnesium deficiency could significantly alter the gut microbiota (only Principal Component Analysis (PCA) analysis results were shown) which may be associated with altered anxiety-like behavior in mice [130,131]. Furthermore, a decrease in the gut microbial diversity was reported with dietary magnesium deficiency [130,131] and an increase in the gut microbial diversity in adult male rats was reported with a magnesium-rich marine mineral blend [132]. More research is needed to further identify the association between magnesium deficiency or magnesium supplementation and the gut microbiota.

Iron supplementation is a common strategy to correct iron-deficiency in clinical settings. However, still no consistent conclusion has been achieved for the effect of iron supplementation on gut microbiota [133]. Both preclinical and clinical studies have shown consistent reductions in the abundance of beneficial microbes and an increased abundance of detrimental microbes after supplementation with Iron. Iron supplementation to anemic Kenyan infants [134,135] and Ivorian children [136] has been suggested to cause gut dysbiosis and inflammation as a result of an increased abundance of pathogenic bacteria and a reduction in beneficial microbiota. In a randomized controlled trial [137], consumption of iron-fortified cereal for 2–4 weeks could lead to a reduction in the median relative abundance of bacteria of the family bifidobacteriacea (declined from 51% to 37%) and an increase in bacteria of the order bacteroidetes (from 5% to 14%) in the stool samples of infants. Furthermore, there was no bacterial richness following the intervention. In a randomized placebo-controlled clinical trial the iron supplementation (50 mg/day, 4 d/week for 38 weeks) did not significantly modify the concentrations of dominant bacterial groups (neither beneficial nor pathogenic) in the gut of children living in rural South Africa. This is in stark contrast to the Ivorian children [136] and may be due to environmental differences between these two cohorts. The former group was living in poverty with poor-quality water and diet and hence had higher pathogenic bacterial load in their gut than the latter group, who had a lower concentration of pathogenic bacteria due to the consumption of good quality water and diet [138]. In a comparative study on infants, two different doses of iron supplementation yielded varying effects on the abundance of beneficial microbiota. In comparison, iron supplementation at a higher dose (6.4 mg/day) significantly reduced the abundance of *Bifidobacterium* levels compared to iron supplementation at a lower dose (1.2 mg/day) in infant gut microbiota. However, the opposite was observed for an abundance of *Lactobacillus,* with an increased abundance with this higher dose than the lower dose [139]. Studies on experimental animals have also demonstrated that excess iron could cause intestinal dysbiosis, which leads to an increase in bacteria of the genera *Defluviitaleaceae*, *Ruminococcaceae*, and *Coprococcus* and a reduction in some members of family *Lachnospiraceae* and genus *Allobaculum* [140]. The same was reflected in in vitro fermentation studies, where it was shown that increased iron concentrations could decrease the number of commensal bacteria, increase the number of toxic metabolites and increase the virulence of pathogenic bacteria [141,142]. It was also reported that iron levels up to 60 mg/d did not significantly alter the composition of the fecal microbiome at any taxonomic level in overweight and obese women in early pregnancy [143]. In contrast, in a cross sectional study, consumption of a diet containing a significantly higher iron concentration could lead to an increase in *Bifidobacterium* levels in Japanese women [144]. However, the results of this study should be interpreted with caution as the diet contained micro and macronutrients other than iron and the bifidogenic response might have come from other ingredients in the diet.

The gut microbiota also responds differently depending upon the chemical form of the dietary iron supplemented. Ferric ethylenediaminetetraacetic acid, compared to ferrous formulations, exacerbated dextran sulfate sodium (DSS)-induced colitis in mice by reducing the abundance of *Roseburia* sp. [145]. In comparison, non-heme iron interventions could increase the abundance of Firmicutes in mice, while heme iron decreased the abundance of Firmicutes, along with decreasing overall microbial diversity, and increased the abundance of Proteobacteria [146–148].

Additionally, the ways of administration of iron have also been reported to have different influences on gut microbiota. Lee et al. (2017) [149] reported that oral administration of iron resulted in a lower abundance of *Fecalibacterium prausnitzii, Ruminococcus bromii, Collinsella aerofaciens,* and *Dorea* when compared with that of the intravenous administration. It was also reported that the administration of iron as drops at the required standard dose could lead to decreased relative abundance of lactobacilli, and potentially increase susceptibility to bacterial infection [139].

Phosphorus is the second most abundant inorganic element in the body and plays an important role in the maintenance of blood systemic acid balance [150]. The recommended intake for phosphorus is 700–1000 mg for adults, but intake levels are commonly exceeded when processed foods such as baked goods and sugar-sweetened beverages are consumed. A study on broiler chickens showed that phosphorus supplementation increased the abundance of the butyrate-producing bacteria Fecalibacterium and Pseudoflavonifractor in the cecal digesta [151]. A dietary intervention study in human with phosphorus supplementation (1000 mg/day) showed that fecal microbial diversity improved and SCFA concentration increased [124]. However, further clinical studies are needed to investigate the actions of magnesium on gut microbial modulation before any conclusions can be made.

Zinc is an essential micronutrient for maintaining epithelial integrity, possibly by modulating the beneficial gut microbiota [152]. Chronic zinc deficiency in broiler chickens reshapes the gut microbiome, with a significant increase in the abundance of Proteobacteria and a decrease in the abundance of Firmicutes [153]. Animal experimentation has suggested that zinc supplementation (120 mg/kg) [154] in a "Salmonella typhimurium-challenged broiler" model increased the number of beneficial bacteria, such as *Lactobacillus* sp., while reducing the number of detrimental bacteria, including *Salmonella* sp. In mice, however, excess dietary zinc alters the diversity and structure of the gut microbiota. In particular, the genera of *Turicibacter* Operational Taxonomic Unit (OTU) 2 and *Clostridium* OTU 11 decreased and the genera of *Enterococcus* OTU 4 and *Clostridium* XI OTU 3 increased. Furthermore, excess zinc rendered the gut microbiota vulnerable to low-level perturbations and decreased the threshold of antibiotics needed to diminish colonization resistance to the nosocomial pathogen *Clostridium difficile* [155]. Chronic zinc deficiency in broiler chickens reshapes the gut microbiome, with a significant increase in the abundance of Proteobacteria and a decrease in the abundance of Firmicutes [153]. However, the clinical data on the modulation of gut microbiota by dietary zinc in humans are lacking.

A deficiency and excess of selenium is related to health conditions, such as increased mortality, type 2 diabetes, and cancer risk [156]; however, there is limited information regarding the effects on the gut microbiota. Dietary selenium supplementation at a dose range of 0.1 ug/g to 2.25 ug/g in mice was shown to increase the microbial diversity [157]. In another mice study, the supplementation of selenium at a concentration of 0.4 mg/kg led to an increase in the abundance of *Akkermansia* and *Turicibacter*, and a decrease in the abundance of *Dorea* and *Mucispirillum* [158].

Although the evidence is limited to only one animal study, it suggests that iodine supplementation is dependent on the levels of fat in the diet and results in differential effects on the gut microbiome [159]. Iodine supplementation in an HFD mouse model improved the thyroid hormone status, but resulted in a gut dysbiosis characterized by an increased abundance of pathogenic microbes and a depletion of beneficial microbes, such as *Fecalibacterium prausnizii* [159]. Alternatively, when the diet was low in fat, the same dose of iodine had beneficial effects on gut microbiota by increasing *Bifidobacterium*, *Lactobacillus*, *Fecalibacterium*, and *Allobaculuum* in the control group [159].

In summary, there is limited evidence supporting specific mechanisms whereby minerals and trace elements modulate the gut microbiome. However, the studies published to date mostly evaluated changes in the microbiome following micronutrient deficiency and supplementation of minerals and trace elements. Calcium supplementation has been shown to modulate *Akkermansia*, *Bifidobcterium*, and *Ruminococcacea* and the ratio of *Bactereoidetes/Prevotella* in experimental animals. The sufficiency/deficiency of Mg in modulating gut microbiome is not clear, as acute deficiency in a mice model seems to modulate health-beneficial gut microbiota. Evidence is inconsistent in iron supplementation and most of the studies show an increase in deleterious microbes and reduction in the abundance of beneficial microbes such as *Bifidobacterium* in human infants, but no influence of iron supplementation on microbiota also been reported in clinical trials. Interestingly, chemical form and route of administration of iron seems to be important in modulating gut microbiome. Limited research has shown that Phosphorus supplementation affects SCFAs, warranting further preclinical/clinical trials to arrive at a conclusion. Zinc supplementation reduced deleterious microbes and increased beneficial microbes in preclinical studies. Selenium supplementation increased the gut microbial diversity and positively modulated health beneficial microbes, such as *Akkermansia* and *Turicibacter*, and negatively modulated the deleterious microbes, such as *Dorea* and *Mucispirillum*, in a mice model. Iodine supplementation has resulted in gut dysbiosis and also reduced the abundance of health beneficial microbes, such as *Fecalibacterium*, in a mice model. There is a clear lack of preclinical/human intervention studies exploring the role of specific minerals and trace elements on modulating gut microbiota, and hence a thorough study in this area is mandated.

3. The role of Dietary Macronutrients in Modulating Gut Microbiota

3.1. Carbohydrates

Carbohydrates are the predominant energy source for the human body and play an important role in modulating and shaping the gut microbiota. Here, we summarize the evidence for how different types of dietary carbohydrates modulate the microbiota at their genus level, the F/B ratio, and the microbial community diversity (Table 3).

Plant-derived carbohydrates that escape digestion in the upper digestive tract are classified as dietary fiber and their structure, along with other undigested nutrients, influences the extent to which they are fermented by the large intestinal microbes. In animal models, the Western-style diet, with relatively lower fiber content, has been shown to reduce the abundance of *Bifidobacterium*, and the diversity of gut microbiota [160]. A chronic lack of dietary fiber could reduce the diversity of gut microbiota [161].A pre-hispanic Mexican diet (high fiber) has been shown to alleviate gut dysbiosis in the rats fed with a sucrose-enriched high-fat diet, as evidenced by reducing the Firmicutes to Bacteroidetes ratio (F/B ratio) and increasing the abundance of *Lactobacillus* sp. [162]. In a preclinical trial, humanized mice were fed a diet rich in fiber and later introduced a feed with low-quality fiber to perturbate their gut microbiome [15]. However, re-introduction of fiber by feeding a plant polysaccharide-rich diet with neutral detergent fiber content of 15% by weight did not restore the microbial composition and diversity in the tested animals. Moreover, this perturbation was observed to continue over multiple generations [15,163]. In clinical trials, studies have consistently demonstrated that high-fiber diet intervention, e.g., whole grain cereal, inulin and fructo-oligosaccharide (1:1) mixed fiber, soluble corn fiber, barley kernel-based bread, increases the fecal abundance of several beneficial microbiota, such as *Bifidobacterium* sp. [164–166], *Lactobacillus* sp. [166], *Akkermansia* sp. [167,168], *Fecalibacterium* sp. [168], *Roseburia* sp. [168], *Bacteroides* sp. [168,169], and *Prevotella* sp. [170,171]. Moreover, fiber-enriched diets reduce the F/B ratio [169,172] and improve gut microbial diversity [168,170,172]. The relative proportion of Bacteroidetes was reported to be lower in obese people compared with that in lean people [35]. The Bacteroidetes proportion increased on a carbohydrate-restricted low-calorie diet for one year and responded to weight loss [35]. Furthermore, the gut microbiome of obese patients was found to show an increase in beneficial members of *Prevotella*, *Parabacteroides distasonis*, and *Fecalibacterium prausnitzii* after consumption of high-complex carbohydrate diet (low-fat, 28% fat) for one year [173].

Arabinoxylans (AX), arabinoxylan-oligosaccharides (AXOS), and xylo-oligosaccharides (XOS) are commonly found in wheat and are classified as prebiotics, as they specifically increase the pool of beneficial microbiota, including *Bifidobacterium* and *Lactobacillus* [174–182]. In a dietary intervention, an AX-enriched diet increased the abundance of *Bifidobacterium* sp. in adults with metabolic syndrome and lowered microbial diversity [174]. AXOS, consisting of arabinoxylooligosaccharides and XOS, can be obtained by enzymatic hydrolysis of AX [183]. AXOS and XOS were shown to increase *Bifidobacterium* sp. and/or *Lactobacillus* sp. [182] in healthy adults [175–180] and children [181].

In vitro fermentation of galacto-oligosaccharides (GOS) [184] has been shown to increase *Bifidobacterium* sp. and *Lactobacillus* sp. [185]. A similar observation was reported in a dietary intervention study using GOS on a specific pathogen-free mice model [186]. In clinical trials, GOS at a dose range of 1.5 to 10 g/day when consumed for up to 12 weeks by healthy adults increased the fecal level of *Bifidobacterium* [187–192]. A similar dietary intervention in teenage girls (10–13 years old) showed that GOS supplementation at 5 or 10 g/day for three weeks increased *Bifidobacterium* sp. population [193]. In healthy elderly volunteers (65–80 years), administration of GOS at 5.5 g/day for 10 weeks increased *Bifidobacterium* and *Bacteroides* [191]. In addition to *Bifidobacterium* sp., an increase in the relative abundance of lactose-fermenting *Fecalibacterium* and *Lactobacillus* was observed when GOS was consumed by lactose-intolerant volunteers, suggesting that administration of GOS promoted a colonic environment that favors the digestion of lactose [192]. Due to its bifidogenic potential, GOS is included in infant formula to promote a healthy gut microbiome which is dominated by *Bifidobacterium* sp. [184,194–198]. Babies receiving an infant formula containing 4 g GOS/L led to an increase in the abundance of beneficial microbiota *Lactobacillus* and reduced *Clostridium* [184,198]. Lactose-containing baby formula specially formulated with GOS showed significant increases in *Bifidobacterium* and *Lactobacillus* [199]. In a clinical trial for healthy adults, raffinose-oligosaccharide was identified to positively modulate *Bifidobacterium*, and negatively modulate *Clostridium*, viz. *Clostridium histolyticum* and *Clostridium lituseburense* group [200]. In addition, the raffinose-oligosaccharide did not have any significant effect on the diversity of the gut microbiota [200].

Inulin-type fructans (including main dietary sources) have been shown to consistently promote Bifidobacteria. Animal studies have shown that inulin or inulin-type fructan (ITF) could alter gut microbial diversity [201,202], and *Bifidobacterium* sp. was further identified to be promoted by ITF in clinical trials [203–208]. Supplementation of ITF at 16 g/day to obese individuals for three months increased the abundance of *Bifidobacterium* [204,207] and *Fecalibacterium* [204], and reduced the abundance of detrimental microbiota of the genus *Bacteroides* [204]. At a lower level of inulin supplementation (10–12 g/day), individuals with mild constipation showed an increase in *Bifidobacterium* [205] or an increase in *Bifidobacterium* and *Fecalibacterium* in healthy adults [203]. In children (mean age 10 years), a similar dose of inulin (10 g/d) for three months only increased the abundance of *Bifidobacterium* but did not affect the level of *Fecalibacterium* or *Bacteroides* [206]. Another study in overweight or obese children (7–12 years, 8 g inulin/day for 16 weeks) showed an increase in *Bifidobacterium* and decrease in *Bacteroides* [208]. Taken together, these studies highlight a range of factors—dosage, inulin type, and other dietary factors (e.g., total fiber intake)—that may contribute to the effectiveness of ITF in modulating key microbes.

Resistant starch is an important substrate for supporting gut health, as it is utilised by a range of beneficial gut microbes [209]. For instance, *Bifidobacterium* sp., *Fecalibacterium* sp., *Eubacterium* sp., and *Ruminococcus* sp. were significantly increased in healthy adults who consumed resistant starch (100 g/day, type 2/ type 4) for three weeks [210]. Individuals with metabolic syndrome demonstrated that resistant starch (type 2), when applied in conjunction with arabinoxylan, could modify gut microbiota towards a beneficial pool (with higher bifidobacterial concentration and less dysbiotic genera), and modified SCFA composition, which resulted in beneficial effects on colonic health and metabolic syndrome [174]. Moreover, a dietary intervention study using resistant starch as a non-digestible carbohydrate confirmed its function to substantially alter the composition of gut microbial species, including *Ruminococcus bromii, Eubacterium rectale, Collinsella aerofaciens,* and uncultured Oscillibacter group [211].

The intervention of butyrylated high-amylose maize starch was reported in a clinical trial to increase the abundance of the beneficial microbiota, such as *Lactobacillus* sp., *Clostridium coccoides*, *C. leptum* group, and *Ruminococcus bromii*, and reduce the abundance of *R. torques* and *R. gnavus* in the participants who had gut dysbiosis caused by red meat-increased O6-methyl-2-deoxyguanosine adduct level [212].

A six-week dietary intervention study with 10% oligofructose in diet-induced obese rats increased the abundance of *Bifidobacterium* sp., *Lactobacillus* sp., and *Roseburia* sp. and decreased *Clostridium leptum* [213]. In healthy infants, the consumption of infant formula containing oligofructose (3 g/L eight weeks) increased the fecal levels of *Bifidobacterium* sp. [214].

In addition, a synthetic polymer of glucose, polydextrose (PDX) provides similar physiological effects as other dietary fibers and has shown prebiotic potential when tested in animals [215]. Dietary intervention with prebiotics has been shown to selectively stimulate the growth and/or activity of one or a limited number of intestinal bacteria associated with several physiological benefits on health. *Clostridium* clusters I, II, and IV and *Ruminococcus intestinalis* were further reported to be promoted by PDX (8 g/day) in clinical trials for healthy subjects aged 18–50 years during a three-week innervation [216].

Dietary carbohydrates have long been shown to modulate health-beneficial microbes in both humans and animals. A high-fiber diet increased the abundance of *Bifidobacterium* and reduced the ratio of Firmicutes/Bacteroidetes in humans and experimental animals. The prebiotic potential of GOS and other carbohydrates is well known and their supplementation has resulted in an abundance of *Bifidobacterium* sp., *Lactobacillus* sp., *Akkermansia* sp., *Fecalibacterium* sp., *Roseburia* sp., *Bacteroides* sp., and *Prevotella*. Arabinoxylan, resistance starch, and inulin type fructans modulate health-beneficial bacteria, such as *Bifidobacterium, Fecalibacterium,* and *Lactobacillus*. Oligofructose and polydextrose were also found to modulate many health beneficial bacteria, such as *Roseburia, Clostridium lepum,* and *Ruminococcus intestinalis*. Studies have also shown the restorative function of certain carbohydrates on dysbiosis, observed in obese individuals, and hence such carbohydrates could be used as a therapeutic intervention for metabolic diseases.

3.2. Fat

A dietary pattern high in saturated and/or total fat is consistently shown to have adverse effects on intestinal microbiome. Fifteen clinical reports (including six randomized controlled interventional studies and nine observational studies) have shown that diets high in total fat and saturated fat have a negative effect on the richness and diversity of gut microbiota [217]. These findings were supported by carefully controlled feeding trials in rodents, which showed that diets containing fat ranging from 44% to 72% increased the F/B ratio of gut microbiota [34,162,218–226]. The influences of HFD on modulating microbial abundance, the F/B ratio, and the overall diversity are summarized in Table 4.

Although it has been indicated that the changes in the F/B ratio in gut microbiota are dependent on the intestinal region and the duration of ingestion [218], changes in the F/B ratio vary with the amount of fat in the diet (Table 4). In rats, the consumption of a mixed HFD (range from 44%–72%) [34,218–226] increases the abundance of *Firmicutes* and decreases the proportion of *Bacteroidetes*, thereby leading to an increased ratio of F/B. These bacterial phyla viz. *Bacteroidetes* and *Firmicutes* are commonly known to predominate in the intestinal tract, however, with varying compositions. For example, the genetic obese ob/ob mice displayed fewer *Bacteroidetes* and more *Firmicutes* [34]. The same research team discovered that the obesity phenotype could be transmitted by gut microbiota transplantation in mice. The obesity increased the F/B ratio, and thereby increased the abundance of Firmicutes. After the colonization of "obese-microbiota", the total body fat in mice significantly increased, and the capacity to harvest energy from the diet was increased as well, thus contributing to the pathophysiology of obesity [227]. However, the amount of dietary fat ranging from 20% to 40% would result in a F/B ratio decrease [228–231], or no significant changes in their ratio [173,230,232,233]. Furthermore, the gut microbial patterns in HFD-induced rat models showed an abundance of microbes of the order Clostridiales and a decrease in abundance of the microbes of the family Lachnospiraceae, possibly due to its association with body fat percentage [53]. The diminution of *Lactobacillus* population was suggested to be correlated with the high fat and its abundance displayed a negative correlation with body weight and fat mass [162,222,226,229]. In a recent randomized, controlled-feeding clinical trial, 40% fat consumption by healthy young adults was reported to be associated with unfavorable changes in gut microbiota, in that the intervention resulted in an increased abundance of detrimental species from the bacteria *Bacteroides* and *Alistipes*, the two species reported to be abundant in patients with Type 2 diabetes mellitus (T2 DM), and decreased abundance of beneficial bacteria of the genus *Fecalibacterium*. However, 20% of fat consumption showed a positive effect in terms of increasing gut microbiota *Fecalibacterium* sp. and *Blautia* sp. [230]. In people who have metabolic disease, obesity, and coronary heart disease, lowering fat intake to less than 35% fat for two years helped restore the gut microbiome [173,231,233]. The results of this study suggested that low-fat diet intervention for people depends on the degree of metabolic dysfunction, as no change was observed in people if they were not diagnosed with metabolic disease [230]. Furthermore, a sex-dependent effect on shaping the gut microbiota according to diet has been reported recently. Researchers observed a higher abundance of *Roseburia, Holdemania,* and *Desulfovibrio* in men with metabolic syndrome (MetS) than in women with MetS after three years of consumption of the low-fat diet, which led to a detrimental effect in men rather than women [234].

Researchers have also explored the role of saturated and unsaturated fat on the modulation and diversity of gut microbiome. Patterson et al. (2014) [235] showed that different types of dietary fats increased overall gut microbiota diversity but were not significantly different from each other in a mouse model. In a dietary intervention study, the mice fed with palm oil, rich in saturated fatty acid, resulted in a decrease of the Bacteroidetes population, and the changing trends in gut microbiota compositions have been confirmed to be positively correlated with the development of obesity. Similar research found that saturated fat (HFD-containing palm oil) intake (45% fat) induced an elevated F/B ratio in a mice model and has a more stimulatory effect on the development of obesity than mice fed unsaturated fat (olive oil or safflower oil) [236]. The saturated dietary fat altered conditions for gut microbial assemblage by promoting changes in host bile composition, resulting in dysbiosis that can perturb immune homeostasis [228]. In contrast, one of the saturated fats, medium-chain fatty acids, has shown antibacterial effects [237]. Olive oil, high in unsaturated fatty acids, increased commensal bacteria, the populations of *Bacteroidaceae*, in the cecum compared with palm oil, flaxseed oil, and fish oil [235]. Flaxseed/fish oil, when administered together with a low-fat diet, imparted a bifidogenic effect on the host intestinal microbiota composition by increasing the levels of *Bifidobacterium* [235]. *Akkermansia* and *Bifidobacterium* were also considered to be associated with prebiotic consumption and they were reported to show a decreasing trend under the influence of HFD [162,238]. Enteral supplementation with polyunsaturated fatty acids (PUFA) was associated with decreased abundance of detrimental bacteria (e.g., *Streptococcus* sp. and *Escherichia* sp.), greater bacterial diversity in premature infants with an enterostomy [239]. It was also reviewed from the clinical studies that a diet rich in monounsaturated fatty acids decreased total bacterial numbers, whereas a diet rich in polyunsaturated fatty acids had no effect on the richness and diversity of gut microbiota [217].

In summary, both quantity and type of fat in the diet can modulate the F/B ratio and affect both detrimental and beneficial microbes in the gut. In particular, saturated fat consistently lowers health-beneficial microbes, such as *Bifidobacterium* and *Fecalibacterium*, whereas unsaturated fat increases the abundance of *Akkermansia* and *Bifidobacterium* and reduces detrimental bacteria such as *Streptococcus* and *Escherichia* sp. Additionally, saturated fat can increase the F/B ratio and unsaturated fat can lower the F/B ratio, and thereby they could have varying effects on human health depending on the fat quality. Clinical studies to date suggest that a high-fat diet is detrimental to gut health, as it reduces the abundance of beneficial microbes, however this can be reversed if a diet lower in fat is followed.

3.3. Protein

Clinical and preclinical studies have suggested that the type and amount of protein in the diet has substantial effects on the gut microbiota (Table 5).

Evidence from animal models suggests that the protein quality affects the composition of gut microbiota. For example, in a preclinical study, it was shown that the cheese whey proteins could act as growth factors for fecal counts of *Lactobacilli* and *Bifidobacteria* compared with Caesin [240]. It was also shown that a whey protein-based diet reduced the abundance of *Clostridium* [241] in the gut. Mung bean protein was shown to reverse the HFD-induced F/B ratio in mice [242]. The mung bean protein also increased the abundance of the family *Ruminococcacea* in an HFD mice model. Based on this observation the authors hypothesized that the bile acid metabolism mediated by *Ruminococcacea* family members would have provided a health benefit in HFD mice [242]. In contrast to the evidence from plant-based protein interventions, diets containing casein increased fecal *Enterobacteriaceae* and decreased fecal *Lactobacilli* in piglets [243]. Furthermore, Bacteroidales and Clostridiales levels were higher in mice when fed a Western diet that contained high levels of meat and seafood [244]. It was also shown that animal-based protein could increase the sensitivity to intestinal inflammation via increasing the potential detrimental gut microbiota (viz. the genera of *Enterococcus*, *Streptococcus*, *Turicibater*, and *Escherichia*, and families Peptostreptococcaceae and Ruminococcaceaea) compared to mice consuming a plant-based protein [245]. A recent clinical study highlighted that casein and soy protein diets should be considered with caution because they appear to disturb normal gene expression in the rectal mucosa of overweight individuals [246]. The authors could not find any changes in microbial diversity or changes in the abundance of specific taxa but could find both beneficial and detrimental metabolites produced by specific microbes. Specifically, amino acid-degrading metabolites were higher, with a reduction in butyrate concentration that the authors found correlated heavily with specific bacteria of the genera *Clostridia*, *Oscilospira*, *Butyricimonas*, and *Odoribacter* [246].

Although it was suggested that the protein source had a large effect on bacterial community composition [245], other studies have shown that the quantity of proteins is also very important in its effect on gut microbial modulation. In one study [241], mice were fed with a low-fat diet (10% fat) or an HFD (45% fat) for 21 weeks, with either casein (20% kJ) or whey protein isolate (WPI) at 20%, 30%, or 40% kJ. The results of this study showed an increase in abundance of the phylum Proteobacteria and Actinobacteria in the gut microbiota for the experimental animal groups that received 20% WPI. When the protein was increased from 20% to 40% the results were opposite for the phylum Actinobacteria compared to that of the HFD group. A 70-day protein supplementation (a blend of whey isolate (10 g) and beef hydrolysate (10 g)) in a healthy athletes diet had a negative impact on gut microbiota, which resulted in a decreased level of the health-beneficial microbiota, viz. *Roseburia, Blautia,* and *Bifidobacterium longum,* and an increase in the microbiota of the phylum Bacteroidetes [247]. The control group, who received maltodextrin, did not show this effect. In addition, different cooking methods of protein could have different effects on gut microbiota. An in vitro study on human gut microbiota showed that the *C.hidtolyticum/perfringens* group, a common food borne pathogen that can produce enterotoxins, causing a wide range of pathologies, was observed in batch fermentations that contained fried meat compared to those containing boiled meat [248], thus suggesting that the cooking method and meat type can influence fermentation profiles within the human gut microbiota.

From the above discussion it is inferred that both the quality and quantity of protein can have effects on the composition and diversity of gut microbiota. Whey protein exerts a bifidogenic effect in HFD mice at a lower concentration and reverses this effect at a higher concentration. Mung bean protein helps to reverse F/B ratio in HFD mice model, and animal-based protein may increase the sensitivity to intestinal inflammation by increasing the potential detrimental gut microbiota. A blend protein supplementation in healthy adults has a negative effect on beneficial microbiota, such as *Roseburia, Blautia,* and *Bifidobacterium longum.* Furthermore, it was shown that different cooking methods have different effects on the gut microbiota. More preclinical/clinical trials are required to conclude the effects of various protein supplementation on gut microbiota.

4. Summary and Future Perspective

Gut dysbiosis is increasingly recognized as a key factor in the development of type 2 diabetes mellitus (T2 DM), cardiovascular disease, childhood allergy/atopy, and many other metabolic and infectious diseases [249,250]. The gut microbiota is a potential target to improve human health [251,252], and dietary components (both micro- and macro-nutrients) are recognized as playing an important role (Figure 1).

There is consistent evidence suggesting that polyphenols have considerable effects on promoting the abundance of beneficial microbes in the gut, which may contribute to favorable health outcome beyond the gut. Specific polyphenols in animal models have been shown to reduce the F/B ratio. In vitro assays have also shown the ability of specific polyphenols to reduce the abundance of detrimental/pathogenic microbes. The major beneficial microbes positively modulated with polyphenols include *Bifidobacterium, Lactobacillus, Akkermansia,* and *Fecalibacterium* sp. Some specific polyphenols modulate other beneficial microbes, such as *Clostridium coccoides-Eubacterium rectale* group, *Eubacterium dolichum, Lactococcus lactis, Ruminococcus torques, Clostridium hathewayi, Bacteroides uniformis, Prevotella sp., Blautia coccoides,* and *Eggerthella lenta* (Table 1 and Figure 1). Vitamins form the second major micronutrient that modulates the health-beneficial gut microbes. Vitamins show a distinct response on modulating health beneficial/detrimental microbes and vitamin A, C, D, and E supplementation has a positive influence on health-beneficial microbes, such as *Bifidobacteria, Akkermansia,* and *Lactobacilli.* The restorative function of normal flora in the dysbiotic gut by vitamin A in ASD patients promises to explore therapeutic potential of vitamin A in ASD and other similar diseases. Vitamin B administration should be cautioned, as it can activate virulence of pathogenic organisms and can also positively modulate some detrimental bacteria. There is an acute scarcity in the literature that explores the role of minerals and trace elements in modulating gut microbiota. However, supplementation of calcium, magnesium, phosphorus, selenium, and zinc has shown that there may be some small effects that support beneficial gut bacteria, which include *Akkermansia, Bifidobacterium,* and *Ruminococcus.* Iron supplementation in iron-deficient infants has been shown to modulate detrimental and potentially pathogenic microbiota. Iodine supplementation leads to a decrease in the abundance of *Fecalibacterium prausnizii* and selenium supplementation leads to a decrease in the abundance of *Dorea* and *Mucisprillum.* More studies are needed to conclude these effects.

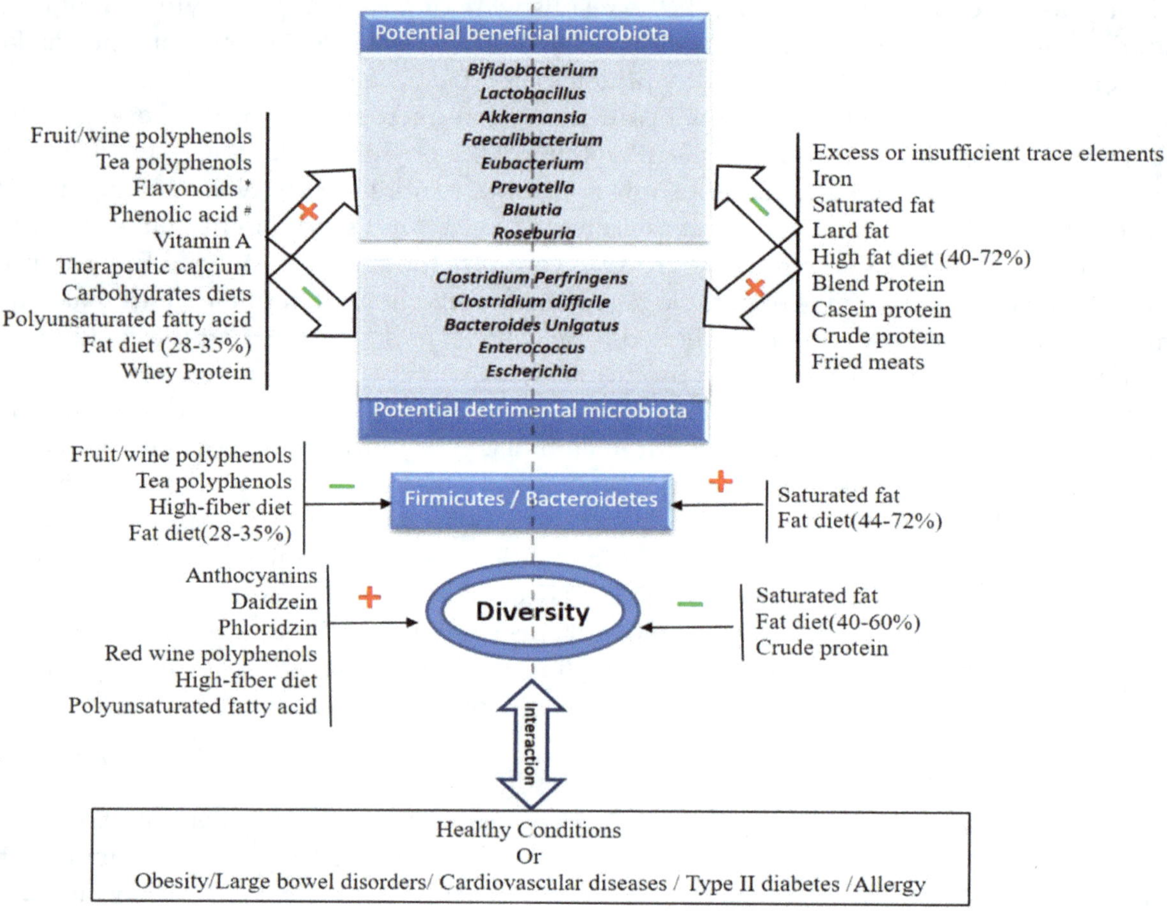

Note: * includes flavonoids: Anthocyanins, Phloridzin, Catechin, Epicatechin, Hesperetin, Naringenin, Quercetin, Rutin, Daidzein, Genistein.
includes Phenolic acid: Chlorogenic acid, Gallic acid, Caffeic acid, 3-O-Methylgallic acid, O-coumaric acid, P-coumaric acid.

Eff

Figure 1. ect of micro-and macro-nutrients on potential beneficial or detrimental gut microbiota.

Under macronutrients, carbohydrates form the major modulator for health-beneficial microbes. Dietary fiber, arabinoxylan, GOS, Inulin type fructan, resistant starch, and polydextran have major bifidogenic effects and can positively modulate health-beneficial microbes in the gut. The major health-beneficial microbes modulated by these major carbohydrates are *Bifidobacterium sp., Lactobacillus sp, Akkermansia sp, Fecalibacterium sp., Roseburia sp., Bacteroides sp. and Prevotella, Roseburia, Clostridium lepum* and *Ruminococcus intestinalis* (Table 4 and Figure 1). Specific carbohydrates are also found to reduce the F/B ratio. Animal experimentation has shown that saturated and unsaturated fats have opposing effects on the modulation of gut microbiota. Compared to saturated fats, diets containing unsaturated fat increase the abundance of beneficial gut microbiota and reduce detrimental gut microbiota (Table 4 and Figure 1). A high-fat diet could lead to gut dysbiosis and thereby increase the F/B ratio. A Mediterranean diet and a low-fat high carbohydrate diet modulated two butyrate producers (*Roseburia* sp. and *Fecalibacterium prausnitzii*) in the gut of an obese population and was associated with insulin sensitivity in these populations [231]. This study further confirmed the health benefits of a low-fat diet via the modulation of gut microbiota. High intake of dietary protein lowers the abundance of microbes that have been associated with beneficial health effects and it is not clear whether this differs between proteins from animal- or plant-based sources. The quality and quantity of the dietary protein influences the gut microbiota. There is an acute scarcity of studies using defined proteins that explore their action on gut microbial modulation. More clinical/preclinical studies are required to make an informed decision on protein supplementation for modulating health-beneficial microbes.

It is further clear in the current review that macro- and micro-nutrients greatly influence the composition and/or diversity of the gut microbiome. For example, fermentable dietary fibers, which include AX, RS, inulin, oligosaccharides, and GOS, increase the abundance of *Bifidobacterium*, *Lactobacillus*, *Roseburia*, *Bacteroides*, *Akkermansia*, butyrate-producing *Fecalibacterium*, and *Ruminococcus* at the genus level, which are associated with various health benefits, whereas diets containing more than 44% energy from fat increase the ratio of F/B, which can be attenuated by red wine/tea-derived polyphenols. High intakes of dietary protein lower the abundance of microbes that have been associated with beneficial health effects and it is not clear whether this differs between proteins from animal- or plant-based sources. Moreover, the role of some micronutrients (e.g., Vitamin D and Calcium) in modulating gut microbiota towards a healthy phenotype by increasing *Bifidobacterium*, *Lactobacillus*, restoring *Ruminococcus* and *Akkermansia* in obese models has indicated that a favorable health outcome could be mediated by dietary intervention studies.

Although this current review summarized key current research outcomes on the effect of specific micro and macro nutrients on modulating gut microbiota, there is a lack of data on how these specific nutrient components alter the gut microbiota in humans. Humanized mouse models and gnotobiotic mouse models could provide further information. Although these models have several limitations, they enable dietary patterns and nutrients to be carefully controlled and microbial changes to be evaluated. Additionally, well-defined dietary intervention studies are needed that utilize a diverse range of individuals to better understand the intra- and inter-individual variability in how individuals and their microbiomes respond differently to dietary patterns and specific food component.

Table 1. Modulations of dietary polyphenols on potentially beneficial and detrimental gut microbiota.

	Dose and Treatment Duration/Test Model	F/B	Potentially Beneficial Microbiota													Potentially Detrimental Microbiota					Species	Diversity
			Bifidobacterium sp.	*Lactobacillus* sp.	*Akkermansia* sp.	*Fecalibacterium* sp.	*Eubacterium* sp.	*Bacteroides* sp.	*Prevotella* sp.	*Blautia* sp.	*Clostridium* sp.	*Ruminococcus* sp.	*Eggerthella* sp.	*Roseburia* sp.	*Coprococcus* sp.	*Ruminococcus* sp.	*Clostridium* sp.	*Bacteroides* sp.	*Enterobacter* sp.	*Enterococcus* sp.		
Anthocyanins																						
Marques et al. (2018)	Standard diet with Blackberry anthocyanin rich extract (25 mg/Kg body weight per day) for 17 weeks and standard diet as reference/rat model [57]																					↑
	High-fat diet (HFD) with blackberry anthocyanin rich extract (25 mg/Kg body weight per day) for 17 weeks and HFD as reference/rat model [57]				↑											↓						↑
Catechin																						
Tzounis et al. (2010)	A high-cocoa flavanol group (21 mg catechin/day) for four weeks of treatment and a low-cocoa flavanol group (3 mg catechin/day) as reference/clinical trials (22 healthy human volunteers) [63]		↑	↑													↓					
Tzounis et al. (2008)	Catechin (150 mg/L) inoculated in stirring batch-culture vessels containing fecal slurry (1:10, w/v), for treatment up to 48 h and incubating flavanol monomers in medium without fecal slurry inoculation as reference/in vitro [48]		↑								↑						↓				*Clostridium coccoides–Eubacterium rectale* group; *C. histolyticum* group	
Caffeic acid																						
Parkar et al. (2013)	Caffeic acid (10 µg/mL) in fermentation medium for 48 h and a control without polyphenol as reference/in vitro [49]	↑	↑					↑														
Chlorogenic acid																						
Parkar et al. (2013)	Chlorogenic acid (30 and 100 µg/mL) in fermentation medium for 48 h and a control without polyphenol as reference/in vitro [49]	↑	↑					↓														
Daidzein																						
Iino et al. (2019)	Diadzin intake (three traditional Japanese soybean products: natto, tofu, and fried tofu) was calculated based on brief self-administered diet history questionnaire/clinical trials (1044 healthy subjects: 411 men and 633 women) [68]																					↑
Epicatechin																						
Tzounis et al. (2008)	Epicatechin (1000 mg/L) inoculated in stirring batch-culture vessels containing fecal slurry (1:10, w/v), for treatment up to 48 h and incubating flavanol monomers in medium without fecal slurry inoculation as reference/in vitro [48]						↑				↑										*E. rectale*; *C.coccoide*	

Table 1. *Cont.*

	Dose and Treatment Duration/Test Model	F/B	Potentially Beneficial Microbiota													Potentially Detrimental Microbiota					Species	Diversity
			Bifidobacterium sp.	*Lactobacillus* sp.	*Akkermansia* sp.	*Fecalibacterium* sp.	*Eubacterium* sp.	*Bacteroides* sp.	*Prevotella* sp.	*Blautia* sp.	*Clostridium* sp.	*Ruminococcus* sp.	*Eggerthella* sp.	*Roseburia* sp.	*Coprococcus* sp.	*Ruminococcus* sp.	*Clostridium* sp.	*Bacteroides* sp.	*Enterobacter* sp.	*Enterococcus* sp.		
Genistein																						
Paul et al. (2017)	Genistein diet (0.25 g/kg) for 4 weeks and the control group without genistein as reference/mice model (humanized germ-free mice that received fecal transplantation from breast cancer patients) [62]			↑	↑		↑				↑	↑						↓			*A. municiphila* *Ruminococcus torques* *Clostridium hatheway* *Bacteroides eggerthii* *Bacteroides ovatus* *Eubacterium dolichum*	
Phloridzin																						
Mei et al. (2016)	Phloridzin (20 mg/kg/day) for 10 weeks and the control (vehicle treated) as reference/mice model (type 2 diabetes mice model) [58]				↑																*A. muciniphila*	↑
Quercetin																						
Etxeberria et al. (2015)	Quercetin supplementation (30 mg/kg body weight/day) for 6 weeks and the control group as reference/rat model (rats fed HFD) [41]	↓																				
Epigallocatechin-3-gallate and resveratrol (EGCG + RES)																						
Most et al. (2017)	EGCG + RES group (282 mg/d, 80 mg/day) for 12 weeks and baseline as reference/clinical trials (19 subjects: overweight, obese females, 37.3 ± 1.6 years, BMI 29.6 ± 0.5 kg/m^2) [72]					↓		↓													*F. prausnitizii*	
Fruit-derived polyphenols																						
Mayta-Apaza et al. (2018)	Tart cherry juice consumption (8 oz/day) for 5 days and baseline as reference/clinical trials (10 healthy participants with low-bacteroides: 5 males, 5 females, aged 23–30 years) [70]		↑					↑	↑							↓						
	Tart cherry juice consumption (8 oz/day) for 5 days and baseline as reference/clinical trials (10 healthy participants with high-bacteroides: 5males, 5females, aged 23–30 years) [70]		↓					↓								↑						
Henning et al. (2017)	Vegetable/fruit juice-based juices (consumed 6 bottles, 16 oz./bottle) for 3 days and baseline as reference/clinical trials (25 healthy subjects: 18–50 years of age with a custom diet including < 3 servings of fruits/vegetables per day) [66]							↑														No significant effect
Li et al. (2015)	Pomegranate (POM) extract (1000 m/d, total phenolic content expressed as gallic acid equivalents of 680 μg/g) for 4 weeks and baseline as reference/clinical trials (20 healthy adults: 9 women and 11 men) [71]			↑	↑				↑												*A. muciniphila*	
Chacar et al. (2018)	Different concentrations of grape phenolic compounds (2.5 and 5 mg/kg/d diluted in 0.1% Dimethyl Sulfoxide) for 14 months and the control group (0.1% Dimethyl Sulfoxide alone) as reference/rat model (30, 2-mo-old rats) [59]		↑																			

Table 1. *Cont.*

	Dose and Treatment Duration/Test Model	F/B	Potentially Beneficial Microbiota													Potentially Detrimental Microbiota					Species	Diversity
			Bifidobacterium sp.	*Lactobacillus* sp.	*Akkermansia* sp.	*Fecalibacterium* sp.	*Eubacterium* sp.	*Bacteroides* sp.	*Prevotella* sp.	*Blautia* sp.	*Clostridium* sp.	*Ruminococcus* sp.	*Eggerthella* sp.	*Roseburia* sp.	*Coprococcus* sp.	*Ruminococcus* sp.	*Clostridium* sp.	*Bacteroides* sp.	*Enterobacter* sp.	*Enterococcus* sp.		
Collins et al. (2016)	A diet of high fat (HF) with an equal combination of the extractable and non-extractable grape-derived polyphenols (EP and NEP) for 16 weeks and the HF diet group as reference/mice model [53]											↑										No significant effect
Taira et al. (2015)	A diet of high fat (HF) with polyphenols from aronia, haskap, and bilerry separately (anthocyanin content was 0.4%) for 4 weeks and the HF diet group as reference/rat model [42]	↓						↓														
Neyrinck et al. (2013)	A diet of high fat (HF) with pomegranate peel-derived polyphenols (6 mg/d per mouse) for 4 weeks and the HF diet group as reference/mice model [54]		↑																			
Viveros et al. (2011)	Antibiotic-free diets containing grape pomace concentrate (60 g/kg) or grape seed extract (7.2 g/kg) for 21 days and the antibiotic-free diets group as reference/broiler chicks model [60]			↑							↑						↓			↑		↑
Mayta-Apaza et al. (2017)	Microbial suspensions (25 mL) of human distal colon compartments cultured with apricots/cherries (5 mL or g), 37 °C for 48 h and stool samples with a low diversity microbiota (dominated by Verrumicrobia and Synergistes) as reference/in vitro (68 human stool samples) [69]							↑														
Red wine-derived polyphenols																						
Moreno-Indias et al. (2016)	Participants drank red wine (272 mL/d) for 30 days and baseline as reference/clinical trials (metabolic syndrome patients) [64]	↓	↑	↑		↑			↑					↑					↓		*F. prausnitzii* *E. cloacae*	↑
Queipo-Ortuño et al. (2012)	Red wine polyphenol (272 mL per day, containing polyphenol of 733–797 mg) for 4 weeks and the baseline as reference/clinical trial (healthy men) [65]		↑				↑	↑	↑	↑			↑							↑	*Bacteroides uniformis* *Eggerthella lenta* *Blautia coccoides* *Eubacterium rectale*	↑
Dolara et al. (2005)	Red wine polyphenols (50 mg/kg) for 16 weeks and the HFD group as reference/rat model [55]		↑	↑													↓					No significant effect
Tea-derived polyphenols																						
Jin et al. (2012)	Green tea (1000 mL/day) for 10 days and baseline as reference/clinical trials [67]		↑																			
Wang et al. (2018)	TP-HFD groups (TP Low- HFD group with 0.05% TP, TP Middle- HFD group with 0.25% TP, TP High- HFD group with 0.8% TP) for 8 weeks and HFD group as reference/mice model [43]	↓																				↑
Seo et al. (2015)	HFD with fermented green tea group for 8 weeks and HFD group as reference/mice model [44]	↓																				

Note: (↑): increased F/B or microbiota population; (↓): reduced F/B or microbiota population; Blank: not reported. The potentially beneficial microbiota and potentially detrimental microbiota listed in the form were based on the information from the literature of the reviewed studies, excluding the taxa without clear description of their functions.

Table 2. Modulations of dietary vitamins, minerals, and trace elements on potentially beneficial and detrimental gut microbiota.

	Does and Treatment Duration/Test Model	F/B	Potentially Beneficial Microbiota											Potentially Detrimental Microbiota												Species	Diversity
			Bifidobacterium sp.	*Lactobacillus* sp.	*Akkermansia* sp.	*Ruminococcus* sp.	*Fecalibacterium* sp.	*Dialister* sp.	*Allobaculum* sp.	*Blautia* sp.	*Clostridium* sp.	*Roseburia* sp.	*Lactococcus* sp.	*Enterobacteria* sp.	*Escherichia* sp.	*Salmonella* sp.	*Bacteroides* sp.	*Ruminococcus* sp.	*Veillonella* sp.	*Clostridium* sp.	*Coprococcus* sp.	*Shigella* sp.	*Oscillibacter* sp.	*Enterococcus* sp.	*Pseudomonas* sp.		
Vitamin A																											
Huda et al. (2019)	One dose of 50,000 IU vitamin A within 48 h of birth and placebo as reference/clinical trial (306 infants in early (6–15 week) or late (2 y) infancy) [81]		↑		↑																						
Liu et al. (2017)	A dose of 200,000 IU vitamin A once orally for a 6-month follow-up intervention and baseline as reference/cinical trial (64 children with autism spectrum disorder, aged 1 to 8 years old) [79]		↓														↑										
Lv et al. (2016)	Vitamin A—deficient and vitamin A—normal as reference/clinical trial (59 pediatric patients with persistent diarrhea aged 1–12 months) [80]										↓													↑		*Clostridium butyricum*	↓
Lee and Ko (2017)	1 mg/kg/day of retinoic acid, the metabolite of dietary vitamin A on murine norovirus infection mice for 8 days and the murine norovirus infection mice as reference/mice model [76]		↑	↑				↑	↑																		

Table 2. *Cont.*

	Does and Treatment Duration/Test Model	F/B	Potentially Beneficial Microbiota											Potentially Detrimental Microbiota												Species	Diversity
			Bifidobacterium sp.	*Lactobacillus* sp.	*Akkermansia* sp.	*Ruminococcus* sp.	*Fecalibacterium* sp.	*Dialister* sp.	*Allobaculum* sp.	*Blautia* sp.	*Clostridium* sp.	*Roseburia* sp.	*Lactococcus* sp.	*Enterobacteria* sp.	*Escherichia* sp.	*Salmonella* sp.	*Bacteroides* sp.	*Ruminococcus* sp.	*Veillonella* sp.	*Clostridium* sp.	*Coprococcus* sp.	*Shigella* sp.	*Oscillibacter* sp.	*Enterococcus* sp.	*Pseudomonas* sp.		
Lee et al. (2016)	1 mg/kg/day of retinoic acid, the metabolite of dietary vitamin A for 8 days and the control group as reference/mice model [75]		↑					↑	↑																		
	1 mg/kg/day of retinoic acid, the metabolite of dietary vitamin A on murine norovirus infection mice for 8 days, and the murine norovirus infection mice as reference/mice model [75]			↑																							
Vitamin B																											
Miki et al. (2017)	Oral gavage with pyridoxine hydrochloride (vitamin B6) at 100 μg/mouse (Sigma) at 1–7 days after infection and baseline as reference/mice model (streptomycin-treated and *Salmonella enterica* serovar Typhimuirum-infected mice) [88]															↓											
Vitamin C																											
Li et al. (2017)	Mean 294.9 mg/d for men and mean 189.8 mg/day for women (3-day food dairy using household measures) and baseline as reference/clinical trial (16 free-living adults with cystic fibrosis) [90]																↓										

Table 2. *Cont.*

	Does and Treatment Duration/Test Model	F/B	Potentially Beneficial Microbiota												Potentially Detrimental Microbiota											Species	Diversity
			Bifidobacterium sp.	*Lactobacillus* sp.	*Akkermansia* sp.	*Ruminococcus* sp.	*Fecalibacterium* sp.	*Dialister* sp.	*Allobaculum* sp.	*Blautia* sp.	*Clostridium* sp.	*Roseburia* sp.	*Lactococcus* sp.	*Enterobacteria* sp.	*Escherichia* sp.	*Salmonella* sp.	*Bacteroides* sp.	*Ruminococcus* sp.	*Veillonella* sp.	*Clostridium* sp.	*Coprococcus* sp.	*Shigella* sp.	*Oscillibacter* sp.	*Enterococcus* sp.	*Pseudomonas* sp.		
Vitamin D																											
Naderpoor et al. (2019)	> 75 nmol/L 25-hydroxyvitamin D (25(OH)D) and vitamin D-deficient (≤ 50 nmol/L) as reference/clinical trial (25 overweight or obese (BMI ≥25 kg/m^2) healthy adults) [111]					↓												↓			↑						No effect
Garg et al. (2018)	A dose of 40,000 IU vitamin D once weekly for 8 weeks using two capsules of 20,000 IU (Plenachol, Encap) and baseline as reference/clinical trial (patients with vitamin D deficiency: 25[OH]D < 50 nmol/L) [107]													↑													No effect
Talsness et al. (2017)	Maternal supplementation of vitamin D was carried out at 0µg/day, <10 µg/day, or ≥ 10 µg/day during pregnancy and the fecal samples from their one-month old babies were tested for gut microbiota/clinical trial [109]		↓								↓						↑			↓						*Bacteroides fragilis; Clostridium difficile*	
Kanhere et al. (2017)	50,000 IU of oral vitamin D3 supplemented for 12 weeks and placebo as reference/clinical trial (Cystic Fibrosis patients as model) [98]												↑						↓								
Luthold et al. (2017)	vitamin D intake ≥ 10 µg/day in three tertiles (tertile 1: 4.21–18.93 ng/mL, tertile 2: 18.93–26.48 ng/mL, tertile 3: 26.48–61.30 ng/mL) and the highest vitamin D intake as reference/clinical trial (150 young healthy adults) [110]		↑																		↑						

Table 2. *Cont.*

	Does and Treatment Duration/Test Model	F/B	Potentially Beneficial Microbiota											Potentially Detrimental Microbiota												Species	Diversity
			Bifidobacterium sp.	*Lactobacillus* sp.	*Akkermansia* sp.	*Ruminococcus* sp.	*Fecalibacterium* sp.	*Dialister* sp.	*Allobaculum* sp.	*Blautia* sp.	*Clostridium* sp.	*Roseburia* sp.	*Lactococcus* sp.	*Enterobacteria* sp.	*Escherichia* sp.	*Salmonella* sp.	*Bacteroides* sp.	*Ruminococcus* sp.	*Veillonella* sp.	*Clostridium* sp.	*Coprococcus* sp.	*Shigella* sp.	*Oscillibacter* sp.	*Enterococcus* sp.	*Pseudomonas* sp.		
Bashir et al. (2016)	Vitamin D3 supplementation with weekly dose of 980 IU/kg bodyweight for 4 weeks, and 490 IU/kg bodyweight for the remaining 4 weeks, the baseline as reference/clinical trial (healthy volunteer) [103]														↓										↓		↑
Ciubotaru et al. (2015)	Vitamin D supplementation with weekly ergocalciferol (50,000 IU) on stable normal glucose tolerance for 12 months and the same treatment on stable prediabetes as reference/clinical trial [97]	↓				↓	↓	↓																			
Vitamin E																											
Tang et al. (2016)	Vitamin E (18 mg/day) added iron therapy (6 mg/kg/d) for 8 weeks and placebo added iron therapy (6 mg/kg/day) as reference/clinical trial (infants and toddlers who were at risk of iron deficiency) [119]											↑															
Choi et al. (2019)	High vitamin E group (0.18 mg/20 g of bw per day) treated by oral gavage for 34 days, the control group (0.2 mL of corn oil) and low vitamin E group (0.06 mg/20 g of bw per day) as reference/mice model [117]	↓																									

Table 2. *Cont.*

	Does and Treatment Duration/Test Model	F/B	Potentially Beneficial Microbiota											Potentially Detrimental Microbiota												Species	Diversity
			Bifidobacterium sp.	*Lactobacillus* sp.	*Akkermansia* sp.	*Ruminococcus* sp.	*Fecalibacterium* sp.	*Dialister* sp.	*Allobaculum* sp.	*Blautia* sp.	*Clostridium* sp.	*Roseburia* sp.	*Lactococcus* sp.	*Enterobacteria* sp.	*Escherichia* sp.	*Salmonella* sp.	*Bacteroides* sp.	*Ruminococcus* sp.	*Veillonella* sp.	*Clostridium* sp.	*Coprococcus* sp.	*Shigella* sp.	*Oscillibacter* sp.	*Enterococcus* sp.	*Pseudomonas* sp.		
Calcium																											
Trautvetter et al. (2018)	Supplementation of 1000 mg calcium +1000 mg phosphorus/day for 8 weeks and the supplementation of 1000 mg phosphorus/day as reference/clinical trials (healthy men) [124]										↑															*Clostridium* XVIII	
	Supplementation of 1000 mg calcium +1000 mg phosphorus/day for 8 weeks and the supplementation of 500 mg calcium + 1000 mg phosphorus/day as reference/clinical trials (healthy men) [124]		↓								↑															*Clostridium* XVIII	
Li et al. (2018)	Maternal insufficient calcium intake (2.5 g/kg) / Maternal excess calcium intake (12 g/kg) for 8 weeks will influence the gut microbiota in the offspring/mice model [126]	↑*																									
Chaplin et al. (2016)	HFD enriched with calcium supplementation (12 g/kg) for 54 days and HFD group (4 g/kg) as reference/mice model [127]		↑	↑																							
Borda-Molina et al. (2016)	Diet mixed with the supplementation of calcium (3 g/kg) for 10 days and diet without calcium group as reference/broiler chickens model [151]																										↓
Aslam et al. (2016)	HFD enriched with calcium supplementation (5.25 g/kg) for 18 months and HFD group (0.41 g/kg) as reference/mice model [125]				↑	↑																					↑

Table 2. *Cont.*

	Does and Treatment Duration/Test Model	F/B	Potentially Beneficial Microbiota											Potentially Detrimental Microbiota												Species	Diversity
			***Bifidobacterium* sp.**	***Lactobacillus* sp.**	***Akkermansia* sp.**	***Ruminococcus* sp.**	***Fecalibacterium* sp.**	***Dialister* sp.**	***Allobaculum* sp.**	***Blautia* sp.**	***Clostridium* sp.**	***Roseburia* sp.**	***Lactococcus* sp.**	***Enterobacteria* sp.**	***Escherichia* sp.**	***Salmonella* sp.**	***Bacteroides* sp.**	***Ruminococcus* sp.**	***Veillonella* sp.**	***Clostridium* sp.**	***Coprococcus* sp.**	***Shigella* sp.**	***Oscillibacter* sp.**	***Enterococcus* sp.**	***Pseudomonas* sp.**		
Magnesium**																											
Jørgensen et al. (2015)	Dietary magnesium deficiency (0.02% magnesium) for 6 weeks and standard diet (0.2% magnesium) group as reference/mice model [130]																										↓
Winther et al. (2015)	Dietary magnesium deficiency (0.02% magnesium) for 6 weeks and standard diet (0.2% magnesium) group as reference / Mice model [131]																										No significant effect
Pachikian et al. (2010)	Magnesium-deficient diet (70 mg/kg) for 4 days and control diet (500 mg/kg) group as reference/mice model [129]		↓																								
	Magnesium-deficient diet (70 mg/kg) for 21 days and control diet (500 mg/kg) group as reference/mice model [129]		↑	↑																							

Table 2. *Cont.*

	Does and Treatment Duration/Test Model	F/B	Potentially Beneficial Microbiota											Potentially Detrimental Microbiota												Species	Diversity
			Bifidobacterium sp.	*Lactobacillus* sp.	*Akkermansia* sp.	*Ruminococcus* sp.	*Fecalibacterium* sp.	*Dialister* sp.	*Allobaculum* sp.	*Blautia* sp.	*Clostridium* sp.	*Roseburia* sp.	*Lactococcus* sp.	*Enterobacteria* sp.	*Escherichia* sp.	*Salmonella* sp.	*Bacteroides* sp.	*Ruminococcus* sp.	*Veillonella* sp.	*Clostridium* sp.	*Coprococcus* sp.	*Shigella* sp.	*Oscillibacter* sp.	*Enterococcus* sp.	*Pseudomonas* sp.		
Iron																											
Kotryna Simonyté Sjodin et al. (2019)	High-iron-fortified formula (6.4 mg Fe/day) for 45 days and the baseline as reference/clinical trials (6-month-old healthy Swedish infants) [139]		↓																								
	High-iron-fortified formula (6.4 mg Fe/day) for 45 days and low-iron-fortified formula (1.2 mg Fe/day) as reference/clinical trials (6-month-old healthy Swedish infants) [139]		↓	↑																							
	High-iron-fortified formula (6.4 mg Fe/day) for 45 days and iron drops (no-added-iron formula with liquid ferrous sulfate supplementation (5.7 mg Fe/day) as reference/clinical trials (6-month-old healthy Swedish infants) [139]			↑													↓										
Tang et al. (2017)	Multiple micronutrient powder containing 12.5 mg iron daily for 3 months and multiple micronutrient powder without the iron as reference/clinical trials (6-month-old Kenyan infants) [135]		↓												↑					↑							
Lee et al. (2017)	Iron therapy via Per Oral over 3 months and via Intravenous as reference/clinical trials (IBD patients with anemia) [149]					↓	↓																			*Fecalibacterium prausnitzii; Ruminococcus bromii*	

Table 2. *Cont.*

	Does and Treatment Duration/Test Model	F/B	Potentially Beneficial Microbiota											Potentially Detrimental Microbiota												Species	Diversity
			Bifidobacterium sp.	*Lactobacillus* sp.	*Akkermansia* sp.	*Ruminococcus* sp.	*Fecalibacterium* sp.	*Dialister* sp.	*Allobaculum* sp.	*Blautia* sp.	*Clostridium* sp.	*Roseburia* sp.	*Lactococcus* sp.	*Enterobacteria* sp.	*Escherichia* sp.	*Salmonella* sp.	*Bacteroides* sp.	*Ruminococcus* sp.	*Veillonella* sp.	*Clostridium* sp.	*Coprococcus* sp.	*Shigella* sp.	*Oscillibacter* sp.	*Enterococcus* sp.	*Pseudomonas* sp.		
Jaeggi et al. (2015)	Home-fortified maize porridge containing 2.5 mg iron daily for 4 months and porridge without the iron as reference/clinical trials (6-month-old Kenyan infants) [134]											↑			↑							↑				*Escherichia coli*	
Jaeggi et al. (2015)	Home-fortified maize porridge containing 12.5 mg iron daily for 4 months and porridge without the iron as reference/clinical trials (6-month-old Kenyan infants) [134]		↓												↑		↑			↑		↑				*Escherichia coli*	
Dostal et al. (2014)	Oral tablets containing 50 mh Fe for 4 d/week, last for 38 weeks, and the placebo as reference/clinical trial (6–11 rural South African children with Fe deficiency) [138]																										
Zimmermann et al. (2010)	Iron-fortified biscuits containing 20 mg Fe/d, and 4 times/week, last for 6 months, and the nonfortified biscuits as reference/clinical trial (6–14 Ivorian children) [136]			↓										↑		↑											↑
Fang et al. (2018)	1 mL liquid iron (Liquid iron preparations were prepared by dissolving $FeSO_4$ salt in 1 mL of 0.01 mol/L HCL) preparation containing 8 mg, 16 mg, or 24 mg of iron for 30 days and control group (0.01 mol/L HCI) as reference/rat model [140]								↓												↑						↑

Table 2. *Cont.*

	Does and Treatment Duration/Test Model	F/B	Potentially Beneficial Microbiota											Potentially Detrimental Microbiota												Species	Diversity
			Bifidobacterium sp.	*Lactobacillus* sp.	*Akkermansia* sp.	*Ruminococcus* sp.	*Fecalibacterium* sp.	*Dialister* sp.	*Allobaculum* sp.	*Blautia* sp.	*Clostridium* sp.	*Roseburia* sp.	*Lactococcus* sp.	*Enterobacteria* sp.	*Escherichia* sp.	*Salmonella* sp.	*Bacteroides* sp.	*Ruminococcus* sp.	*Veillonella* sp.	*Clostridium* sp.	*Coprococcus* sp.	*Shigella* sp.	*Oscillibacter* sp.	*Enterococcus* sp.	*Pseudomonas* sp.		
Constante et al. (2017)	Iron-sufficient diet (50 mg/kg) for 4 weeks and iron-deficient diet (5 mg/kg) as reference/mice model [145]												↓				↑							↑		*Bacteroides caccae*	
	Iron-supplemented diet (500 mg/kg) for 4 weeks and iron-sufficient diet (50 mg/kg) as reference/mice model [145]																							↑			
	Ferrous bisglycinate (FBG) (50 mg/kg) for 4 weeks and ferrous sulfate (FS) (50 mg/kg) as reference/mice model [145]																										
	Ferric ethylenediaminetetraacetic acid (FEDTA) for 4 weeks and ferrous sulfate (FS) (50 mg/kg) as reference/mice model [145]										↓	↓								↓						
Kortman et al. (2016)	Medium with iron (50 or 250 µmol/l ferrous sulfate, 50 or 250 µmol/l ferric citrate, or 50 umol/L hemin) incubated for 44 h at 37 °C and medium without supplementary iron as reference/in vitro (Human fecal sample) [141]																										
Phosphorus																											
Borda-Molina et al. (2016)	Diet mixed with the supplementation of Phosphorus (3 g/kg) for 10 days and diet without calcium group as reference/broiler chickens model [151]			↑↓#			↑																			*Lactobacillus taiwanensis*	↑↓

Table 2. *Cont.*

	Does and Treatment Duration/Test Model	F/B	Potentially Beneficial Microbiota										Potentially Detrimental Microbiota													Species	Diversity
			Bifidobacterium sp.	*Lactobacillus* sp.	*Akkermansia* sp.	*Ruminococcus* sp.	*Fecalibacterium* sp.	*Dialister* sp.	*Allobaculum* sp.	*Blautia* sp.	*Clostridium* sp.	*Roseburia* sp.	*Lactococcus* sp.	*Enterobacteria* sp.	*Escherichia* sp.	*Salmonella* sp.	*Bacteroides* sp.	*Ruminococcus* sp.	*Veillonella* sp.	*Clostridium* sp.	*Coprococcus* sp.	*Shigella* sp.	*Oscillibacter* sp.	*Enterococcus* sp.	*Pseudomonas* sp.		
Witzig et al. (2015)	Diet mixed with the supplementation of phosphorus for 10 days and diet without phosphorus group as reference/broiler chickens model [253]			↑ ↓#																						*Lactobacillus taiwanensis; Lactobacillus salivarius; Lactobacillus crispatus; Lactobacillus reuteri*	↑↓
Zinc																											
Zackular et al. (2016)	High Zn diet (1000 mg/kg) for 5 weeks and control diet (29 mg/kg) as reference/mice model [155]																			↑				↑		*Clostridium* XI	↓
Reed et al. (2015)	Zn diet (42 ug/g) for 28 days and Zn deficiency diet (2.5 ug/g) as reference/chicks model [153]													↓										↓			↑
Shao et al. (2014)	Supplemental Zn (120 mg/kg) diet for 42 days and diet without Zn as reference/Salmonella Typhimurium-challenged Broiler chicken model [154]			↑												↓											↑
Selenium																											
Zhai et al. (2018)	Selenium diet (added amounts of Se 0.4 mg/kg) for 8 weeks and Se-deficient diet (Se level < 0.01 mg /kg) as reference/mice model [158]				↑																						Not significant effect

Table 2. *Cont.*

	Does and Treatment Duration/Test Model	F/B	Potentially Beneficial Microbiota										Potentially Detrimental Microbiota													Species	Diversity
			Bifidobacterium sp.	*Lactobacillus* sp.	*Akkermansia* sp.	*Ruminococcus* sp.	*Fecalibacterium* sp.	*Dialister* sp.	*Allobaculum* sp.	*Blautia* sp.	*Clostridium* sp.	*Roseburia* sp.	*Lactococcus* sp.	*Enterobacteria* sp.	*Escherichia* sp.	*Salmonella* sp.	*Bacteroides* sp.	*Ruminococcus* sp.	*Veillonella* sp.	*Clostridium* sp.	*Coprococcus* sp.	*Shigella* sp.	*Oscillibacter* sp.	*Enterococcus* sp.	*Pseudomonas* sp.		
Kasaikina et al. (2011)	Selenium diet (added amounts of Se 0, 0.1, 0.4, and 2.25 ppm) for 10 weeks and Se-deficient diet (0 ppm Se diet) as reference/mice model [157]																										↑
Iodine																											
Shen et al. (2019)	18µg/kg/d iodine for 8 weeks and un-treated obese mice as reference/HFD-induced obesity mice model [159]								↑	↓										↑			↑	↑			
	18µg/kg/d iodine for 8 weeks and control group as reference/mice model [159]		↑	↑			↑		↑	↓		↑														*Fecalibacterium prausnizii*	

* Insufficient calcium for mother mice leads to change in their offspring; ** Magnesium deficient; # Changes in different sections of gastrointestinal tract of broiler chickens. Note: (↑): increased F/B or microbiota population; (↓): reduced F/B or microbiota population; Blank: not reported. The potentially beneficial microbiota and potentially detrimental microbiota listed in the form were based on the information from the literature of the reviewed studies, excluding the taxa without a clear description of their functions.

Table 3. Modulations of dietary carbohydrates on potentially beneficial and detrimental gut microbiota.

	Dose and Treatment Duration/Test Model	F/B	Potentially Beneficial Microbiota										Potentially Detrimental Microbiota					Species	Diversity
			Bifidobacterium sp.	*Lactobacillus* sp.	*Akkermansia* sp.	*Fecalibacterium* sp.	*Roseburia* sp.	*Eubacterium* sp.	*Bacteroides* sp.	*Prevotella* sp.	*Clostridium* sp.	*Runinococcus* sp.	*Eggerthella* sp.	*Ruminococcus* sp.	*Clostridium* sp.	*Bacteroides* sp.	*Enterococcus* sp.		
Arabinoxylan																			
Hald et al. (2016)	Arabinoxylan (AX)-enriched diet (whole-grain rye and enzyme-treated wheat bran) for 4 weeks and baseline as reference/clinical trials (24 subjects: 39–75 years with metabolic syndrome) [174]		↑																↓
	Arabinoxylan (AX)-enriched diet (whole-grain rye and enzyme-treated wheat bran) for 4 weeks and a low-fiber western-style diet (refined grains and a minimal concentration dietary fiber) as reference/clinical trials (24 subjects: 39–75 years with metabolic syndrome) [174]		↑																↓
Arabinoxylan-oligosaccharides																			
Windey et al. (2015)	Wheat bran extract (10 g/day) containing arabinoxylan-oligosaccharides for 3 weeks and placebo (maltodextrin, 10 g/day) as reference/clinical trials (20 healthy subjects: 17 women and 3 men; age range 19–44 years; BMI range 18.7–24.3 kg/m^2) [182]			↑														*Bifidobacterium adolescentis*	
François et al. (2014)	WBE (enriched AXOS) at 5 g/day for 3 weeks and placebo as reference/clinical trials (29 healthy children, age range of 8–12 years) [181]		↑																
Walton et al. (2012)	AXOS treatment (2.2 g) for 21 days and placebo as reference/clinical trials (40 healthy adults: 20 males and 20 females, mean age 31.4 years (± 8.9), average BMI 23.3 kg/m^2 (± 2.8)) [178]		↑																
François et al. (2012)	Wheat bran extract (WBE, 10 g/day)-enriched AXOS for 3 weeks; both WBE (3 g/day) group and placebo group as references/clinical trials (63 healthy adults) [176]		↑																
Cloetens et al. (2010)	Arabinoxylan-oligosaccharides (AXOS, 10 g/d) for 3 weeks and placebo as reference/clinical trials (20 healthy subjects: 14 women, 6 men; mean age 24 (sd 5) years, mean BMI 20.9 (sd 2.3) kg/m^2) [175]		↑																
Xylo-oligosaccharide																			
Childs et al. (2014)	XOS (8 g/day) for 21 days and placebo as reference/clinical trials (44 healthy adults, 25–65 years) [179]		↑																
Finegold et al. (2014)	XOS (1.4 g/day or 2.8 g/day) for 8 weeks and the placebo as reference/clinical trials (32 healthy adults) [180]		↑																
Lecerf et al. (2012)	Xylo-oligosaccharide (XOS, 5 g/d) for 4 weeks and placebo (wheat maltodextrin, 5 g/day) as reference/clinical trials (60 healthy volunteers) [177]		↑																

Table 3. *Cont.*

	Dose and Treatment Duration/Test Model	F/B	Potentially Beneficial Microbiota											Potentially Detrimental Microbiota				Species	Diversity
			Bifidobacterium sp.	*Lactobacillus* sp.	*Akkermansia* sp.	*Fecalibacterium* sp.	*Roseburia* sp.	*Eubacterium* sp.	*Bacteroides* sp.	*Prevotella* sp.	*Clostridium* sp.	*Ruminococcus* sp.	*Eggerthella* sp.	*Ruminococcus* sp.	*Clostridium* sp.	*Bacteroides* sp.	*Enterococcus* sp.		
Galacto-oligosaccharides																			
Azcarate-Peril et al. (2017)	GOS (> 95% purity) treatment in 5 d increments according to a fixed schedule from 1.5 g/day to 15 g/day up to 36 days and placebo (Sweetose) as reference/clinical trials (52 lactose-intolerant individuals, mean age of 41 year, mean BMI of 27.1) [192]		↑	↑		↑									↓				
Civardi et al. (2017)	GOS (7 g/L) for 60 ± 5 days and standard formula without GOS as reference/clinical trials (117 healthy infants: formula milk supplemented with functional ingredients (n = 55), or a standard formula (n = 62)) [197]		↑																
Paganini et al. (2017)	Iron-containing micronutrient powders (MNPs) with GOS (7.5 g/day) for 4 months; MNPs without iron and MNPs with 5 mg iron as references/clinical trials (Kenyan infants aged 6.5–9.5 months (n = 155)) [198]		↑	↑											↓				
Musilova et al. (2015)	GOS (9 g/day) and maltodextrins (1 g/d) for 5 days and baseline as reference/clinical trials (fecal samples of 11 healthy adults: 6 women and 5 men; mean age, 35.18 ± 10.91 years) [190]		↑																
Vulevic et al. (2015)	GOS (5.5 g/day) for 10 weeks and placebo (maltodextrin) as reference/clinical trials (40 elderly volunteers: 25 women and 15 men; range age of 65–80 years) [191]		↑						↑										
Sierra et al. (2015)	GOS (0.44 g/day) for 6 months with additional feeding of GOS (0.5 g/dl) for 6 months and placebo as reference/clinical trials (365 healthy infants had a gestational age of 37–42 weeks and a birth weight greater than 2500 g) [196]		↑																
Giovannini et al. (2014)	GOS-supplemented formula (0.4 g/100 mL) for up to 70 days and the identical formula without GOS as reference/clinical trials (160 healthy infants: gestational age from 37 to 42 completed weeks; birth weight ≥ 2500 g) [134]		↑	↑											↓				
Whisner et al. (2013)	Smoothie drinks with daily GOS intake 0 g, 5 g, and 10 g for three 3-week periods in a random order and baseline as reference/clinical trials (31 healthy adolescent girls: age 10–13 years) [193]		↑																
Westerbeek et al. (2013)	Mixture of neutral and acidic oligosaccharides (scGOS/lcFOS/pAOS) in increasing doses between days 3 and 30 of life to 1.5 g/kg/day, and the placebo as reference/clinical trials (113 healthy infants) [195]		↑																↓
Scalabrin et al. (2012)	Formula with polydextrose (PDX) and galacto-oligosaccharides (GOS) (4 g/L, 1:1 ratio) for 60 days and control formula (Enfamil Lipil) as reference/clinical trials (230 healthy infants: 21- to 30-days-old with 37 to 42 weeks of gestational age, birth weight ≥2500 g) [194]		↑																
Walton et al. (2012 b)	GOS (4 g) twice/d for 3 weeks and placebo as reference/clinical trials (39 volunteers: age 50–81 years, BMI of 19.7–38.4 kg/m^2) [189]		↑																

Table 3. *Cont.*

	Dose and Treatment Duration/Test Model	F/B	Potentially Beneficial Microbiota											Potentially Detrimental Microbiota				Species	Diversity
			Bifidobacterium sp.	*Lactobacillus* sp.	*Akkermansia* sp.	*Fecalibacterium* sp.	*Roseburia* sp.	*Eubacterium* sp.	*Bacteroides* sp.	*Prevotella* sp.	*Clostridium* sp.	*Ruminococcus* sp.	*Eggerthella* sp.	*Ruminococcus* sp.	*Clostridium* sp.	*Bacteroides* sp.	*Enterococcus* sp.		
Davis et al. (2011)	GOS with four dosages (0, 2.5, 5, and 10 g/d) for 3 eewks each (12 weeks in total) and baseline as reference/clinical trials (18 healthy volunteers) [188]		↑																
Davis et al. (2010)	GOS-containing chocolate chews with dosage levels (5.0 g and 10.0 g) for 3 weeks and baseline as reference/clinical trials (18 subjects: 13 males and 5 females, ages of 19 to 50 years old) [187]		↑																
Monteagudo-Mera et al. (2016)	GOS (90% purity, 40 mL/day equivalent of 0.26 g/kg bodyweight of GOS) for 14 days and baseline as reference/mice model (four pathogen-free mice) [186]		↑	↑					↑		↑				↓				
Ladirat et al. (2014)	GOS (4.2 mg/mL) and 4 antibiotics (1 or 10 μg/mL) in the medium for healthy adult fecal sample fermentation for up to 48 h and antibiotic-treated samples as reference/in vitro (8 healthy adult fecal samples) [185]		↑	↑															
Raffinose-oligosaccharide																			
Fernando et al. (2010)	Diet fortified with canned chickpeas (200 g/day) or raffinose oligosaccharide (5 g/day) for 3 weeks and control diet as reference/clinical trials (12 healthy adults: 18–65 years) [200]		↑												↓			*Clostridium* clusters I/II and XI; *Clostridium histolyticum; Clostridium lituseburense* group	No significant effect
Lactose																			
Francavilla et al. (2012)	Formula with no lactose for 2 months followed by an identical lactose-containing (3.8% lactose) formula for an additional 2 months to infants with cow's milk protein allergy (CMA), and the formula with no-lactose as reference/clinical trials (28 infants with CMA) [199]		↑	↑															
Inulin/inulin-type fructans																			
Drabinska et al. (2018)	Oligofructose-enriched inulin (Synergy 1) (10 g/d) for 3 months and placebo (maltodextrin; 7 g/day) as reference/clinical trials (34 pediatric celiac disease patients, mean age 10 years, 62% females, on a gluten-free diet) [206]		↑																
Vandeputte et al. (2017)	Chicory-derived Orafti inulin (12 g/day) for 4 weeks and placebo as reference/clinical trials (42 healthy adults with mild constipation) [205]		↑																No significant effect
Nicolucci et al. (2017)	Oligofructose-enriched inulin (8 g/day) for 16 wks and placebo (maltodextrin) as reference/clinical trials (42 healthy children, 7–12 years, overweight or obese >85 th percentile of body mass index) [208]		↑													↓		*Bacteroides vulgatus*	
Salazar et al. (2014)	ITF (16 g/day) for 3 months and the placebo maltodextrin group as reference/clinical trials (30 obese women, BMI > 30 kg/m^2, age range of 18 to 65 years) [207]		↑															*Bifidobacterium longum, B. pseudocatenulatum; B. adolescentis*	

Table 3. *Cont.*

	Dose and Treatment Duration/Test Model	F/B	Potentially Beneficial Microbiota											Potentially Detrimental Microbiota				Species	Diversity
			Bifidobacterium sp.	*Lactobacillus* sp.	*Akkermansia* sp.	*Fecalibacterium* sp.	*Roseburia* sp.	*Eubacterium* sp.	*Bacteroides* sp.	*Prevotella* sp.	*Clostridium* sp.	*Ruminococcus* sp.	*Eggerthella* sp.	*Ruminococcus* sp.	*Clostridium* sp.	*Bacteroides* sp.	*Enterococcus* sp.		
Dewulf et al. (2013)	ITF (Synergy 1, inulin/ oligofructose 50/50 mix, 16 g/day) for 3 months and placebo (maltodextrin, 16 g/d) as reference/clinical trials (30 obese women, BMI > 30 kg/m^2, age range of 18 to 65 years) [204]		↑			↑										↓		*Fecalibacterium prausnitzii*; *Bacteroides intestinalis*; *B. vulgatus*	
Ramirez-Farias et al. (2008)	Inulin (10 g/day) for 16 days and a control period without any supplement intake as reference/clinical trials (12 human volunteers) [203]		↑			↑													
Catry et al. (2017)	*n*-3 polyunsaturated fatty acid-depleted diet for 12 weeks with inulin-type fructans (ITF) (250 mg/mouse/d) for the last 15 days and group without ITF as reference/mice model (*n*-3 PUFA-depleted Apoe−/− mice) [202]				↑														No significant effect
Licht et al. (2006)	Inulin (150 g/kg) in diet for 5 weeks and baseline as reference/Rats model (8 rats with western type diet) [201]																↓		
High-fiber diet																			
Dao et al. (2016)	Calorie-restricted diet (enriched with fiber and protein) for 6 weeks and baseline as reference/clinical trials (49 overweight and obese adults) [167]				↑													*Akkermansia muciniphila*	
Candela et al. (2016)	Fiber-rich macrobiotic Ma-Pi 2 diet and a diet recommended by Italian professional societies for type 2 diabetes (T2 D) treatment, baseline as reference/clinical trials (40 overweight T2 D patients, aged 50–77 years) [168]				↑	↑	↑		↑										↑
Holscher et al. (2014)	Soluble corn fiber (21 g/day) for 21 days and no supplemental fiber placebo as reference/clinical trials (14 healthy adult men) [169]	↓							↑										
Tap et al. (2015)	A basal diet supplemented with dietary fiber (40 g/day) for 5 days and diet with dietary fiber (10 g/day) as reference/clinical trials (19 healthy adults: 9 males and 10 females, aged 19–25 years) [170]									↑									↑
Kovatcheva-Datchary et al. (2015)	Barley kernel-based bread consumption for 3 days and white wheat flour bread group as reference/clinical trials (39 healthy subjects: 6 men and 33 women, age 50–70 years, BMI 18–28 kg/m^2) [171]									↑								*Prevotella copri*	
García-Peris et al. (2012)	Mixture of fiber (6 g twice daily, 50% inulin and 50% fructo-oligosaccharide) from one week before to three weeks after radiotherapy and the placebo (maltodextrin, 6 g twice daily) as reference/clinical trials (≥ 18-year-old female patients with gynecological cancer who received radiotherapy after surgery) [166]		↑	↑															
De Filippo et al. (2010)	High-fiber diet represented by the one of children in a rural African village of Burkina Faso (BF) and a diet represented by the one of European (EU) children as reference/clinical trials (15 healthy children in BF, additional 15 healthy children in EU, age range of 1–6 years) [172]	↓																	↑

Table 3. *Cont.*

	Dose and Treatment Duration/Test Model	F/B	Potentially Beneficial Microbiota										Potentially Detrimental Microbiota					Species	Diversity
			Bifidobacterium sp.	*Lactobacillus* sp.	*Akkermansia* sp.	*Fecalibacterium* sp.	*Roseburia* sp.	*Eubacterium* sp.	*Bacteroides* sp.	*Prevotella* sp.	*Clostridium* sp.	*Ruminococcus* sp.	*Eggerthella* sp.	*Ruminococcus* sp.	*Clostridium* sp.	*Bacteroides* sp.	*Enterococcus* sp.		
Benus et al. (2010)	Dietary fiber formula (dietary fiber 19.6 and 18.0 g/day) for 14 days and the fiber-free diet as reference/clinical trials (10 healthy subjects: 6 women and 4 men, age range of 21–34 years) [164]		↑																
Carvalho-Wells et al. (2010)	Maize-derived whole grain cereal (48 g/day) for 21 days and the same dose of placebo cereal as reference/clinical trials (28 healthy volunteers: 7 males and 21 females, age range 20–51 years, BMI 20–30 kg/m^2) [165]		↑																
Avila-Nava et al. (2017)	Pre-hispanic Mexican diet (PMD: containing corn flour, black beans concentrate, nopal, chia and pumpkin seed, with 8 g fiber/100 g diet) for 3 months and control diet (AIN-93) as reference/rats model (18 rats sucrose-enriched high-fat diet caused gut microbiota dysbiosis) [162]	↓		↑															
Resistant Starch																			
Martínez et al. (2010)	Crackers (100 g/day) containing native starch for 3 weeks and the baseline as references/clinical trials (10 subjects: age range of 23–38 years) [210]					↑												*Fecalibacterium prausnitzii*	
	Crackers (100 g/day) containing 33 g type 2 resistant starch (RS) for 3 wks and RS type 4 as references /Clinical trials (10 subjects: age range of 23–38 years) [210]							↑				↑						*Ruminococcus bromii* *Eubacterium rectale*	
	Crackers (100 g/d) containing 33 g type 4 RS for 3 weeks and the baseline as references/clinical trials (10 subjects: age range of 23–38 years) [210]	↓	↑															*Bifidobacterium adolescentis*	
Butyrylated Starch																			
Hald et al. (2016)	Resistant starch (type 2) and arabinoxylan enriched diet for 4 weeks and the baseline as reference/clinical trials (19 subjects: 39–75 years, with metabolic syndrome) [174]		↑																↓
	Resistant starch (type 2) and arabinoxylan enriched diet for 4 weeks and a low-fiber western-style diet group as reference/clinical trials (19 subjects: 39–75 years, with metabolic syndrome) [174]		↑																↓
Le Leu et al. (2015)	Butyrylated high-amylose maize starch (HAMSB, 40 g/d) with a high red meat diet (HRM, cooked red meat 300 g/d) for 4 weeks and baseline as reference/clinical trials (23 individuals with red meat-increased O6-methyl-2-deoxyguanosine adduct level) [212]			↑							↑	↑		↓				*Clostridium coccoides* *C. leptum* group *Ruminococcus bromii*; *R. torques*; *R. gnavus*	

Table 3. *Cont.*

	Dose and Treatment Duration/Test Model	F/B	Potentially Beneficial Microbiota											Potentially Detrimental Microbiota				Species	Diversity
			Bifidobacterium sp.	*Lactobacillus* sp.	*Akkermansia* sp.	*Fecalibacterium* sp.	*Roseburia* sp.	*Eubacterium* sp.	*Bacteroides* sp.	*Prevotella* sp.	*Clostridium* sp.	*Ruminococcus* sp.	*Eggerthella* sp.	*Ruminococcus* sp.	*Clostridium* sp.	*Bacteroides* sp.	*Enterococcus* sp.		
Oligofructose																			
Wernimont et al. (2015)	Formula with oligofructose (OF, 3.0 g/L) for 8 weeks and identical formula without OF but enriched with α-lactalbumin (3.0 g/L) as reference/clinical trials (48 healthy infants) [214]		↑																
Cluny et al. (2015)	High-fat/high-sucrose (HFS) diet with 10% oligofructose for 6 weeks and HFS diet group as reference/rats model (46 rats with diet-induced obesity (23) and diet-resistant (23)) [213]		↑	↑			↑								↓			*Clostridium leptum*	
Polydextrose																			
Costabile et al. (2012)	Polydextrose (PDX; 8 g/d) for 3 weeks and the equivalent placebo (maltodextrin powder, 8 g/d) as reference/clinical trials (31 healthy subjects: age 18–50 years, BMI 19–25 kg/m^2) [216]										↑	↑						*Ruminococcus intestinalis* *Clostridium* clusters I, II and IV	
High/low carbohydrate diet																			
Haro et al. (2016)	High-complex carbohydrate diet with low fat (28% fat, 12% monounsaturated) for 1 year and the baseline group as reference/clinical trials (20 obese patients (men) with coronary heart disease) [173]					↑	↓			↑								*Fecalibacterium prausnitzii*	
Ley et al. (2006)	Carbohydrate-restricted low-calorie diet for 1 year with obese people and a lean people group as reference/clinical trials (12 obese people) [35]	↓							↑										

Note: (↑): increased F/B or microbiota population; (↓): reduced F/B or microbiota population; Blank: not reported. The potentially beneficial microbiota and potentially detrimental microbiota listed in the form were based on the information from the literature of the reviewed studies, excluding the taxa without clear description of their function.

Table 4. Modulations of dietary fat on potentially beneficial and detrimental gut microbiota.

	Dose and Treatment Duration/Test Model	F/B	Potentially Beneficial Microbiota										Potentially Detrimental Microbiota													Species	Diversity
			Bifidobacterium sp.	*Lactobacillus* sp.	*Akkermansia* sp.	*Fecalibacterium* sp.	*Roseburia* sp.	*Eubacterium* sp.	*Bacteroides* sp.	*Prevotella* sp.	*Blautia* sp.	*Parabacteroides* sp.	*Ruminococcus* sp.	*Oscillospira* sp.	*Allobaculum* sp.	*Clostridium* sp.	*Enterococcus* sp.	*Escherichia* sp.	*Bilophila* sp.	*Streptococcus* sp.	*Alistipes* sp.	*Bacteroides* sp.	*Serratia* sp.	*Pantoea* sp.	*Citrobacter* sp.		
Saturated fat																											
Patterson et al. (2014)	High-palm oil (45% energy from fat) for 16 weeks and compared with low-fat diet (12% energy from fat)/mice model [235]	↑																									
De Wit et al. (2012)	High-palm oil (45% energy from fat) for 8 weeks and low-palm oil diet (10% energy from fat) as reference/mice model [236]	↑														↑										*Clostridium XI*	↓
Devkota et al. (2012)	Lard-based fat (37% energy from fat) for 24 weeks and low-fat diet (5% energy from fat) as reference/mice model [228]	↑																									
	Milk-derived fat (37% energy from fat) for 24 weeks and low-fat diet (5% energy from fat) as reference/mice model [228]	↓																	↑							*B. wadsworthia*	↓
Zentek et al. (2012)	Diet with medium-chain fatty acids uncoated (MCFA) for 4 weeks and the diet without MCFA as reference/piglets model [237]			↑				↑																		*L. johnsonii*; *L. amylovorus*	
Polyunsaturated fatty acid (PUFA)																											
Younge et al. (2017)	Early enteral supplementation with a high fat-PUFA blend of fish oil and safflower oil up to 10 weeks and the standard nutritional therapy as reference/clinical trial (premature infants with an enterostomy) [239]															↓		↓		↓			↓	↓	↓		↑
Patterson et al. (2014)	High flaxseed/fish oil (45% energy from fat) for 16 weeks and compared with a low-fat diet (12% energy from fat)/mice model [235]		↑												↑												↑
Devkota et al. (2012)	High safflower oil (37% energy from fat) for 24 weeks and low-fat diet (5% energy from fat) as reference/mice model [228]	↓																									↓
Fat diet (17% lard)																											
Avila-Nava et al. (2017)	HFD (17% lard fat and 7% soy oil) for 6 months and control diet (7% soy oil) as reference/rat model [162]	↑	↓	↓	↓																						
Fat diet (20–21.45% fat)																											
Wan et al. (2019)	Fat diet (20%) for 6 months and the baseline as reference/clinical trial (healthy young adults) [230]					↑					↑																
Lecomte et al. (2015)	HFD (21.45% fat) for 16 weeks and normal diet (12% fat) as reference/rat model [229]	↓		↓																							↑
Qiao et al. (2013)	HFD (21.45% mixed fat) for 8 weeks and normal diet (4.89% fat) as reference/mice model [233]																↑	↑								*Escherichia coli*	

Table 4. *Cont.*

	Dose and Treatment Duration/Test Model	F/B	Potentially Beneficial Microbiota											Potentially Detrimental Microbiota												Species	Diversity
			Bifidobacterium sp.	*Lactobacillus* sp.	*Akkermansia* sp.	*Fecalibacterium* sp.	*Roseburia* sp.	*Eubacterium* sp.	*Bacteroides* sp.	*Prevotella* sp.	*Blautia* sp.	*Parabacteroides* sp.	*Ruminococcus* sp.	*Oscillospira* sp.	*Allobaculum* sp.	*Clostridium* sp.	*Enterococcus* sp.	*Escherichia* sp.	*Bilophila* sp.	*Streptococcus* sp.	*Alistipes* sp.	*Bacteroides* sp.	*Serratia* sp.	*Pantoea* sp.	*Citrobacter* sp.		
Fat diet (28–35%)																											
Wan et al. (2019)	Moderate fat diet (30%) for 6 months and the baseline as reference/clinical trial (healthy young adults) [230]	↓																									
Haro et al. (2017)	Dietary intervention of < 30% total fat for 2 years and the baseline as reference/clinical trial (male patients with coronary heart disease, who are obese and also with severe metabolic disease) [231]	↓				↑			↑	↑						↓				↓							
Haro et al. (2017)	Dietary intervention of minimum 35% fat for 2 years and the baseline as reference/clinical trial (male patients with coronary heart disease) [231]	↓				↑	↑		↑	↑		↑	↑													*Parabacteroides distasonis* *Fecalibacterium prausnitzii*	
Haro et al. (2016)	Dietary intervention of 28% fat for 1 years and the baseline as reference/clinical trial (male obese patients with coronary heart disease) [173]						↓			↑																*Fecalibacterium prausnitzii*	
	Dietary intervention of 35% fat for 1 years and the baseline as reference/clinical trial (male obese patients with coronary heart disease) [173]						↑			↓		↑		↑												*Parabacteroides distasonis*	
Fat diet (40%)																											
Wan et al. (2019)	High-fat diet (40%) for 6 months and the baseline as reference/clinical trial (healthy young adults) [230]	↓				↓															↑	↑					
	High-fat diet (40%) for 6 months and the lower-fat diet (20%) as reference/clinical trial (healthy young adults) [230]	↓				↓					↓										↑	↑					↓
HFD (44–45% fat)																											
Chen et al. (2018)	HFD (45% fat) for 8 weeks and control diet (10% fat) as reference/mice model [220]	↑																									
Collins et al. (2016)	HFD (44% mixed fat) for 16 weeks and low-fat diet (10% fat) as reference/mice model [53]																										↓
Hamilton et al. (2015)	HFD (45% mixed fat) for 1, 3, 6 weeks and normal diet (13% fat) as reference/rat model [218]	↑																									↓
Murphy et al. (2010)	HFD (45% fat) for 8 weeks and low-fat diet (10% fat) as reference/mice model [221]	↑																									
Hildebrandt et al. (2009)	HFD (45% fat) for 1 month and standard diet (12% fat) as reference/mice model [219]	↑																									

Table 4. *Cont.*

	Dose and Treatment Duration/Test Model	F/B	Potentially Beneficial Microbiota									Potentially Detrimental Microbiota														Species	Diversity
			Bifidobacterium sp.	*Lactobacillus* sp.	*Akkermansia* sp.	*Fecalibacterium* sp.	*Roseburia* sp.	*Eubacterium* sp.	*Bacteroides* sp.	*Prevotella* sp.	*Blautia* sp.	*Parabacteroides* sp.	*Ruminococcus* sp.	*Oscillospira* sp.	*Allobaculum* sp.	*Clostridium* sp.	*Enterococcus* sp.	*Escherichia* sp.	*Bilophila* sp.	*Streptococcus* sp.	*Alistipes* sp.	*Bacteroides* sp.	*Serratia* sp.	*Pantoea* sp.	*Citrobacter* sp.		
HFD (60% fat)																											
Ojo et al. (2016)	HFD (60% fat) for 12 weeks and control diet (10% fat) as reference/mice model [238]		↓		↓																						
Cowan et al. (2014)	HFD (60% fat) for 10 weeks and control diet (12% fat) as reference/rat model [224]	↑	↑													↑										*Clostridium leptum*	
Mujico et al. (2013)	HFD (60% fat) for 19 weeks and maintenance diet (12% fat) as reference/mice model [225]	↑	↓																								
Lam et al. (2012)	HFD (60% mixed fat) for 8, 12 weeks and control diet (10% fat) as reference/mice model [222]	↑		↓																							↓
Kim et al. (2012)	HFD (60% fat) for 8 weeks and low-fat diet (10% fat) as reference/mice model [223]	↑																									
HFD (72% fat)																											
Cani et al. (2008)	HFD (72% fat) for 4 weeks and standard A04 diet as reference/mice model [226]	↑		↓																							
Ley et al. (2005)	HFD (72% fat) for 19 weeks and maintenance diet (12% fat) as reference/mice model [34]	↑																									

Note: (↑): increased F/B or microbiota population; (↓): reduced F/B or microbiota population; Blank: not reported. The potentially beneficial microbiota and potentially detrimental microbiota listed in the form were based on the information from the literature of the reviewed studies, excluding the taxa without clear description of their functions.

Table 5. Modulations of dietary protein on potentially beneficial and detrimental gut microbiota.

	Dose and Treatment Duration/Test Model	F/B	Potentially Beneficial Microbiota									Potentially Detrimental Microbiota														Species	Diversity
			Bifidobacterium sp.	*Lactobacillus* sp.	*Desulfovibrio* sp.	*Robinsoniella* sp.	*Barnesiella* sp.	*Allobaculum* sp.	*Akkermansia* sp.	*Roseburia* sp.	*Blautia* sp.	*Fecalibacterium* sp.	*Bacteroides* sp.	*Clostridium* sp.	*Enterorhabdus* sp.	*Clostridium* sp.	*Alloprevotella* sp.	*Haemophilus* sp.	*Ethanoligenens* sp.	*Klebsiella* sp.	*Porphyromonas* sp.	*Escherichia* sp.	*Turicibacter* sp.	*Staphylococcus* sp.	*Enterococcus* sp.		
												Blend protein															
Moreno-Pérez et al. (2018)	Protein group (20 g/day) for 10 weeks and control group (no protein) as reference/clinical trials [247]	↓								↓	↓																No significant effect
	Protein group (20 g//day) for 70 days and before protein treatment group as reference/clinical trials [247]	↓								↓	↓																No significant effect
												Casein protein															
Rist et al. (2014)	Casein-based group/CAS (85–335 g/kg) for 3 experimental periods (7 days/period) and Soybean meal-based group/SBM (85–335 g/kg) as reference/piglet model [243]		↓	↓																							↓
												Soybean protein															
Rist et al. (2014)	SBM group (85–335 g/kg) for 3 experimental periods (7 days/period) and the CAS (85–335 g/kg) as reference/piglet model [243]																										↑
												Crude protein															
Kostovcikova et al. (2019)	High animal protein-based diet (514 g/kg) for 3 weeks and control group (176 g/kg) as reference/mice model [245]								↑													↑		↑		*A. muciniphila*	↓
	High animal protein-based diet (514 g/kg) for 3 weeks and baseline as reference/mice model [245]																					↑		↑	↑	*Escherichia coli*	
	Animal protein-based control diet (176 g/kg) for 3 weeks and baseline as reference/mice model [245]																					↑	↑	↑	↑		
	High plant protein-based diet (500 g/kg) for 3 weeks and control group (173 g/kg) as reference/mice model [245]																					↑		↑		*Escherichia coli*	
	High plant protein-based diet (514 g/kg) for 3 weeks and baseline as reference/mice model [245]																					↑			↑	*Escherichia coli*	
	Plant protein-based control diet (176 g/kg) for 3 weeks and baseline as reference/mice model [245]																								↑		
Hang et al. (2012)	High protein group (crude protein 609 g/kg) for 28 days and dry commercial group (264 g/kg) as reference/dog model [254]																										↓
Lubbs et al. (2009)	High protein group (crude protein 50%) for 8 weeks and moderate-protein group (crude protein 30%) as reference/cat model [255]		↓													↑										*C. perfringens*	↑

Table 5. *Cont.*

	Dose and Treatment Duration/Test Model	F/B	Potentially Beneficial Microbiota												Potentially Detrimental Microbiota											Species	Diversity
			Bifidobacterium sp.	*Lactobacillus* sp.	*Desulfovibrio* sp.	*Robinsoniella* sp.	*Barnesiella* sp.	*Allobaculum* sp.	*Akkermansia* sp.	*Roseburia* sp.	*Blautia* sp.	*Fecalibacterium* sp.	*Bacteroides* sp.	*Clostridium* sp.	*Enterorhabdus* sp.	*Clostridium* sp.	*Alloprevotella* sp.	*Haemophilus* sp.	*Ethanoligenens* sp.	*Klebsiella* sp.	*Porphyromonas* sp.	*Escherichia* sp.	*Turicibacter* sp.	*Staphylococcus* sp.	*Enterococcus* sp.		
Milk protein																											
Vidal-Lletjós et al. (2019)	Isocaloric diets with 53% protein for 3 days and the diets with 30% protein as reference/DDS-treated mice model [256]				↓								↑				↑	↑		↑							↓
	Isocaloric diets with 53% protein for 3 days and the diets with 14% protein as reference/DDS-treated mice model [256]				↓												↑	↑		↑							
	Isocaloric diets with 30% protein for 3 days and the diets with 14% protein as reference/DDS-treated mice model [256]												↓														↑
	Isocaloric diets with 53% protein for 6 days and the diets with 30% protein as reference/DDS-treated mice model [256]				↓							↓		↓												*Clostridium* XI	↓
	Isocaloric diets with 53% protein for 6 days and the diets with 14% protein as reference/DDS-treated mice model [256]														↑			↑									
	Isocaloric diets with 30% protein for 6 days and the diets with 14% protein as reference/DDS-treated mice model [256]												↑														
	Isocaloric diets with 53% protein for 21 days and the diets with 30% protein as reference/DDS-treated mice model [256]									↓		↓	↓					↑	↑	↑	↑						
	Isocaloric diets with 53% protein for 21 days and the diets with 14% protein as reference/DDS-treated mice model [256]												↓					↑	↑		↑						
	Isocaloric diets with 30% protein for 21 days and the diets with 14% protein as reference/DDS-treated mice model [256]									↑																	
Mung bean protein																											
Nakatani et al. (2018)	HFD-mung bean protein isolate (MPI) group (205.3 g MPI) for 4 weeks and HFD group (casein 200 g rather than MPI) as reference/mice model [242]	↓		↓																							
Seafood protein																											
Holm et al. (2016)	Seafood western diet (exchange casein with seafood powder) for 12 weeks and meat western diet (exchange casein with lean meat powder) as reference/mice model [244]			↓		↑	↑	↑	↓																		
Whey Protein																											
McAllan et al. (2014)	HFD-whey protein isolate (WPI) group (HFD with 20% WPI) for 21 weeks and HFD group as reference/mice model [241]		↑	↑	↑											↓											
Fried meats																											
Shen et al. (2010)	Fried meats (fry without oil at 300°C for 15 min, then ground, frozen, and freeze-dried) for fermentation over 48 h./in vitro, human fecal sample [248]															↑										*Clostridium perfringens*	

Note: (↑): increased F/B or microbiota population; (↓): reduced F/B or microbiota population; Blank: not reported. The potentially beneficial microbiota and potentially detrimental microbiota listed in the form were based on the information from the literature of the reviewed studies, excluding the taxa without clear description of their functions.

Author Contributions: Writing—original draft preparation, Q.Y., Q.L.; writing—review and editing, Q.Y., Q.L., B.B., D.P.B., Q.-J.F. and W.Z.; supervision, W.Z. and D.B. All authors have read and agreed to the published version of the manuscript.

Acknowledgments: The authors acknowledge the support from Centre for Marine Bioproducts Development (CMBD) in Flinders University. Authors are thankful to the Shanxi Tianzhirun Jujube Co Ltd., China for its collaboration with the CMBD and financial support.

References

1. Schmidt, T.S.; Raes, J.; Bork, P. The human gut microbiome: From association to modulation. *Cell* **2018**, *172*, 1198–1215. [CrossRef] [PubMed]
2. Jackson, M.A.; Verdi, S.; Maxan, M.-E.; Shin, C.M.; Zierer, J.; Bowyer, R.C.; Martin, T.; Williams, F.M.; Menni, C.; Bell, J.T. Gut microbiota associations with common Dis. and prescription medications in a population-based cohort. *Nat. Commun.* **2018**, *9*, 2655. [CrossRef] [PubMed]
3. Valdes, A.M.; Walter, J.; Segal, E.; Spector, T.D. Role of the gut microbiota in Nutr. and health. *Br. Med J.* **2018**, *361*, k2179. [CrossRef] [PubMed]
4. Berg, R.D. The indigenous gastrointestinal microflora. *Trends Microbiol.* **1996**, *4*, 430–435. [CrossRef]
5. Savage, D.C. Microbial ecology of the gastrointestinal tract. *Annu. Rev. Microbiol.* **1977**, *31*, 107–133. [CrossRef]
6. Sender, R.; Fuchs, S.; Milo, R. Are we really vastly outnumbered? Revisiting the ratio of bacterial to host cells in humans. *Cell* **2016**, *164*, 337–340. [CrossRef]
7. Rosner, J. Ten times more microbial cells than body cells in humans. *Microbe* **2014**, *9*, 47. [CrossRef]
8. McFall-Ngai, M.; Hadfield, M.G.; Bosch, T.C.; Carey, H.V.; Domazet-Lošo, T.; Douglas, A.E.; Dubilier, N.; Eberl, G.; Fukami, T.; Gilbert, S.F. Animals in a bacterial world, a new imperative for the life Sci.s. *Proc. Natl. Acad. Sci.* **2013**, *110*, 3229–3236. [CrossRef]
9. Abreu, C.; Lopez, A.O.; Gore, J. Pairing off: A bottom-up approach to the human gut microbiome. *Mol. Syst. Biol.* **2018**, *14*, e8425. [CrossRef]
10. Consortium, H.M.J.R.S. A catalog of reference genomes from the human microbiome. *Science* **2010**, *328*, 994–999.
11. Methé, B.A.; Nelson, K.E.; Pop, M.; Creasy, H.H.; Giglio, M.G.; Huttenhower, C.; Gevers, D.; Petrosino, J.F.; Abubucker, S.; Badger, J.H. A framework for human microbiome research. *Nature* **2012**, *486*, 215.
12. Qin, J.; Li, R.; Raes, J.; Arumugam, M.; Burgdorf, K.S.; Manichanh, C.; Nielsen, T.; Pons, N.; Levenez, F.; Yamada, T. A human gut microbial gene catalogue established by metagenomic sequencing. *Nature* **2010**, *464*, 59. [CrossRef] [PubMed]
13. Li, J.; Jia, H.; Cai, X.; Zhong, H.; Feng, Q.; Sunagawa, S.; Arumugam, M.; Kultima, J.R.; Prifti, E.; Nielsen, T. An integrated catalog of reference genes in the human gut microbiome. *Nat. Biotechnol.* **2014**, *32*, 834. [CrossRef] [PubMed]
14. Odamaki, T.; Kato, K.; Sugahara, H.; Hashikura, N.; Takahashi, S.; Xiao, J.Z.; Abe, F.; Osawa, R. Age-related changes in gut microbiota composition from newborn to centenarian: A cross-sectional study. *BMC Microbiol.* **2016**, *16*, 90. [CrossRef] [PubMed]
15. Sonnenburg, E.D.; Smits, S.A.; Tikhonov, M.; Higginbottom, S.K.; Wingreen, N.S.; Sonnenburg, J.L. Diet-induced extinctions in the gut microbiota compound over generations. *Nature* **2016**, *529*, 212. [CrossRef] [PubMed]
16. Ma, J.; Prince, A.L.; Bader, D.; Hu, M.; Ganu, R.; Baquero, K.; Blundell, P.; Harris, R.A.; Frias, A.E.; Grove, K.L. High-fat maternal diet during pregnancy persistently alters the offspring microbiome in a primate model. *Nat. Commun.* **2014**, *5*, 3889. [CrossRef]
17. Paul, H.A.; Bomhof, M.R.; Vogel, H.J.; Reimer, R.A. Diet-induced changes in maternal gut microbiota and metabolomic profiles influence programming of offspring obesity risk in rats. *Sci. Rep.* **2016**, *6*, 20683. [CrossRef]
18. Biasucci, G.; Benenati, B.; Morelli, L.; Bessi, E.; Boehm, G. Cesarean delivery may affect the early biodiversity of intestinal bacteria. *J. Nutr.* **2008** *138*, 1796S–1800S. [CrossRef]

19. Neu, J.; Rushing, J. Cesarean versus vaginal delivery: Long-term infant outcomes and the hygiene hypothesis. *Clin. Perinatol.* **2011**, *38*, 321–331. [CrossRef]
20. Friedman, N.J.; Zeiger, R.S. The role of breast-feeding in the development of allergies and asthma. *J. Allergy Clin. Immunol.* **2005**, *115*, 1238–1248. [CrossRef]
21. Harmsen, H.J.; Wildeboer–Veloo, A.C.; Raangs, G.C.; Wagendorp, A.A.; Klijn, N.; Bindels, J.G.; Welling, G.W. Analysis of intestinal flora development in breast-fed and formula-fed infants by using Mol. identification and detection methods. *J. Pediatric Gastroenterol. Nutr.* **2000**, *30*, 61–67. [CrossRef] [PubMed]
22. Rogers, M.A.; Aronoff, D.M. The influence of non-steroidal anti-inflammatory drugs on the gut microbiome. *Clin. Microbiol. Infect.* **2016**, *22*, e171–e178. [CrossRef] [PubMed]
23. Jernberg, C.; Löfmark, S.; Edlund, C.; Jansson, J.K. Long-term impacts of antibiotic exposure on the human intestinal microbiota. *Microbiol.* **2010**, *156*, 3216–3223. [CrossRef] [PubMed]
24. Suzuki, T.A.; Worobey, M. Geographical variation of human gut microbial composition. *Biol. Lett.* **2014**, *10*, 20131037. [CrossRef] [PubMed]
25. Heiman, M.L.; Greenway, F.L. A healthy gastrointestinal microbiome is dependent on dietary diversity. *Mol. Metab.* **2016**, *5*, 317–320. [CrossRef] [PubMed]
26. Zhernakova, A.; Kurilshikov, A.; Bonder, M.J.; Tigchelaar, E.F.; Schirmer, M.; Vatanen, T.; Mujagic, Z.; Vila, A.V.; Falony, G.; Vieira-Silva, S. Population-based metagenomics analysis reveals markers for gut microbiome composition and diversity. *Science* **2016**, *352*, 565–569. [CrossRef]
27. Zhang, N.; Ju, Z.; Zuo, T. Time for food: The impact of diet on gut microbiota and human health. *Nutrition* **2018**, *51–52*, 80–85. [CrossRef]
28. Hiippala, K.; Jouhten, H.; Ronkainen, A.; Hartikainen, A.; Kainulainen, V.; Jalanka, J.; Satokari, R. The potential of gut commensals in reinforcing intestinal barrier Funct. and alleviating inflammation. *Nutrition* **2018**, *10*, 988.
29. Cancello, R.; Turroni, S.; Rampelli, S.; Cattaldo, S.; Candela, M.; Cattani, L.; Mai, S.; Vietti, R.; Scacchi, M.; Brigidi, P. Effect of short-term dietary intervention and probiotic mix supplementation on the gut microbiota of elderly obese women. *Nutrition* **2019**, *11*, 3011. [CrossRef]
30. O'Callaghan, A.A.; Corr, S.C. Establishing boundaries: The relationship that exists between intestinal epithelial cells and gut-dwelling bacteria. *Microorg.* **2019**, *7*, 663. [CrossRef]
31. Gagniere, J.; Raisch, J.; Veziant, J.; Barnich, N.; Bonnet, R.; Buc, E.; Bringer, M.A.; Pezet, D.; Bonnet, M. Gut microbiota imbalance and colorectal cancer. *World J. Gastroenterol.* **2016**, *22*, 501–518. [CrossRef] [PubMed]
32. Kowalska-Duplaga, K.; Gosiewski, T.; Kapusta, P.; Sroka-Oleksiak, A.; Wedrychowicz, A.; Pieczarkowski, S.; Ludwig-Slomczynska, A.H.; Wolkow, P.P.; Fyderek, K. Differences in the intestinal microbiome of healthy children and patients with newly diagnosed crohn's disease. *Sci. Rep.* **2019**, *9*, 18880. [CrossRef] [PubMed]
33. Alhinai, E.A.; Walton, G.E.; Commane, D.M. The role of the gut microbiota in colorectal cancer causation. *Int. J. Mol. Sci.* **2019**, *20*, 5295. [CrossRef] [PubMed]
34. Ley, R.E.; Bäckhed, F.; Turnbaugh, P.; Lozupone, C.A.; Knight, R.D.; Gordon, J.I. Obesity alters gut microbial ecology. *Proc. Nat. Acad. Sci.* **2005**, *102*, 11070–11075. [CrossRef] [PubMed]
35. Ley, R.E.; Turnbaugh, P.J.; Klein, S.; Gordon, J.I. Microbial ecology: Human gut microbes associated with obesity. *Nature* **2006**, *444*, 1022. [CrossRef]
36. Williamson, G. The role of polyphenols in modern. *Nutr. Bull.* **2017**, *42*, 226–235. [CrossRef] [PubMed]
37. Puupponen-Pimiä, R.; Aura, A.-M.; Oksman-Caldentey, K.-M.; Myllärinen, P.; Saarela, M.; Mattila-Sandholm, T.; Poutanen, K. Development of Functional ingredients for gut health. *Trends Food Sci.Technol.* **2002**, *13*, 3–11. [CrossRef]
38. Han, X.; Shen, T.; Lou, H. Dietary polyphenols and their biological significance. *Int. J. Mol. Sci.s* **2007**, *8*, 950–988. [CrossRef]
39. Selma, M.V.; Espin, J.C.; Tomas-Barberan, F.A. Interaction between phenolics and gut microbiota: Role in human health. *J. Agric. Food Chem.* **2009**, *57*, 6485–6501. [CrossRef]
40. Parkar, S.G.; Stevenson, D.E.; Skinner, M.A. The potential influence of fruit polyphenols on colonic microflora and human gut health. *Int. J. Food Microbiol.* **2008**, *124*, 295–298. [CrossRef]
41. Etxeberria, U.; Arias, N.; Boqué, N.; Macarulla, M.; Portillo, M.; Martínez, J.; Milagro, F. Reshaping faecal gut microbiota composition by the intake of trans-resveratrol and quercetin in high-fat sucrose diet-fed rats. *J. Nutr.Biochem.* **2015**, *26*, 651–660. [CrossRef] [PubMed]

42. Taira, T.; Yamaguchi, S.; Takahashi, A.; Okazaki, Y.; Yamaguchi, A.; Sakaguchi, H.; Chiji, H. Dietary polyphenols increase fecal mucin and immunoglobulin a and ameliorate the disturbance in gut microbiota caused by a high fat diet. *J. Clin. Biochem.Nutr.* **2015**, *57*, 212–216. [CrossRef] [PubMed]
43. Wang, L.; Zeng, B.; Liu, Z.; Liao, Z.; Zhong, Q.; Gu, L.; Wei, H.; Fang, X. Green tea polyphenols modulate colonic microbiota diversity and lipid Metab. in high-fat diet treated hfa mice. *J. Food Sci.* **2018**, *83*, 864–873. [CrossRef] [PubMed]
44. Seo, D.-B.; Jeong, H.W.; Cho, D.; Lee, B.J.; Lee, J.H.; Choi, J.Y.; Bae, I.-H.; Lee, S.-J. Fermented green tea extract alleviates obesity and related complications and alters gut microbiota composition in diet-induced obese mice. *J. Med. Food* **2015**, *18*, 549–556. [CrossRef] [PubMed]
45. Santino, A.; Scarano, A.; De Santis, S.; De Benedictis, M.; Giovinazzo, G.; Chieppa, M. Gut microbiota modulation and anti-inflammatory properties of dietary polyphenols in ibd: New and consolidated perspectives. *Curr. Pharm. Des.* **2017**, *23*, 2344–2351. [CrossRef] [PubMed]
46. Lee, Y.-L.; Cesario, T.; Wang, Y.; Shanbrom, E.; Thrupp, L. Antibacterial activity of vegetables and juices. *Nutrition* **2003**, *19*, 994–996. [CrossRef]
47. Tabasco, R.; Sánchez-Patán, F.; Monagas, M.; Bartolomé, B.; Moreno-Arribas, M.V.; Peláez, C.; Requena, T. Effect of grape polyphenols on lactic acid bacteria and bifidobacteria growth: Resistance and Metab. *Food Microbiol.* **2011**, *28*, 1345–1352. [CrossRef]
48. Tzounis, X.; Vulevic, J.; Kuhnle, G.G.; George, T.; Leonczak, J.; Gibson, G.R.; Kwik-Uribe, C.; Spencer, J.P. Flavanol monomer-induced changes to the human faecal microflora. *Br. J. Nutr.* **2008**, *99*, 782–792. [CrossRef]
49. Parkar, S.G.; Trower, T.M.; Stevenson, D.E. Fecal microbial Metab. of polyphenols and its effects on human gut microbiota. *Anaerobe* **2013**, *23*, 12–19. [CrossRef]
50. Topping, D.L.; Clifton, P.M. Short-chain fatty acids and human colonic Funct.: Roles of resistant starch and nonstarch polysaccharides. *Physiol. Rev.* **2001**, *81*, 1031–1064. [CrossRef]
51. Firrman, J.; Liu, L.; Argoty, G.A.; Zhang, L.; Tomasula, P.; Wang, M.; Pontious, S.; Kobori, M.; Xiao, W. Analysis of temporal changes in growth and gene expression for commensal gut microbes in response to the polyphenol naringenin. *Microbiol. Insights* **2018**, *11*, 1178636118775100. [CrossRef] [PubMed]
52. Lee, H.C.; Jenner, A.M.; Low, C.S.; Lee, Y.K. Effect of tea phenolics and their aromatic fecal bacterial metabolites on intestinal microbiota. *Res. Microbiol.* **2006**, *157*, 876–884. [CrossRef] [PubMed]
53. Collins, B.; Hoffman, J.; Martinez, K.; Grace, M.; Lila, M.A.; Cockrell, C.; Nadimpalli, A.; Chang, E.; Chuang, C.-C.; Zhong, W. A polyphenol-rich fraction obtained from table grapes decreases adiposity, insulin resistance and markers of inflammation and impacts gut microbiota in high-fat-fed mice. *J. Nutr.Biochem.* **2016**, *31*, 150–165. [CrossRef] [PubMed]
54. Neyrinck, A.M.; Van Hée, V.F., Bindels, L.B.; De Backer, F.; Cani, P.D.; Delzenne, N.M. Polyphenol-rich extract of pomegranate peel alleviates tissue inflammation and hypercholesterolaemia in high-fat diet-induced obese mice: Potential implication of the gut microbiota. *Br. J. Nutr.* **2013**, *109*, 802–809. [CrossRef] [PubMed]
55. Dolara, P.; Luceri, C.; De Filippo, C.; Femia, A.P.; Giovannelli, L.; Caderni, G.; Cecchini, C.; Silvi, S.; Orpianesi, C.; Cresci, A. Red wine polyphenols influence carcinogenesis, intestinal microflora, oxidative damage and gene expression profiles of colonic mucosa in f344 rats. *Mutat. Res./Fundam. Mol. Mech. Mutagenesis* **2005**, *591*, 237–246. [CrossRef]
56. Axling, U.; Olsson, C.; Xu, J.; Fernandez, C.; Larsson, S.; Ström, K.; Ahrné, S.; Holm, C.; Molin, G.; Berger, K. Green tea powder and lactobacillus plantarum affect gut microbiota, lipid Metab. and inflammation in high-fat fed c57bl/6j mice. *Nutr. Metab.* **2012**, *9*, 105.
57. Marques, C.; Fernandes, I.; Meireles, M.; Faria, A.; Spencer, J.P.; Mateus, N.; Calhau, C. Gut microbiota modulation accounts for the neuroprotective properties of anthocyanins. *Sci. Rep.* **2018**, *8*, 11341. [CrossRef]
58. Mei, X.; Zhang, X.; Wang, Z.; Gao, Z.; Liu, G.; Hu, H.; Zou, L.; Li, X. Insulin sensitivity-enhancing activity of phlorizin is associated with lipopolysaccharide decrease and gut microbiota changes in obese and type 2 diabetes (db/db) mice. *J. Agric. Food Chem.* **2016**, *64*, 7502–7511. [CrossRef]
59. Chacar, S.; Itani, T.; Hajal, J.; Saliba, Y.; Louka, N.; Faivre, J.F.; Maroun, R.; Fares, N. The impact of long-term intake of phenolic compounds-rich grape pomace on rat gut microbiota. *J. Food Sci.* **2018**, *83*, 246–251. [CrossRef]
60. Viveros, A.; Chamorro, S.; Pizarro, M.; Arija, I.; Centeno, C.; Brenes, A. Effects of dietary polyphenol-rich grape products on intestinal microflora and gut morphology in broiler chicks. *Poult. Sci.* **2011**, *90*, 566–578. [CrossRef]

61. Ohno, M.; Nishida, A.; Sugitani, Y.; Nishino, K.; Inatomi, O.; Sugimoto, M.; Kawahara, M.; Andoh, A. Nanoparticle curcumin ameliorates experimental colitis via modulation of gut microbiota and induction of regulatory t cells. *PLoS ONE* **2017**, *12*, e0185999. [CrossRef] [PubMed]
62. Paul, B.; Royston, K.J.; Li, Y.; Stoll, M.L.; Skibola, C.F.; Wilson, L.S.; Barnes, S.; Morrow, C.D.; Tollefsbol, T.O. Impact of genistein on the gut microbiome of humanized mice and its role in breast tumor inhibition. *PLoS ONE* **2017**, *12*, e0189756. [CrossRef] [PubMed]
63. Tzounis, X.; Rodriguez-Mateos, A.; Vulevic, J.; Gibson, G.R.; Kwik-Uribe, C.; Spencer, J.P. Prebiotic evaluation of cocoa-derived flavanols in healthy humans by using a randomized, controlled, double-blind, crossover intervention study. *The Am. J. Clin. Nutr.* **2010**, *93*, 62–72. [CrossRef] [PubMed]
64. Moreno-Indias, I.; Sánchez-Alcoholado, L.; Pérez-Martínez, P.; Andrés-Lacueva, C.; Cardona, F.; Tinahones, F.; Queipo-Ortuño, M.I. Red wine polyphenols modulate fecal microbiota and reduce markers of the metabolic syndrome in obese patients. *Food Funct.* **2016**, *7*, 1775–1787.
65. Queipo-Ortuño, M.I.; Boto-Ordóñez, M.; Murri, M.; Gomez-Zumaquero, J.M.; Clemente-Postigo, M.; Estruch, R.; Cardona Diaz, F.; Andres-Lacueva, C.; Tinahones, F.J. Influence of red wine polyphenols and ethanol on the gut microbiota ecology and Biochem.ical biomarkers. *Am. J. Clin. Nutr.* **2012**, *95*, 1323–1334. [CrossRef] [PubMed]
66. Henning, S.M.; Yang, J.; Shao, P.; Lee, R.-P.; Huang, J.; Ly, A.; Hsu, M.; Lu, Q.-Y.; Thames, G.; Heber, D. Health benefit of vegetable/fruit juice-based diet: Role of microbiome. *Sci. Rep.* **2017**, *7*, 2167. [CrossRef] [PubMed]
67. Jin, J.S.; Touyama, M.; Hisada, T.; Benno, Y. Effects of green tea consumption on human fecal microbiota with special reference to bifidobacterium species. *Microbiol. Immunol.* **2012**, *56*, 729–739. [CrossRef]
68. Iino, C.; Shimoyama, T.; Iino, K.; Yokoyama, Y.; Chinda, D.; Sakuraba, H.; Fukuda, S.; Nakaji, S. Daidzein intake is associated with equol producing status through an increase in the intestinal bacteria responsible for equol production. *Nutrition* **2019**, *11*, 433. [CrossRef]
69. Mayta-Apaza, A.C. Evaluation of the impact of tart cherries polyphenols on the human gut microbiota and phenolic metabolites in vitro and in vivo. Master's Thesis, Food Sci., University of Arkansas, Fayetteville, AR, USA, 2017.
70. Mayta-Apaza, A.C.; Pottgen, E.; De Bodt, J.; Papp, N.; Marasini, D.; Howard, L.; Abranko, L.; Van de Wiele, T.; Lee, S.-O.; Carbonero, F. Impact of tart cherries polyphenols on the human gut microbiota and phenolic metabolites in vitro and in vivo. *J. Nutr.Biochem..* **2018**, *59*, 160–172. [CrossRef]
71. Li, Z.; Henning, S.M.; Lee, R.-P.; Lu, Q.-Y.; Summanen, P.H.; Thames, G.; Corbett, K.; Downes, J.; Tseng, C.-H.; Finegold, S.M. Pomegranate extract induces ellagitannin metabolite formation and changes stool microbiota in healthy volunteers. *Food Funct.* **2015**, *6*, 2487–2495.
72. Most, J.; Penders, J.; Lucchesi, M.; Goossens, G.; Blaak, E. Gut microbiota composition in relation to the metabolic response to 12-week combined polyphenol supplementation in overweight men and women. *Eur. J. Clin. Nutr.* **2017**, *71*, 1040. [CrossRef] [PubMed]
73. Haro, C.; Rangel-Zuniga, O.A.; Alcala-Diaz, J.F.; Gomez-Delgado, F.; Perez-Martinez, P.; Delgado-Lista, J.; Quintana-Navarro, G.M.; Landa, B.B.; Navas-Cortes, J.A.; Tena-Sempere, M.; et al. Intestinal microbiota is influenced by gender and body mass index. *PLoS ONE* **2016**, *11*, e0154090. [CrossRef] [PubMed]
74. Rowland, I.; Gibson, G.; Heinken, A.; Scott, K.; Swann, J.; Thiele, I.; Tuohy, K. Gut microbiota Funct.s: Metab. of Nutr. and other food components. *Eur. J. Nutr.* **2018**, *57*, 1–24. [CrossRef] [PubMed]
75. Lee, H.; Ko, G. Antiviral effect of vitamin A on norovirus Infect. via modulation of the gut microbiome. *Sci. Rep.* **2016**, *6*, 25835. [CrossRef]
76. Lee, H.; Ko, G. New perspectives regarding the antiviral effect of vitamin A on norovirus using modulation of gut microbiota. *Gut Microbes* **2017**, *8*, 616–620. [CrossRef]
77. Long, K.Z.; García, C.; Santos, J.I.; Rosado, J.L.; Hertzmark, E.; DuPont, H.L.; Ko, G. Vitamin A supplementation has divergent effects on norovirus Infect.s and Clin. symptoms among mexican children. *J. Infect. Dis.* **2007**, *196*, 978–985. [CrossRef]
78. Thornton, K.A.; Mora-Plazas, M.; Marín, C.; Villamor, E. Vitamin A deficiency is associated with gastrointestinal and respiratory morbidity in school-age children. *J. Nutr.* **2014**, *144*, 496–503. [CrossRef] [PubMed]
79. Liu, J.; Liu, X.; Xiong, X.-Q.; Yang, T.; Cui, T.; Hou, N.-L.; Lai, X.; Liu, S.; Guo, M.; Liang, X.-H.; et al. Effect of vitamin A supplementation on gut microbiota in children with autism spectrum disorders - a pilot study. *BMC Microbiol.* **2017**, *17*, 204. [CrossRef]

80. Lv, Z.; Wang, Y.; Yang, T.; Zhan, X.; Li, Z.; Hu, H.; Li, T.; Chen, J. Vitamin A deficiency impacts the structural segregation of gut microbiota in children with persistent diarrhea. *J. Clin. Biochem. Nutr.* **2016**, *59*, 113–121. [CrossRef]
81. Huda, M.N.; Ahmad, S.M.; Kalanetra, K.M.; Taft, D.H.; Alam, M.J.; Khanam, A.; Raqib, R.; Underwood, M.A.; Mills, D.A.; Stephensen, C.B. Neonatal vitamin a supplementation and vitamin A status are associated with gut microbiome composition in bangladeshi infants in early infancy and at 2 years of age. *J. Nutr.* **2019**, *149*, 1075–1088. [CrossRef]
82. Sperandio, V. Take your pick: Vitamins and microbiota facilitate pathogen clearance. *Cell Host Microbe* **2017**, *21*, 130–131.
83. Degnan, P.H.; Barry, N.A.; Mok, K.C.; Taga, M.E.; Goodman, A.L. Human gut microbes use multiple transporters to distinguish vitamin B12 analogs and compete in the gut. *Cell Host Microbe* **2014**, *15*, 47–57. [CrossRef] [PubMed]
84. Anderson, C.J.; Clark, D.E.; Adli, M.; Kendall, M.M. Ethanolamine signaling promotes salmonella niche recognition and adaptation during Infect. *Plos Pathog.* **2015**, *11*, e1005278.
85. Thiennimitr, P.; Winter, S.E.; Winter, M.G.; Xavier, M.N.; Tolstikov, V.; Huseby, D.L.; Sterzenbach, T.; Tsolis, R.M.; Roth, J.R.; Bäumler, A.J. Intestinal inflammation allows *salmonella* to use ethanolamine to compete with the microbiota. *Proc. Natl. Acad. Sci.* **2011**, *108*, 17480–17485. [CrossRef] [PubMed]
86. Magnúsdóttir, S.; Ravcheev, D.; de Crécy-Lagard, V.; Thiele, I. Systematic genome assessment of B-vitamin biosynthesis suggests co-operation among gut microbes. *Front. Genet.* **2015**, *6*, 148. [CrossRef] [PubMed]
87. Harbige, L.S. Nutrition and immunity with emphasis on Infect. and autoimmune disease. *Nutr. Health* **1996**, *10*, 285–312. [CrossRef]
88. Miki, T.; Goto, R.; Fujimoto, M.; Okada, N.; Hardt, W.D. The bactericidal lectin regiiibeta prolongs gut colonization and enteropathy in the streptomycin mouse model for salmonella diarrhea. *Cell Host Microbe* **2017**, *21*, 195–207.
89. Subramanian, V.S.; Srinivasan, P.; Wildman, A.J.; Marchant, J.S.; Said, H.M. Mol. mechanism (s) involved in differential expression of vitamin c transporters along the intestinal tract. *Am. J. Physiol. -Gastrointest. Liver Physiol.* **2016**, *312*, G340–G347. [CrossRef]
90. Li, L.; Krause, L.; Somerset, S. Associations between micronutrient intakes and gut microbiota in a group of adults with cystic fibrosis. *Clin. Nutr.* **2017**, *36*, 1097–1104. [CrossRef]
91. Wilson, R.; Willis, J.; Gearry, R.; Hughes, A.; Lawley, B.; Skidmore, P.; Frampton, C.; Fleming, E.; Anderson, A.; Jones, L. Sungold kiwifruit supplementation of individuals with prediabetes alters gut microbiota and improves vitamin c status, anthropometric and Clinical markers. *Nutrients* **2018**, *10*, 895. [CrossRef]
92. Xu, J.; Xu, C.; Chen, X.; Cai, X.; Yang, S.; Sheng, Y.; Wang, T. Regulation of an antioxidant blend on intestinal redox status and major microbiota in early weaned piglets. *Nutrition* **2014**, *30*, 584–589. [CrossRef] [PubMed]
93. Wang, H.; Chen, W.; Li, D.; Yin, X.; Zhang, X.; Olsen, N.; Zheng, S.G. Vitamin D and chronic Dis. *Aging Dis.* **2017**, *8*, 346. [CrossRef] [PubMed]
94. Jeffery, L.E.; Qureshi, O.S.; Gardner, D.; Hou, T.Z.; Briggs, Z.; Soskic, B.; Baker, J.; Raza, K.; Sansom, D.M. Vitamin D antagonises the suppressive effect of inflammatory cytokines on ctla-4 expression and regulatory Funct. *PLoS ONE* **2015**, *10*, e0131539. [CrossRef] [PubMed]
95. Kesby, J.P.; Eyles, D.W.; Burne, T.H.; McGrath, J.J. The effects of vitamin D on brain development and adult brain Funct. *Mol. Cell. Endocrinol.* **2011**, *347*, 121–127. [CrossRef]
96. Bertone-Johnson, E.R.; Powers, S.I.; Spangler, L.; Brunner, R.L.; Michael, Y.L.; Larson, J.C.; Millen, A.E.; Bueche, M.N.; Salmoirago-Blotcher, E.; Liu, S. Vitamin D intake from foods and supplements and depressive symptoms in a diverse population of older women. *Am. J. of Clin. Nutr.* **2011**, *94*, 1104–1112. [CrossRef]
97. Ciubotaru, I.; Green, S.J.; Kukreja, S.; Barengolts, E. Significant differences in fecal microbiota are associated with various stages of glucose tolerance in african Am. male veterans. *Transl. Res.* **2015**, *166*, 401–411. [CrossRef]
98. Kanhere, M.; He, J.; Hanfelt, J.; Gewirtz, A.T.; Chassaing, B.; Ivie, E.A.; Alvarez, J.A.; Hao, L.; Ziegler, T.R.; Tangpricha, V. Bolus weekly vitamin D3 supplementation impacts gut and airway microbiota in adults with cystic fibrosis: A double-blind, randomized, placebo-controlled Clin. trial. *J. Clin. Endocrinol. Metab.* **2017**, *103*, 564–574.
99. Jacobs, C.; Hutton, B.; Ng, T.; Shorr, R.; Clemons, M. Is there a role for oral or intravenous ascorbate (vitamin C) in treating patients with cancer? A systematic review. *Oncol.* **2015** *20*, 210–223. [CrossRef]

100. Iniesta, R.R.; Rush, R.; Paciarotti, I.; Rhatigan, E.; Brougham, F.; McKenzie, J.; Wilson, D. Systematic review and meta-analysis: Prevalence and possible causes of vitamin D deficiency and insufficiency in pediatric cancer patients. *Clin. Nutr.* **2016**, *35*, 95–108. [CrossRef]
101. Meeker, S.; Seamons, A.; Maggio-Price, L.; Paik, J. Protective links between vitamin D, inflammatory bowel disease and colon cancer. *World J. Gastroenterol.* **2016**, *22*, 933. [CrossRef]
102. Ardesia, M.; Ferlazzo, G.; Fries, W. Vitamin D and inflammatory bowel disease. *BioMed Res. Int.* **2015**, *2015*, 470805. [CrossRef] [PubMed]
103. Bashir, M.; Prietl, B.; Tauschmann, M.; Mautner, S.I.; Kump, P.K.; Treiber, G.; Wurm, P.; Gorkiewicz, G.; Högenauer, C.; Pieber, T.R. Effects of high doses of vitamin D3 on mucosa-associated gut microbiome vary between regions of the human gastrointestinal tract. *Eur. J. of Nutr.* **2016**, *55*, 1479–1489. [CrossRef] [PubMed]
104. Tabatabaeizadeh, S.-A.; Tafazoli, N.; Ferns, G.A.; Avan, A.; Ghayour-Mobarhan, M. Vitamin D, the gut microbiome and inflammatory bowel disease. *J. of Res. in Medical Sci. Off. J. Isfahan Univ. Med Sci.* **2018**, *23*, 75.
105. Sun, J. Dietary vitamin D, vitamin D receptor, and microbiome. *Curr. Opinion in Clin. Nutr. Metab. Care* **2018**, *21*, 471–474. [CrossRef]
106. Clark, A.; Mach, N. Role of vitamin d in the hygiene hypothesis: The interplay between vitamin D, vitamin D receptors, gut microbiota, and immune response. *Front. Immunol.* **2016**, *7*, 627. [CrossRef]
107. Garg, M.; Hendy, P.; Ding, J.N.; Shaw, S.; Hold, G.; Hart, A. The effect of vitamin D on intestinal inflammation and faecal microbiota in patients with ulcerative colitis. *J. Crohn's Colitis* **2018**, *12*, 963–972. [CrossRef]
108. Schäffler, H.; Herlemann, D.P.; Klinitzke, P.; Berlin, P.; Kreikemeyer, B.; Jaster, R.; Lamprecht, G. Vitamin D administration leads to a shift of the intestinal bacterial composition in crohn's disease patients, but not in healthy controls. *J. Dig. Dis.* **2018**, *19*, 225–234. [CrossRef]
109. Talsness, C.E.; Penders, J.; Jansen, E.H.J.M.; Damoiseaux, J.; Thijs, C.; Mommers, M. Influence of vitamin D on key bacterial taxa in infant microbiota in the koala birth cohort study. *PLoS ONE* **2017**, *12*, e0188011. [CrossRef]
110. Luthold, R.V.; Fernandes, G.R.; Franco-de-Moraes, A.C.; Folchetti, L.G.; Ferreira, S.R.G. Gut microbiota interactions with the immunomodulatory role of vitamin D in normal individuals. *Metabolism* **2017**, *69*, 76–86. [CrossRef]
111. Naderpoor, N.; Mousa, A.; Fernanda Gomez Arango, L.; Barrett, H.L.; Dekker Nitert, M.; de Courten, B. Effect of vitamin D supplementation on faecal microbiota: A randomised Clin. trial. *Nutrition* **2019**, *11*, 2888. [CrossRef]
112. Zuo, K.; Li, J.; Xu, Q.; Hu, C.; Gao, Y.; Chen, M.; Hu, R.; Liu, Y.; Chi, H.; Yin, Q. Dysbiotic gut microbes may contribute to hypertension by limiting vitamin D production. *Clin. Cardiol.* **2019**, *42*, 710–719. [CrossRef] [PubMed]
113. Yan, H.; Wang, H.; Zhang, X.; Li, X.; Yu, J. Ascorbic acid ameliorates oxidative stress and inflammation in dextran sulfate sodium-induced ulcerative colitis in mice. *Int. J. Clin. Exp. Med.* **2015**, *8*, 20245. [PubMed]
114. Tahan, G.; Aytac, E.; Aytekin, H.; Gunduz, F.; Dogusoy, G.; Aydin, S.; Tahan, V.; Uzun, H. Vitamin e has a dual effect of anti-inflammatory and antioxidant activities in acetic acid–induced ulcerative colitis in rats. *Can. J. Surg.* **2011**, *54*, 333. [CrossRef] [PubMed]
115. Maggini, S.; Wintergerst, E.S.; Beveridge, S.; Hornig, D.H. Selected vitamins and trace elements support immune Funct. by strengthening epithelial barriers and cellular and humoral immune responses. *Br. J. Nutr.* **2007**, *98*, S29–S35. [CrossRef]
116. Pierre, J.F.; Hinterleitner, R.; Bouziat, R.; Hubert, N.A.; Leone, V.; Miyoshi, J.; Jabri, B.; Chang, E.B. Dietary antioxidant microNutr. alter mucosal inflammatory risk in a murine model of genetic and microbial susceptibility. *J. Nutr. Biochem.* **2018**, *54*, 95–104. [CrossRef] [PubMed]
117. Choi, Y.; Lee, S.; Kim, S.; Lee, J.; Ha, J.; Oh, H.; Lee, Y.; Kim, Y.; Yoon, Y. Vitamin e (α-tocopherol) consumption influences gut microbiota composition. *Int. J. Food Sci.s Nutr.* **2019**, 1–5. [CrossRef]
118. Mandal, S.; Godfrey, K.M.; McDonald, D.; Treuren, W.V.; Bjørnholt, J.V.; Midtvedt, T.; Moen, B.; Rudi, K.; Knight, R.; Brantsæter, A.L. Fat and vitamin intakes during pregnancy have stronger relations with a pro-inflammatory maternal microbiota than does carbohydrate intake. *Microbiome* **2016**, *4*, 55. [CrossRef]
119. Tang, M.; Frank, D.N.; Sherlock, L.; Ir, D.; Robertson, C.E.; Krebs, N.F. Effect of vitamin e with therapeutic iron supplementation on iron repletion and gut microbiome in us iron deficient infants and toddlers. *J. Pediatric Gastroenterol. Nutr.* **2016**, *63*, 379–385.

120. Skrypnik, K.; Suliburska, J. Association between the gut microbiota and mineral Metab. *J. Sci. Food Agric.* **2018**, *98*, 2449–2460. [CrossRef]
121. Gîlcă-Blanariu, G.-E.; Diaconescu, S.; Ciocoiu, M.; Ştefănescu, G. New insights into the role of trace elements in IBD. *BioMed. Res. Int.* **2018**, *2018*, 1813047. [CrossRef]
122. Zhang, F.; Ye, J.; Zhu, X.; Wang, L.; Gao, P.; Shu, G.; Jiang, Q.; Wang, S. Anti-obesity effects of dietary calcium: The evidence and possible mechanisms. *Int. J. Mol. Sci.s* **2019**, *20*, 3072. [CrossRef] [PubMed]
123. Gomes, J.; Costa, J.; Alfenas, R. Could the beneficial effects of dietary calcium on obesity and diabetes control be mediated by changes in intestinal microbiota and integrity? *Br. J. Nutr.* **2015**, *114*, 1756–1765. [CrossRef] [PubMed]
124. Trautvetter, U.; Camarinha-Silva, A.; Jahreis, G.; Lorkowski, S.; Glei, M. High phosphorus intake and gut-related parameters–results of a randomized placebo-controlled human intervention study. *Nutr. J.* **2018**, *17*, 23. [CrossRef] [PubMed]
125. Aslam, M.N.; Bassis, C.M.; Zhang, L.; Zaidi, S.; Varani, J.; Bergin, I.L. Calcium reduces liver injury in mice on a high-fat diet: Alterations in microbial and bile acid profiles. *PLoS ONE* **2016**, *11*, e0166178. [CrossRef]
126. Li, P.; Tang, T.; Chang, X.; Fan, X.; Chen, X.; Wang, R.; Fan, C.; Qi, K. Abnormality in maternal dietary calcium intake during pregnancy and lactation promotes body weight gain by affecting the gut microbiota in mouse offspring. *Mol. Nutr. Food Res.* **2018**, *63*, 1800399.
127. Chaplin, A.; Parra, P.; Laraichi, S.; Serra, F.; Palou, A. Calcium supplementation modulates gut microbiota in a prebiotic manner in dietary obese mice. *Mol. Nutr. Food Res.* **2016**, *60*, 468–480.
128. Gröber, U.; Schmidt, J.; Kisters, K. Magnesium in prevention and therapy. *Nutrition* **2015**, *7*, 8199–8226. [CrossRef]
129. Pachikian, B.D.; Neyrinck, A.M.; Deldicque, L.; De Backer, F.C.; Catry, E.; Dewulf, E.M.; Sohet, F.M.; Bindels, L.B.; Everard, A.; Francaux, M. Changes in intestinal bifidobacteria levels are associated with the inflammatory response in magnesium-deficient mice. *J. Nutr.* **2010**, *140*, 509–514. [CrossRef]
130. Jørgensen, B.P.; Winther, G.; Kihl, P.; Nielsen, D.S.; Wegener, G.; Hansen, A.K.; Sørensen, D.B. Dietary magnesium deficiency affects gut microbiota and anxiety-like behaviour in c57bl/6n mice. *Acta Neuropsychiatr.* **2015**, *27*, 307–311. [CrossRef]
131. Winther, G.; Jørgensen, B.M.P.; Elfving, B.; Nielsen, D.S.; Kihl, P.; Lund, S.; Sørensen, D.B.; Wegener, G. Dietary magnesium deficiency alters gut microbiota and leads to depressive-like behaviour. *Acta Neuropsychiatr.* **2015**, *27*, 168–176. [CrossRef]
132. Crowley, E.; Long-Smith, C.; Murphy, A.; Patterson, E.; Murphy, K.; O'Gorman, D.; Stanton, C.; Nolan, Y. Dietary supplementation with a magnesium-rich marine mineral blend enhances the diversity of gastrointestinal microbiota. *Mar. Drugs* **2018**, *16*, 216. [CrossRef] [PubMed]
133. Lönnerdal, B. Excess iron intake as a factor in growth, Infect.s, and development of infants and young children. *Am. J. Clin. Nutr.* **2017**, *106*, 1681S–1687S. [CrossRef] [PubMed]
134. Jaeggi, T.; Kortman, G.A.; Moretti, D.; Chassard, C.; Holding, P.; Dostal, A.; Boekhorst, J.; Timmerman, H.M.; Swinkels, D.W.; Tjalsma, H. Iron fortification adversely affects the gut microbiome, increases pathogen abundance and induces intestinal inflammation in kenyan infants. *Gut* **2015**, *64*, 731–742. [CrossRef] [PubMed]
135. Tang, M.; Frank, D.N.; Hendricks, A.E.; Ir, D.; Esamai, F.; Liechty, E.; Hambidge, K.M.; Krebs, N.F. Iron in micronutrient powder promotes an unfavorable gut microbiota in kenyan infants. *Nutrition* **2017**, *9*, 776. [CrossRef]
136. Zimmermann, M.B.; Chassard, C.; Rohner, F.; N'Goran, E.K.; Nindjin, C.; Dostal, A.; Utzinger, J.; Ghattas, H.; Lacroix, C.; Hurrell, R.F. The effects of iron fortification on the gut microbiota in african children: A randomized controlled trial in cote d'ivoire. *Am. J. Clin. Nutr.* **2010**, *92*, 1406–1415. [CrossRef]
137. Qasem, W.; Azad, M.B.; Hossain, Z.; Azad, E.; Jorgensen, S.; San Juan, S.C.; Cai, C.; Khafipour, E.; Beta, T.; Roberts, L.J. Assessment of complementary feeding of canadian infants: Effects on microbiome oxidative stress, a randomized controlled trial. *BMC Pediatrics* **2017**, *17*, 54.
138. Dostal, A.; Baumgartner, J.; Riesen, N.; Chassard, C.; Smuts, C.M.; Zimmermann, M.B.; Lacroix, C. Effects of iron supplementation on dominant bacterial groups in the gut, faecal scfa and gut inflammation: A randomised, placebo-controlled intervention trial in south african children. *Br. J. Nutr.* **2014**, *112*, 547–556. [CrossRef]

139. Sjödin, K.S.; Domellöf, M.; Lagerqvist, C.; Hernell, O.; Lönnerdal, B.; Szymlek-Gay, E.A.; Sjödin, A.; West, C.E.; Lind, T. Administration of ferrous sulfate drops has significant effects on the gut microbiota of iron-sufficient infants: A randomised controlled study. *Gut* **2019**, *68*, 2095–2097.
140. Fang, S.; Zhuo, Z.; Yu, X.; Wang, H.; Feng, J. Oral administration of liquid iron preparation containing excess iron induces intestine and liver injury, impairs intestinal barrier Funct. and alters the gut microbiota in rats. *J. of Trace Elem. Med. Biol.* **2018**, *47*, 12–20. [CrossRef]
141. Kortman, G.A.; Dutilh, B.E.; Maathuis, A.J.; Engelke, U.F.; Boekhorst, J.; Keegan, K.P.; Nielsen, F.G.; Betley, J.; Weir, J.C.; Kingsbury, Z. Microbial Metab. shifts towards an adverse profile with supplementary iron in the tim-2 in vitro model of the human colon. *Front. Microbiol.* **2016**, *6*, 1481. [CrossRef]
142. Vazquez-Gutierrez, P.; Lacroix, C.; Jaeggi, T.; Zeder, C.; Zimmerman, M.B.; Chassard, C. Bifidobacteria strains isolated from stools of iron deficient infants can efficiently sequester iron. *BMC Microbiol.* **2015**, *15*, 3. [CrossRef] [PubMed]
143. Nitert, M.D.; Gomez-Arango, L.F.; Barrett, H.L.; McIntyre, H.D.; Anderson, G.J.; Frazer, D.M.; Callaway, L.K. Iron supplementation has minor effects on gut microbiota composition in overweight and obese women in early pregnancy. *Br. J. Nutr.* **2018**, *120*, 283–289. [CrossRef] [PubMed]
144. Seura, T.; Yoshino, Y.; Fukuwatari, T. The relationship between habitual dietary intake and gut microbiota in young japanese women. *J. Nutr. Sci. Vitaminol.* **2017**, *63*, 396–404. [CrossRef] [PubMed]
145. Constante, M.; Fragoso, G.; Lupien-Meilleur, J.; Calvé, A.; Santos, M.M. Iron supplements modulate colon microbiota composition and potentiate the protective effects of probiotics in dextran sodium sulfate-induced colitis. *Inflamm. Bowel Dis.* **2017**, *23*, 753–766. [CrossRef] [PubMed]
146. Ijssennagger, N.; Belzer, C.; Hooiveld, G.J.; Dekker, J.; van Mil, S.W.; Müller, M.; Kleerebezem, M.; van der Meer, R. Gut microbiota facilitates dietary heme-induced epithelial hyperproliferation by opening the mucus barrier in colon. *Proc. Natl. Acad. Sci.s* **2015**, *112*, 10038–10043. [CrossRef]
147. IJssennagger, N.; Derrien, M.; van Doorn, G.M.; Rijnierse, A.; van den Bogert, B.; Müller, M.; Dekker, J.; Kleerebezem, M.; van der Meer, R. Dietary heme alters microbiota and mucosa of mouse colon without Functional changes in host-microbe cross-talk. *PLoS ONE* **2012**, *7*, e49868. [CrossRef]
148. Martin, O.C.; Olier, M.; Ellero-Simatos, S.; Naud, N.; Dupuy, J.; Huc, L.; Taché, S.; Graillot, V.; Levêque, M.; Bézirard, V. Haem iron reshapes colonic luminal environment: Impact on mucosal homeostasis and microbiome through aldehyde formation. *Microbiome* **2019**, *7*, 72. [CrossRef]
149. Lee, T.; Clavel, T.; Smirnov, K.; Schmidt, A.; Lagkouvardos, I.; Walker, A.; Lucio, M.; Michalke, B.; Schmitt-Kopplin, P.; Fedorak, R.; et al. Oral versus intravenous iron replacement therapy distinctly alters the gut microbiota and metabolome in patients with ibd. *Gut* **2017**, *66*, 863–871. [CrossRef]
150. Capra, S. Nutrient Reference Values for Australia and New Zealand: Including Recommended Dietary Intakes. Available online: https://www.nhmrc.gov.au/about-us/publications/nutrient-reference-values-australia-and-new-zealand-including-recommended-dietary-intakes (accessed on 21 January 2020).
151. Borda-Molina, D.; Vital, M.; Sommerfeld, V.; Rodehutscord, M.; Camarinha-Silva, A. Insights into broilers' gut microbiota fed with phosphorus, calcium, and phytase supplemented diets. *Front.Microbiol.* **2016**, *7*, 2033. [CrossRef]
152. Ohashi, W.; Fukada, T. Contribution of zinc and zinc transporters in the pathogenesis of inflammatory bowel Dis. *J. Immunol. Res.* **2019**, *2019*, 8396878. [CrossRef]
153. Reed, S.; Neuman, H.; Moscovich, S.; Glahn, R.; Koren, O.; Tako, E. Chronic zinc deficiency alters chick gut microbiota composition and Funct. *Nutrition* **2015**, *7*, 9768–9784.
154. Shao, Y.; Lei, Z.; Yuan, J.; Yang, Y.; Guo, Y.; Zhang, B. Effect of zinc on growth performance, gut morphometry, and cecal microbial community in broilers challenged with salmonella enterica serovar typhimurium. *J. Microbiol.* **2014**, *52*, 1002–1011. [CrossRef] [PubMed]
155. Zackular, J.P.; Moore, J.L.; Jordan, A.T.; Juttukonda, L.J.; Noto, M.J.; Nicholson, M.R.; Crews, J.D.; Semler, M.W.; Zhang, Y.; Ware, L.B. Dietary zinc alters the microbiota and decreases resistance to clostridium difficile Infect. *Nat. Med.* **2016**, *22*, 1330. [CrossRef]
156. Rayman, M.P. Selenium intake, status, and health: A complex relationship. *Horm.* **2019**, 1–6. [CrossRef] [PubMed]
157. Kasaikina, M.V.; Kravtsova, M.A.; Lee, B.C.; Seravalli, J.; Peterson, D.A.; Walter, J.; Legge, R.; Benson, A.K.; Hatfield, D.L.; Gladyshev, V.N. Dietary selenium affects host selenoproteome expression by influencing the gut microbiota. *FASEB J.* **2011**, *25*, 2492–2499. [CrossRef]

158. Zhai, Q.; Cen, S.; Li, P.; Tian, F.; Zhao, J.; Zhang, H.; Chen, W. Effects of dietary selenium supplementation on intestinal barrier and immune responses associated with its modulation of gut microbiota. *Environ. Sci. Technol. Lett.* **2018**, *5*, 724–730. [CrossRef]
159. Shen, H.; Han, J.; Li, Y.; Lu, C.; Zhou, J.; Li, Y.; Su, X. Different host-specific responses in thyroid Funct. and gut microbiota modulation between diet-induced obese and normal mice given the same dose of iodine. *Appl. Microbiol. BioTechnol.* **2019**, *103*, 3537–3547. [CrossRef]
160. Schroeder, B.O.; Birchenough, G.M.; Ståhlman, M.; Arike, L.; Johansson, M.E.; Hansson, G.C.; Bäckhed, F. Bifidobacteria or fiber protects against diet-induced microbiota-mediated colonic mucus deterioration. *Cell Host Microbe* **2018**, *23*, 27–40.
161. Prajapati, B.; Rajput, P.; Kumar Jena, P.; Seshadri, S. Investigation of chitosan for prevention of diabetic progression through gut microbiota alteration in sugar rich diet induced diabetic rats. *Curr. Pharm. BioTechnol.* **2016**, *17*, 173–184. [CrossRef] [PubMed]
162. Avila-Nava, A.; Noriega, L.G.; Tovar, A.R.; Granados, O.; Perez-Cruz, C.; Pedraza-Chaverri, J.; Torres, N. Food combination based on a pre-hispanic mexican diet decreases metabolic and cognitive abnormalities and gut microbiota dysbiosis caused by a sucrose-enriched high-fat diet in rats. *Mol. Nutr. Food Res.* **2017**, *61*. [CrossRef]
163. Martens, E.C. Microbiome: Fibre for the future. *Nature* **2016**, *529*, 158. [CrossRef] [PubMed]
164. Benus, R.F.; van der Werf, T.S.; Welling, G.W.; Judd, P.A.; Taylor, M.A.; Harmsen, H.J.; Whelan, K. Association between faecalibacterium prausnitzii and dietary fibre in colonic fermentation in healthy human subjects. *Br. J. Nutr.* **2010**, *104*, 693–700. [CrossRef] [PubMed]
165. Carvalho-Wells, A.L.; Helmolz, K.; Nodet, C.; Molzer, C.; Leonard, C.; McKevith, B.; Thielecke, F.; Jackson, K.G.; Tuohy, K.M. Determination of the in vivo prebiotic potential of a maize-based whole grain breakfast cereal: A human feeding study. *Br. J. Nutr.* **2010**, *104*, 1353–1356. [CrossRef] [PubMed]
166. García-Peris, P.; Velasco, C.; Lozano, M.; Moreno, Y.; Paron, L.; De la Cuerda, C.; Bretón, I.; Camblor, M.; García-Hernández, J.; Guarner, F. Effect of a mixture of inulin and fructo-oligosaccharide on lactobacillus and bifidobacterium intestinal microbiota of patients receiving radiotherapy; a randomised, double-blind, placebo-controlled trial. *Nutr. Hosp.* **2012**, *27*, 1908–1915.
167. Dao, M.C.; Everard, A.; Aron-Wisnewsky, J.; Sokolovska, N.; Prifti, E.; Verger, E.O.; Kayser, B.D.; Levenez, F.; Chilloux, J.; Hoyles, L. Akkermansia muciniphila and improved metabolic health during a dietary intervention in obesity: Relationship with gut microbiome richness and ecology. *Gut* **2016**, *65*, 426–436. [CrossRef]
168. Candela, M.; Biagi, E.; Soverini, M.; Consolandi, C.; Quercia, S.; Severgnini, M.; Peano, C.; Turroni, S.; Rampelli, S.; Pozzilli, P. Modulation of gut microbiota dysbioses in type 2 diabetic patients by macrobiotic ma-pi 2 diet. *Br. J. Nutr.* **2016**, *116*, 80–93. [CrossRef]
169. Holscher, H.D.; Caporaso, J.G.; Hooda, S.; Brulc, J.M.; Fahey Jr, G.C.; Swanson, K.S. Fiber supplementation influences phylogenetic structure and Functional capacity of the human intestinal microbiome: Follow-up of a randomized controlled trial. *Am. J. Clin. Nutr.* **2014**, *101*, 55–64. [CrossRef]
170. Tap, J.; Furet, J.P.; Bensaada, M.; Philippe, C.; Roth, H.; Rabot, S.; Lakhdari, O.; Lombard, V.; Henrissat, B.; Corthier, G. Gut microbiota richness promotes its stability upon increased dietary fibre intake in healthy adults. *Environ. Microbiol.* **2015**, *17*, 4954–4964. [CrossRef]
171. Kovatcheva-Datchary, P.; Nilsson, A.; Akrami, R.; Lee, Y.S.; De Vadder, F.; Arora, T.; Hallen, A.; Martens, E.; Björck, I.; Bäckhed, F. Dietary fiber-induced improvement in glucose Metab. is associated with increased abundance of prevotella. *Cell Metab.* **2015**, *22*, 971–982. [CrossRef]
172. De Filippo, C.; Cavalieri, D.; Di Paola, M.; Ramazzotti, M.; Poullet, J.B.; Massart, S.; Collini, S.; Pieraccini, G.; Lionetti, P. Impact of diet in shaping gut microbiota revealed by a comparative study in children from europe and rural africa. *Proc. Natl. Acad. Sci.s* **2010**, *107*, 14691–14696. [CrossRef]
173. Haro, C.; Montes-Borrego, M.; Rangel-Zúñiga, O.A.; Alcalá-Díaz, J.F.; Gómez-Delgado, F.; Pérez-Martínez, P.; Delgado-Lista, J.; Quintana-Navarro, G.M.; Tinahones, F.J.; Landa, B.B. Two healthy diets modulate gut microbial community improving insulin sensitivity in a human obese population. *J. Clin. Endocrinol.* **2016**, *101*, 233–242. [CrossRef] [PubMed]
174. Hald, S.; Schioldan, A.G.; Moore, M.E.; Dige, A.; Lærke, H.N.; Agnholt, J.; Knudsen, K.E.B.; Hermansen, K.; Marco, M.L.; Gregersen, S. Effects of arabinoxylan and resistant starch on intestinal microbiota and short-chain fatty acids in subjects with metabolic syndrome: A randomised crossover study. *PLoS ONE* **2016**, *11*, e0159223. [CrossRef] [PubMed]

175. Cloetens, L.; Broekaert, W.F.; Delaedt, Y.; Ollevier, F.; Courtin, C.M.; Delcour, J.A.; Rutgeerts, P.; Verbeke, K. Tolerance of arabinoxylan-oligosaccharides and their prebiotic activity in healthy subjects: A randomised, placebo-controlled cross-over study. *Br. J. Nutr.* **2010**, *103*, 703–713. [CrossRef] [PubMed]
176. François, I.E.; Lescroart, O.; Veraverbeke, W.S.; Marzorati, M.; Possemiers, S.; Evenepoel, P.; Hamer, H.; Houben, E.; Windey, K.; Welling, G.W. Effects of a wheat bran extract containing arabinoxylan oligosaccharides on gastrointestinal health parameters in healthy adult human volunteers: A double-blind, randomised, placebo-controlled, cross-over trial. *Br. J. Nutr.* **2012**, *108*, 2229–2242. [CrossRef] [PubMed]
177. Lecerf, J.-M.; Dépeint, F.; Clerc, E.; Dugenet, Y.; Niamba, C.N.; Rhazi, L.; Cayzeele, A.; Abdelnour, G.; Jaruga, A.; Younes, H. Xylo-oligosaccharide (xos) in combination with inulin modulates both the intestinal environment and immune status in healthy subjects, while xos alone only shows prebiotic properties. *Br. J. Nutr.* **2012**, *108*, 1847–1858. [CrossRef]
178. Walton, G.E.; Lu, C.; Trogh, I.; Arnaut, F.; Gibson, G.R. A randomised, double-blind, placebo controlled cross-over study to determine the gastrointestinal effects of consumption of arabinoxylan-oligosaccharides enriched bread in healthy volunteers. *Nutr. J.* **2012**, *11*, 36. [CrossRef] [PubMed]
179. Childs, C.E.; Röytiö, H.; Alhoniemi, E.; Fekete, A.A.; Forssten, S.D.; Hudjec, N.; Lim, Y.N.; Steger, C.J.; Yaqoob, P.; Tuohy, K.M. Xylo-oligosaccharides alone or in synbiotic combination with bifidobacterium animalis subsp. Lactis induce bifidogenesis and modulate markers of immune Funct. in healthy adults: A double-blind, placebo-controlled, randomised, factorial cross-over study. *Br. J. Nutr.* **2014**, *111*, 1945–1956. [CrossRef]
180. Finegold, S.M.; Li, Z.; Summanen, P.H.; Downes, J.; Thames, G.; Corbett, K.; Dowd, S.; Krak, M.; Heber, D. Xylooligosaccharide increases bifidobacteria but not lactobacilli in human gut microbiota. *Food Funct.* **2014**, *5*, 436–445. [CrossRef]
181. François, I.E.; Lescroart, O.; Veraverbeke, W.S.; Marzorati, M.; Possemiers, S.; Hamer, H.; Windey, K.; Welling, G.W.; Delcour, J.A.; Courtin, C.M. Effects of wheat bran extract containing arabinoxylan oligosaccharides on gastrointestinal parameters in healthy preadolescent children. *J. Pediatric Gastroenterol. Nutr.* **2014**, *58*, 647–653. [CrossRef]
182. Windey, K.; De Preter, V.; Huys, G.; Broekaert, W.F.; Delcour, J.A.; Louat, T.; Herman, J.; Verbeke, K. Wheat bran extract alters colonic fermentation and microbial composition, but does not affect faecal water toxicity: A randomised controlled trial in healthy subjects. *Br. J. Nutr.* **2015**, *113*, 225–238. [CrossRef]
183. Broekaert, W.F.; Courtin, C.M.; Verbeke, K.; Van de Wiele, T.; Verstraete, W.; Delcour, J.A. Prebiotic and other health-related effects of cereal-derived arabinoxylans, arabinoxylan-oligosaccharides, and xylooligosaccharides. *Crit. Rev.Food Sci. Nutr.* **2011**, *51*, 178–194. [CrossRef] [PubMed]
184. Giovannini, M.; Verduci, E.; Gregori, D.; Ballali, S.; Soldi, S.; Ghisleni, D.; Riva, E.; Group, P.T.S. Prebiotic effect of an infant formula supplemented with galacto-oligosaccharides: Randomized multicenter trial. *J. Am. Coll. Nutr.* **2014**, *33*, 385–393. [CrossRef] [PubMed]
185. Ladirat, S.E.; Schuren, F.H.; Schoterman, M.H.; Nauta, A.; Gruppen, H.; Schols, H.A. Impact of galacto-oligosaccharides on the gut microbiota composition and metabolic activity upon antibiotic treatment during in vitro fermentation. *FEMS Microbiol. Ecol.* **2014**, *87*, 41–51. [CrossRef] [PubMed]
186. Monteagudo-Mera, A.; Arthur, J.; Jobin, C.; Keku, T.; Bruno-Barcena, J.; Azcarate-Peril, M. High purity galacto-oligosaccharides enhance specific bifidobacterium species and their metabolic activity in the mouse gut microbiome. *Benef. Microbes* **2016**, *7*, 247–264. [CrossRef] [PubMed]
187. Davis, L.; Martinez, I.; Walter, J.; Hutkins, R. A dose dependent impact of prebiotic galactooligosaccharides on the intestinal microbiota of healthy adults. *Int. J. Food Microbiol.* **2010**, *144*, 285–292. [CrossRef] [PubMed]
188. Davis, L.M.; Martínez, I.; Walter, J.; Goin, C.; Hutkins, R.W. Barcoded pyrosequencing reveals that consumption of galactooligosaccharides results in a highly specific bifidogenic response in humans. *PLoS ONE* **2011**, *6*, e25200. [CrossRef] [PubMed]
189. Walton, G.E.; van den Heuvel, E.G.; Kosters, M.H.; Rastall, R.A.; Tuohy, K.M.; Gibson, G.R. A randomised crossover study investigating the effects of galacto-oligosaccharides on the faecal microbiota in men and women over 50 years of age. *Br. J. Nutr.* **2012**, *107*, 1466–1475. [CrossRef]
190. Musilova, S.; Rada, V.; Marounek, M.; Nevoral, J.; Dušková, D.; Bunesova, V.; Vlkova, E.; Zelenka, R. Prebiotic effects of a novel combination of galactooligosaccharides and maltodextrins. *J. Med. Food* **2015**, *18*, 685–689. [CrossRef]

191. Vulevic, J.; Juric, A.; Walton, G.E.; Claus, S.P.; Tzortzis, G.; Toward, R.E.; Gibson, G.R. Influence of galacto-oligosaccharide mixture (b-gos) on gut microbiota, immune parameters and metabonomics in elderly persons. *Br. J. Nutr.* **2015**, *114*, 586–595. [CrossRef]
192. Azcarate-Peril, M.A.; Ritter, A.J.; Savaiano, D.; Monteagudo-Mera, A.; Anderson, C.; Magness, S.T.; Klaenhammer, T.R. Impact of short-chain galactooligosaccharides on the gut microbiome of lactose-intolerant individuals. *Proc. Natl. Acad. Sci.s* **2017**, *114*, E367–E375. [CrossRef]
193. Whisner, C.M.; Martin, B.R.; Schoterman, M.H.; Nakatsu, C.H.; McCabe, L.D.; McCabe, G.P.; Wastney, M.E.; Van Den Heuvel, E.G.; Weaver, C.M. Galacto-oligosaccharides increase calcium absorption and gut bifidobacteria in young girls: A double-blind cross-over trial. *Br. J. Nutr.* **2013**, *110*, 1292–1303. [CrossRef] [PubMed]
194. Scalabrin, D.M.; Mitmesser, S.H.; Welling, G.W.; Harris, C.L.; Marunycz, J.D.; Walker, D.C.; Bos, N.A.; Tölkkö, S.; Salminen, S.; Vanderhoof, J.A. New prebiotic blend of polydextrose and galacto-oligosaccharides has a bifidogenic effect in young infants. *J. Pediatric Gastroenterol. Nutr.* **2012**, *54*, 343–352. [CrossRef] [PubMed]
195. Westerbeek, E.; Slump, R.; Lafeber, H.; Knol, J.; Georgi, G.; Fetter, W.; van Elburg, R. The effect of enteral supplementation of specific neutral and acidic oligosaccharides on the faecal microbiota and intestinal microenvironment in preterm infants. *Eur. J. Clin. Microbiol. Infect. Dis.* **2013**, *32*, 269–276. [CrossRef] [PubMed]
196. Sierra, C.; Bernal, M.-J.; Blasco, J.; Martínez, R.; Dalmau, J.; Ortuno, I.; Espín, B.; Vasallo, M.-I.; Gil, D.; Vidal, M.-L. Prebiotic effect during the first year of life in healthy infants fed formula containing gos as the only prebiotic: A multicentre, randomised, double-blind and placebo-controlled trial. *Eur. J. Nutr.* **2015**, *54*, 89–99. [CrossRef] [PubMed]
197. Civardi, E.; Garofoli, F.; Longo, S.; Mongini, M.E.; Grenci, B.; Mazzucchelli, I.; Angelini, M.; Castellazzi, A.; Fasano, F.; Grinzato, A. Safety, growth, and support to healthy gut microbiota by an infant formula enriched with Functional compounds. *Clin. Nutr.* **2017**, *36*, 238–245. [CrossRef] [PubMed]
198. Paganini, D.; Uyoga, M.A.; Kortman, G.A.M.; Cercamondi, C.I.; Moretti, D.; Barth-Jaeggi, T.; Schwab, C.; Boekhorst, J.; Timmerman, H.M.; Lacroix, C.; et al. Prebiotic galacto-oligosaccharides mitigate the adverse effects of iron fortification on the gut microbiome: A randomised controlled study in kenyan infants. *Gut* **2017**, *66*, 1956–1967. [CrossRef]
199. Francavilla, R.; Calasso, M.; Calace, L.; Siragusa, S.; Ndagijimana, M.; Vernocchi, P.; Brunetti, L.; Mancino, G.; Tedeschi, G.; Guerzoni, E. Effect of lactose on gut microbiota and metabolome of infants with cow's milk allergy. *Pediatric Allergy Immunol.* **2012**, *23*, 420–427. [CrossRef]
200. Fernando, W.; Hill, J.; Zello, G.; Tyler, R.; Dahl, W.; Van Kessel, A. Diets supplemented with chickpea or its main oligosaccharide component raffinose modify faecal microbial composition in healthy adults. *Benef. Microbes* **2010**, *1*, 197–207. [CrossRef]
201. Licht, T.R.; Hansen, M.; Poulsen, M.; Dragsted, L.O. Dietary carbohydrate source influences Mol. fingerprints of the rat faecal microbiota. *BMC Microbiol.* **2006**, *6*, 98. [CrossRef]
202. Catry, E.; Bindels, L.B.; Tailleux, A.; Lestavel, S.; Neyrinck, A.M.; Goossens, J.-F.; Lobysheva, I.; Plovier, H.; Essaghir, A.; Demoulin, J.-B. Targeting the gut microbiota with inulin-type fructans: PreClin. demonstration of a novel approach in the management of endothelial dysFunct. *Gut* **2018**, *67*, 271–283. [CrossRef]
203. Ramirez-Farias, C.; Slezak, K.; Fuller, Z.; Duncan, A.; Holtrop, G.; Louis, P. Effect of inulin on the human gut microbiota: Stimulation of bifidobacterium adolescentis and faecalibacterium prausnitzii. *Br. J. Nutr.* **2008**, *101*, 541–550. [CrossRef] [PubMed]
204. Dewulf, E.M.; Cani, P.D.; Claus, S.P.; Fuentes, S.; Puylaert, P.G.; Neyrinck, A.M.; Bindels, L.B.; de Vos, W.M.; Gibson, G.R.; Thissen, J.-P. Insight into the prebiotic concept: Lessons from an exploratory, double blind intervention study with inulin-type fructans in obese women. *Gut* **2013**, *62*, 1112–1121. [CrossRef] [PubMed]
205. Vandeputte, D.; Falony, G.; Vieira-Silva, S.; Wang, J.; Sailer, M.; Theis, S.; Verbeke, K.; Raes, J. Prebiotic inulin-type fructans induce specific changes in the human gut microbiota. *Gut* **2017**, *66*, 1968–1974. [CrossRef] [PubMed]
206. Drabińska, N.; Jarocka-Cyrta, E.; Markiewicz, L.H.; Krupa-Kozak, U. The effect of oligofructose-enriched inulin on faecal bacterial counts and microbiota-associated characteristics in celiac disease children following a gluten-free diet: Results of a randomized, placebo-controlled trial. *Nutrition* **2018**, *10*, 201. [CrossRef]

207. Salazar, N.; Dewulf, E.M.; Neyrinck, A.M.; Bindels, L.B.; Cani, P.D.; Mahillon, J.; de Vos, W.M.; Thissen, J.-P.; Gueimonde, M.; Clara, G. Inulin-type fructans modulate intestinal bifidobacterium species populations and decrease fecal short-chain fatty acids in obese women. *Clin. Nutr.* **2015**, *34*, 501–507. [CrossRef]
208. Nicolucci, A.C.; Hume, M.P.; Martinez, I.; Mayengbam, S.; Walter, J.; Reimer, R.A. Prebiotics reduce body fat and alter intestinal microbiota in children who are overweight or with obesity. *Gastroenterol.* **2017**, *153*, 711–722. [CrossRef]
209. Yang, X.; Darko, K.O.; Huang, Y.; He, C.; Yang, H.; He, S.; Li, J.; Li, J.; Hocher, B.; Yin, Y. Resistant starch regulates gut microbiota: Structure, Biochem. and cell signalling. *Cell. Physiol. Biochem.* **2017**, *42*, 306–318. [CrossRef]
210. Martínez, I.; Kim, J.; Duffy, P.R.; Schlegel, V.L.; Walter, J. Resistant starches types 2 and 4 have differential effects on the composition of the fecal microbiota in human subjects. *PLoS ONE* **2010**, *5*, e15046. [CrossRef]
211. Walker, A.W.; Ince, J.; Duncan, S.H.; Webster, L.M.; Holtrop, G.; Ze, X.; Brown, D.; Stares, M.D.; Scott, P.; Bergerat, A. Dominant and diet-responsive groups of bacteria within the human colonic microbiota. *ISME J.* **2011**, *5*, 220. [CrossRef]
212. Le Leu, R.K.; Winter, J.M.; Christophersen, C.T.; Young, G.P.; Humphreys, K.J.; Hu, Y.; Gratz, S.W.; Miller, R.B.; Topping, D.L.; Bird, A.R. Butyrylated starch intake can prevent red meat-induced o 6-methyl-2-deoxyguanosine adducts in human rectal tissue: A randomised Clin. trial. *Br. J. Nutr.* **2015**, *114*, 220–230. [CrossRef]
213. Cluny, N.L.; Eller, L.K.; Keenan, C.M.; Reimer, R.A.; Sharkey, K.A. Interactive effects of oligofructose and obesity predisposition on gut hormones and microbiota in diet-induced obese rats. *Obes.* **2015**, *23*, 769–778. [CrossRef]
214. Wernimont, S.; Northington, R.; Kullen, M.J.; Yao, M.; Bettler, J. Effect of an α-lactalbumin-enriched infant formula supplemented with oligofructose on fecal microbiota, stool characteristics, and hydration status: A randomized, double-blind, controlled trial. *Clin. Pediatrics* **2015**, *54*, 359–370. [CrossRef]
215. Raninen, K.; Lappi, J.; Mykkänen, H.; Poutanen, K. Dietary fiber type reflects Physiol. Functionality: Comparison of grain fiber, inulin, and polydextrose. *Nutr. Rev.* **2011**, *69*, 9–21. [CrossRef] [PubMed]
216. Costabile, A.; Fava, F.; Röytiö, H.; Forssten, S.D.; Olli, K.; Klievink, J.; Rowland, I.R.; Ouwehand, A.C.; Rastall, R.A.; Gibson, G.R. Impact of polydextrose on the faecal microbiota: A double-blind, crossover, placebo-controlled feeding study in healthy human subjects. *Br. J. Nutr.* **2012**, *108*, 471–481. [CrossRef] [PubMed]
217. Wolters, M.; Ahrens, J.; Perez, M.R.; Watkins, C.; Sanz, Y.; Benítez-Páez, A.; Stanton, C.; Günther, K. Dietary fat, the gut microbiota, and metabolic health–a systematic review conducted within the mynewgut project. *Clin. Nutr.* **2019**, *38*, 2504–2520. [CrossRef] [PubMed]
218. Hamilton, M.K.; Boudry, G.; Lemay, D.G.; Raybould, H.E. Changes in intestinal barrier Funct. and gut microbiota in high-fat diet-fed rats are dynamic and region dependent. *Am. J. Physiol. -Gastrointest. Liver Physiol.* **2015**, *308*, G840–G851. [CrossRef]
219. Hildebrandt, M.A.; Hoffmann, C.; Sherrill–Mix, S.A.; Keilbaugh, S.A.; Hamady, M.; Chen, Y.Y.; Knight, R.; Ahima, R.S.; Bushman, F.; Wu, G.D. High-fat diet determines the composition of the murine gut microbiome independently of obesity. *Gastroenterol.* **2009**, *137*, 1716–1724. [CrossRef]
220. Chen, G.; Xie, M.; Wan, P.; Chen, D.; Dai, Z.; Ye, H.; Hu, B.; Zeng, X.; Liu, Z. Fuzhuan brick tea polysaccharides attenuate metabolic syndrome in high-fat diet induced mice in association with modulation in the gut microbiota. *J. Agric. Food Chem.* **2018**, *66*, 2783–2795. [CrossRef]
221. Murphy, E.; Cotter, P.; Healy, S.; Marques, T.M.; O'sullivan, O.; Fouhy, F.; Clarke, S.; O'toole, P.; Quigley, E.M.; Stanton, C. Composition and energy harvesting capacity of the gut microbiota: Relationship to diet, obesity and time in mouse models. *Gut* **2010**, *59*, 1635–1642. [CrossRef]
222. Lam, Y.Y.; Ha, C.W.; Campbell, C.R.; Mitchell, A.J.; Dinudom, A.; Oscarsson, J.; Cook, D.I.; Hunt, N.H.; Caterson, I.D.; Holmes, A.J. Increased gut permeability and microbiota change associate with mesenteric fat inflammation and metabolic dysFunct. in diet-induced obese mice. *PLoS ONE* **2012**, *7*, e34233. [CrossRef]
223. Kim, K.-A.; Gu, W.; Lee, I.-A.; Joh, E.-H.; Kim, D.-H. High fat diet-induced gut microbiota exacerbates inflammation and obesity in mice via the tlr4 signaling pathway. *PLoS ONE* **2012**, *7*, e47713. [CrossRef] [PubMed]

224. Cowan, T.E.; Palmnäs, M.S.; Yang, J.; Bomhof, M.R.; Ardell, K.L.; Reimer, R.A.; Vogel, H.J.; Shearer, J. Chronic coffee consumption in the diet-induced obese rat: Impact on gut microbiota and serum metabolomics. *J. Nutr. Biochem.* **2014**, *25*, 489–495. [CrossRef] [PubMed]
225. Mujico, J.R.; Baccan, G.C.; Gheorghe, A.; Díaz, L.E.; Marcos, A. Changes in gut microbiota due to supplemented fatty acids in diet-induced obese mice. *Br. J. Nutr.* **2013**, *110*, 711–720. [CrossRef] [PubMed]
226. Cani, P.D.; Bibiloni, R.; Knauf, C.; Waget, A.; Neyrinck, A.M.; Delzenne, N.M.; Burcelin, R. Changes in gut microbiota control metabolic endotoxemia-induced inflammation in high-fat diet–induced obesity and diabetes in mice. *Diabetes* **2008**, *57*, 1470–1481. [CrossRef] [PubMed]
227. Turnbaugh, P.J.; Ley, R.E.; Mahowald, M.A.; Magrini, V.; Mardis, E.R.; Gordon, J.I. An obesity-associated gut microbiome with increased capacity for energy harvest. *Nature* **2006**, *444*, 1027. [CrossRef] [PubMed]
228. Devkota, S.; Wang, Y.; Musch, M.W.; Leone, V.; Fehlner-Peach, H.; Nadimpalli, A.; Antonopoulos, D.A.; Jabri, B.; Chang, E.B. Dietary-fat-induced taurocholic acid promotes pathobiont expansion and colitis in il10−/− mice. *Nature* **2012**, *487*, 104. [CrossRef]
229. Lecomte, V.; Kaakoush, N.O.; Maloney, C.A.; Raipuria, M.; Huinao, K.D.; Mitchell, H.M.; Morris, M.J. Changes in gut microbiota in rats fed a high fat diet correlate with obesity-associated metabolic parameters. *PLoS ONE* **2015**, *10*, e0126931. [CrossRef]
230. Wan, Y.; Wang, F.; Yuan, J.; Li, J.; Jiang, D.; Zhang, J.; Li, H.; Wang, R.; Tang, J.; Huang, T.; et al. Effects of dietary fat on gut microbiota and faecal metabolites, and their relationship with cardiometabolic risk factors: A 6-month randomised controlled-feeding trial. *Gut* **2019**, *68*, 1417–1429. [CrossRef]
231. Haro, C.; Garcia-Carpintero, S.; Rangel-Zuniga, O.A.; Alcala-Diaz, J.F.; Landa, B.B.; Clemente, J.C.; Perez-Martinez, P.; Lopez-Miranda, J.; Perez-Jimenez, F.; Camargo, A. Consumption of two healthy dietary patterns restored microbiota dysbiosis in obese patients with metabolic dysFunct. *Mol. Nutr. Food Res.* **2017**, *61*. [CrossRef]
232. Lee, S.; Keirsey, K.I.; Kirkland, R.; Grunewald, Z.I.; Fischer, J.G.; de La Serre, C.B. Blueberry supplementation influences the gut microbiota, inflammation, and insulin resistance in high-fat-diet–fed rats. *J. Nutr.* **2018**, *148*, 209–219. [CrossRef]
233. Qiao, Y.; Sun, J.; Ding, Y.; Le, G.; Shi, Y. Alterations of the gut microbiota in high-fat diet mice is strongly linked to oxidative stress. *Appl. Microbiol. BioTechnol.* **2013**, *97*, 1689–1697. [CrossRef] [PubMed]
234. Santos-Marcos, J.A.; Haro, C.; Vega-Rojas, A.; Alcala-Diaz, J.F.; Molina-Abril, H.; Leon-Acuña, A.; Lopez-Moreno, J.; Landa, B.B.; Tena-Sempere, M.; Perez-Martinez, P. Sex differences in the gut microbiota as potential determinants of gender predisposition to disease. *Mol. Nutr. Food Res.* **2019**, *63*, 1800870. [CrossRef] [PubMed]
235. Patterson, E.; O'Doherty, R.M.; Murphy, E.F.; Wall, R.; O'Sullivan, O.; Nilaweera, K.; Fitzgerald, G.F.; Cotter, P.D.; Ross, R.P.; Stanton, C. Impact of dietary fatty acids on metabolic activity and host intestinal microbiota composition in c57bl/6j mice. *Br. J. Nutr.* **2014**, *111*, 1905–1917. [CrossRef] [PubMed]
236. De Wit, N.; Derrien, M.; Bosch-Vermeulen, H.; Oosterink, E.; Keshtkar, S.; Duval, C.; de Vogel-van den Bosch, J.; Kleerebezem, M.; Müller, M.; van der Meer, R. Saturated fat stimulates obesity and hepatic steatosis and affects gut microbiota composition by an enhanced overflow of dietary fat to the distal intestine. *Am. J. Physiol. -Gastrointest. Liver Physiol.* **2012**, *303*, G589–G599. [CrossRef] [PubMed]
237. Zentek, J.; Buchheit-Renko, S.; Männer, K.; Pieper, R.; Vahjen, W. Intestinal concentrations of free and encapsulated dietary medium-chain fatty acids and effects on gastric microbial ecology and bacterial metabolic products in the digestive tract of piglets. *Arch. Anim. Nutr.* **2012**, *66*, 14–26. [CrossRef] [PubMed]
238. Ojo, B.; El-Rassi, G.D.; Payton, M.E.; Perkins-Veazie, P.; Clarke, S.; Smith, B.J.; Lucas, E.A. Mango supplementation modulates gut microbial dysbiosis and short-chain fatty acid production independent of body weight reduction in c57bl/6 mice fed a high-fat diet–3. *J. Nutr.* **2016**, *146*, 1483–1491. [CrossRef]
239. Younge, N.; Yang, Q.; Seed, P.C. Enteral high fat-polyunsaturated fatty acid blend alters the pathogen composition of the intestinal microbiome in premature infants with an enterostomy. *J. Pediatrics* **2017**, *181*, 93–101. [CrossRef]
240. Sprong, R.; Schonewille, A.; Van der Meer, R. Dietary cheese whey protein protects rats against mild dextran sulfate sodium–induced colitis: Role of mucin and microbiota. *J. Dairy Sci.* **2010**, *93*, 1364–1371. [CrossRef]
241. McAllan, L.; Skuse, P.; Cotter, P.D.; O'Connor, P.; Cryan, J.F.; Ross, R.P.; Fitzgerald, G.; Roche, H.M.; Nilaweera, K.N. Protein quality and the protein to carbohydrate ratio within a high fat diet influences energy balance and the gut microbiota in c57bl/6j mice. *PLoS ONE* **2014**, *9*, e88904. [CrossRef]

242. Nakatani, A.; Li, X.; Miyamoto, J.; Igarashi, M.; Watanabe, H.; Sutou, A.; Watanabe, K.; Motoyama, T.; Tachibana, N.; Kohno, M. Dietary mung bean protein reduces high-fat diet-induced weight gain by modulating host bile acid Metab. in a gut microbiota-dependent manner. *Biochem. Biophys. Res. Commun.* **2018**, *501*, 955–961. [CrossRef]
243. Rist, V.T.; Weiss, E.; Sauer, N.; Mosenthin, R.; Eklund, M. Effect of dietary protein supply originating from soybean meal or casein on the intestinal microbiota of piglets. *Anaerobe* **2014**, *25*, 72–79. [CrossRef] [PubMed]
244. Holm, J.B.; Rønnevik, A.; Tastesen, H.S.; Fjære, E.; Fauske, K.R.; Liisberg, U.; Madsen, L.; Kristiansen, K.; Liaset, B. Diet-induced obesity, energy Metab. and gut microbiota in c57bl/6j mice fed western diets based on lean seafood or lean meat mixtures. *J. Nutr. Biochem.* **2016**, *31*, 127–136. [CrossRef] [PubMed]
245. Kostovcikova, K.; Coufal, S.; Galanova, N.; Fajstova, A.; Hudcovic, T.; Kostovcik, M.; Prochazkova, P.; Zakostelska, Z.J.; Cermakova, M.; Sediva, B. Diet rich in animal protein promotes pro-inflammatory macrophage response and exacerbates colitis in mice. *Front. Immunol.* **2019**, *10*, 919. [CrossRef] [PubMed]
246. Beaumont, M.; Portune, K.J.; Steuer, N.; Lan, A.; Cerrudo, V.; Audebert, M.; Dumont, F.; Mancano, G.; Khodorova, N.; Andriamihaja, M. Quantity and source of dietary protein influence metabolite production by gut microbiota and rectal mucosa gene expression: A randomized, parallel, double-blind trial in overweight humans. *Am. J. Clin. Nutr.* **2017**, *106*, 1005–1019. [CrossRef] [PubMed]
247. Moreno-Pérez, D.; Bressa, C.; Bailén, M.; Hamed-Bousdar, S.; Naclerio, F.; Carmona, M.; Pérez, M.; González-Soltero, R.; Montalvo-Lominchar, M.G.; Carabaña, C. Effect of a protein supplement on the gut microbiota of endurance athletes: A randomized, controlled, double-blind pilot study. *Nutrition* **2018**, *10*, 337. [CrossRef] [PubMed]
248. Shen, Q.; Chen, Y.A.; Tuohy, K.M. A comparative in vitro investigation into the effects of cooked meats on the human faecal microbiota. *Anaerobe* **2010**, *16*, 572–577. [CrossRef]
249. Harris, V.C.; Haak, B.W.; Boele van Hensbroek, M.; Wiersinga, W.J. The intestinal microbiome in infectious Dis.: The Clin. relevance of a rapidly emerging field. *Open Forum Infect. Dis.* **2017**, *4*, ofx144. [CrossRef]
250. Harsch, I.; Konturek, P. The role of gut microbiota in obesity and type 2 and type 1 diabetes mellitus: New insights into "old" Dis. *Med Sci.s* **2018**, *6*, 32. [CrossRef]
251. Koropatkin, N.M.; Cameron, E.A.; Martens, E.C. How glycan Metab. shapes the human gut microbiota. *Nat. Rev. Microbiol.* **2012**, *10*, 323. [CrossRef]
252. David, L.A.; Maurice, C.F.; Carmody, R.N.; Gootenberg, D.B.; Button, J.E.; Wolfe, B.E.; Ling, A.V.; Devlin, A.S.; Varma, Y.; Fischbach, M.A. Diet rapidly and reproducibly alters the human gut microbiome. *Nature* **2014**, *505*, 559. [CrossRef]
253. Witzig, M.; da Silva, A.C.; Green-Engert, R.; Hoelzle, K.; Zeller, E.; Seifert, J.; Hoelzle, L.E.; Rodehutscord, M. Spatial variation of the gut microbiota in broiler chickens as affected by dietary available phosphorus and assessed by t-rflp analysis and 454 pyrosequencing. *PLoS ONE* **2015**, *10*, e0143442.
254. Hang, I.; Rinttila, T.; Zentek, J.; Kettunen, A.; Alaja, S.; Apajalahti, J.; Harmoinen, J.; de Vos, W.M.; Spillmann, T. Effect of high contents of dietary animal-derived protein or carbohydrates on canine faecal microbiota. *BMC Vet. Res.* **2012**, *8*, 90. [CrossRef] [PubMed]
255. Lubbs, D.; Vester, B.; Fastinger, N.; Swanson, K. Dietary protein concentration affects intestinal microbiota of adult cats: A study using dgge and qpcr to evaluate differences in microbial populations in the feline gastrointestinal tract. *J. Anim. Physiol. Anim. Nutr.* **2009**, *93*, 113–121. [CrossRef] [PubMed]
256. Vidal-Lletjós, S.; Andriamihaja, M.; Blais, A.; Grauso, M.; Lepage, P.; Davila, A.-M.; Viel, R.; Gaudichon, C.; Leclerc, M.; Blachier, F. Dietary protein intake level modulates mucosal healing and mucosa-adherent microbiota in mouse model of colitis. *Nutrition* **2019**, *11*, 514. [CrossRef] [PubMed]

2

Soluble Fiber with High Water-Binding Capacity, Swelling Capacity, and Fermentability Reduces Food Intake by Promoting Satiety Rather Than Satiation in Rats

Chengquan Tan [1], Hongkui Wei [1], Xichen Zhao [1], Chuanhui Xu [1], Yuanfei Zhou [1,*] and Jian Peng [1,2,*]

1 Department of Animal Nutrition and Feed Science, College of Animal Science and Technology, Huazhong Agricultural University, Wuhan 430070, China; cooper2005@163.com (C.T.); weihongkui@mail.hzau.edu.cn (H.W.); FenziYY@126.com (X.Z.); xuchuanhui001@hzau.edu.cn (C.X.)

2 The Cooperative Innovation Center for Sustainable Pig Production, Wuhan 430070, China

* Correspondence: zhuoyuanfei@mail.hzau.edu.cn (Y.Z.); pengjian@mail.hzau.edu.cn (J.P.);

Abstract: To understand whether soluble fiber (SF) with high water-binding capacity (WBC), swelling capacity (SC) and fermentability reduces food intake and whether it does so by promoting satiety or satiation or both, we investigated the effects of different SFs with these properties on the food intake in rats. Thirty-two male Sprague-Dawley rats were randomized to four equal groups and fed the control diet or diet containing 2% *konjac* flour (KF), pregelatinized waxy maize starch (PWMS) plus guar gum (PG), and PWMS starch plus xanthan gum (PX) for three weeks, with the measured values of SF, WBC, and SC in the four diets following the order of PG > KF > PX > control. Food intake, body weight, meal pattern, behavioral satiety sequence, and short-chain fatty acids (SCFAs) in cecal content were evaluated. KF and PG groups reduced the food intake, mainly due to the decreased feeding behavior and increased satiety, as indicated by decreased meal numbers and increased inter-meal intervals. Additionally, KF and PG groups increased concentrations of acetate acid, propionate acid, and SCFAs in the cecal contents. Our results indicate that SF with high WBC, SC, and fermentability reduces food intake—probably by promoting a feeling of satiety in rats to decrease their feeding behavior.

Keywords: guar gum; water binding capacity; meal pattern; food intake; satiety

---

1. Introduction

Satiation and satiety are part of the body's appetite control system involved in limiting food intake. Satiation is reflected in meal size and meal duration, while satiety is reflected in meal number and inter-meal intervals [1]. Modulation of food intake by consuming foods with a high satiety or satiation value may be one of the approaches to help reduce obesity. The efficacy by which different types of dietary fibers promote satiety or satiation is varied [2,3]. This issue can be explored first by using laboratory animals due to the advantages of a complete control over the diet, facile collection of gut samples, and systematic observation of behaviors.

Growing evidence showed that the physicochemical properties of dietary fiber such as viscosity, water-binding capacity, and fermentability may contribute to decrease the food intake in human beings and rodents [3–5]. Viscous fibers increase chewing activity and saliva production in the mouth [6], which could result in early satiation and reduced food intake [7,8]. However, dietary fiber with high water-binding capacity may increase gastric distension by expanding their volume up to eight-fold in the stomach [9], which will increase feelings of satiety [10], probably via afferent vagal signals of fullness [6]. Moreover, a delay in gastric emptying accompanied by an increase in gastric distension is often associated with enhanced satiety between meals [11]. In addition, dietary fiber is also fermented by intestinal microbiota, contributing to the increase of short-chain fatty acids (SCFAs). Furthermore, SCFAs could stimulate the release of satiety-related peptides, such as peptide tyrosine-tyrosine (PYY) and glucagon-like peptide-1 (GLP-1) from entero-endocrine cells, which may promote feelings of satiety [12].

Konjac flour (KF) is a water soluble, viscous dietary fiber with a high water-binding capacity (15.5 mL H_2O/g) [13,14]. KF mainly contains *konjac* glucomannan (KGM), which is composed of β-1,4-linked D-mannosyl and D-glucosyl residues at a molar ratio of 1.6:1.0 as the main chain with a small number of branches through β-1,3 mannosyl units [15]. KGM is considered a functional fiber of food ingredient and has been consumed in the form of rubbery jelly, noodles, and other food products by humans in Asia for centuries [16]. KGM has been known to be helpful in lowering cholesterol levels, reducing weight in human beings [17], and modifying intestinal microbial metabolism in sows [18,19]. Our previous study indicated that dietary inclusion of KF with higher water-binding capacity (1.97 vs. 1.78 g/g) and swelling capacity (2.14 vs. 1.62 mL/g) than inclusion of wheat bran promoted the satiety of gestating sow [20]. However, the tuber is usually grown in Asian countries and the resources for commercial production are limited, suggesting the necessity to develop novel dietary fibers with functional properties similar to those of KF, as well as similar effects on food intake reduction by promoting satiety or satiation.

Pregelatinized waxy maize starch, a fermentable resistant starch composed mainly of highly branched amorphous amylopectin, has many specific food attributes [21]. Dietary supplementation with modified waxy maize starch lowers glucose-dependent insulinotropic polypeptides and has beneficial implications in weight management [22]. Guar and xanthan gums with high viscosity and hydrating properties are used as stabilizer and thickener in various food products [23,24]. A previous study reported that the digesta viscosity of subjects was increased after consuming cookies containing 2.5% guar gum alone for 42 days, without any effect on their food intake [3]. The consumption of beverages enriched with dietary fibers and xanthan gum (0.22%) for one week also had no influence on the appetite sensations in healthy men [25]. Our previous results showed that the combined fiber materials (pregelatinized waxy maize starch plus guar gum (PG) and pregelatinized waxy maize starch plus xanthan gum (PX)) had higher or similar water-binding capacity or swelling capacity than the KF [26]. Therefore, we hypothesized that the combination of pregelatinized waxy maize starch with guar gum or xanthan gum inclusion in diet may have a similar effect to that of KF on physicochemical properties (water-binding capacity and swelling capacity) and fermentability, as well as food intake reduction by promoting satiety or satiation. The objective of the present study was to investigate whether dietary fibers with high water-binding capacity, swelling capacity, and fermentability reduce food intake by promoting satiety or satiation as well as the mechanism underlying it by evaluating their effects on plasma concentrations of GLP-1 and PYY, SCFAs in cecal contents, meal pattern, feeding behavior, food intake, and body weight in rats.

2. Experimental Section

2.1. Animals and Diets

A total of 32 male Sprague-Dawley rats (average initial body weight of 377.10 ± 3.43 g; 10 weeks of age) (Hunan SJA Laboratory Animal Co., Ltd., Changsha, China) were housed individually in standard cages that allowed recording of food intake. The cages were placed in a temperature-and humidity-controlled room (21 ± 2 °C, 55% ± 10% humidity) with a 12:12 light/dark cycle (lights off at 8:30 p.m.). The animals were acclimatized for one week with the control diet fed prior to the experiment. Rats were given free access to water and food. All the experiment protocols were approved by the animal care and use committee of Huazhong Agriculture University and were in accordance with the

National Research Council's Guide for the Care and Use of Laboratory Animals. Sprague-Dawley rats were used because they are reported to have a good consistency in meal patterns [27].

Rats were divided randomly to four dietary treatment groups (8 rats/treatment): the control fed control diet with wheat bran as a fiber source (Control); a positive control fed the control diet with 2% *konjac* flour (Qingjiang Konjac Products Co., Ltd., Wuhan, China) to replace 2% wheat bran (KF); a treatment fed the control diet with 2% pregelatinized waxy maize starch (Hangzhou Puluoxiang Starch Corp., Ltd., Hangzhou, China) plus guar gum (Shangdong Yunzhou Science and Technology Corp., Ltd., Yunzhou, China) to replace 2% wheat bran (PG) (PG; 85.7% pregelatinized waxy maize starch and 14.3% guar gum); and a treatment fed the control diet with 2% pregelatinized waxy maize starch plus xanthan gum (Shangdong Yunzhou Science and Technology Corp., Ltd., Yunzhou, China) to replace 2% wheat bran (PX) (PX; 95% pregelatinized waxy maize starch and 5% xanthan gum). The ingredient and chemical composition of the diets are listed in Table 1. The experiment lasted 21 days, during which food intake was determined daily and body weights were measured.

Table 1. Ingredient and composition of experimental diets.

Ingredient (% *w/w*)	Control [1]	KF [1]	PG [1]	PX [1]
Corn	52.2	52.2	52.2	52.2
Soybean meal	15.9	15.9	15.9	15.9
Fish meal	10.0	10.0	10.0	10.0
Wheat bran	12.0	10.0	10.0	10.0
Sucrose	5.0	5.0	5.0	5.0
Fiber source		2.0	2.0	2.0
AIN-93 Mineral mix [2]	3.5	3.5	3.5	3.5
AIN-93 Vitamin mix [3]	1.0	1.0	1.0	1.0
Composition				
Crude protein (%)	20.04	19.94	19.78	19.90
Energy (kcal/g)	3.81	3.83	3.76	3.74
Soluble fiber (%)	1.91	2.89	3.09	2.57
Insoluble fiber (%)	10.46	10.58	10.61	11.10
Viscosity (mPa/s)	1.53	1.66	1.60	1.57
Swelling (mL/g)	1.81	2.63	3.03	2.18
Water-binding capacity (g/g)	2.05	2.58	2.87	2.26

[1] Diets were control or supplemented with 2% fiber of *konjac* flour (KF), 2% pregelatinized waxy maize starch plus guar gum (PG) or 2% pregelatinized waxy maize starch plus xanthan gum (PX); [2] AIN-93 Mineral mix according to Reeves (1997), per kg mix: Calcium carbonate, 357.00; Potassium phosphate, 196.00; Potassium citrate, 70.78; Sodium chloride, 74.00; Potassium sulfate, 46.60; Magnesium oxide, 24.00; Ferric citrate, 6.06; Zinc carbonate, 1.65; Sodium meta-silicate, 1.45; Manganous carbonate, 0.63; Cupric carbonate, 0.30; Chromium potassium sulfate, 0.28; Boric acid, 0.08; Sodium fluoride, 0.06; Nickel carbonate, 0.03; Lithium chloride, 0.02; Sodium selenate, 0.01; Potassium iodate, 0.01; Ammonium paramolybdate, 0.008; Ammonium vanadate, 0.007; Powdered sucrose, 221.03; [3] AIN-93 Vitamin mix according to Reeves (1997). Vitamin (mg/kg) (except as noted): Nicotinic acid, 3.00; Ca pantothenate, 1.60; Pyridoxine, 0.70; Thiamin, 0.60; Folic acid, 0.20; Biotin, 0.02; Vitamin B_{12}, 2.50; Vitamin E (500 IU/g), Vitamin A (500,000 IU/g), 0.80; Vitamin D_3 (400,000 IU/g), 0.25; Vitamin K, 0.08; Powdered sucrose, 974.65.

2.2. *Behavioral Satiety Sequence*

The analysis of the behavioral satiety sequence was performed on day 15 of dietary treatment essentially as described by Halford et al. [28]. Rats were housed individually in transparent observational cages and fasted overnight for 12 h. Water was available ad libitum. The following morning (8:30–9:30), rats were given a pre-weighed amount of food and their behaviors were monitored. For all rats, behavior was recorded every 30 s for 1 h as reported previously [29] and food intake was calculated. Feeding and non-feeding behaviors were continuously scored using a video system connected with a computer in a nearby room by a highly trained experimenter blind to the dietary treatment of the animals. Behaviors were categorized as: feeding (animal at hopper trying to obtain food, chewing, gnawing, or holding food in paws), drinking (animal licking spout of water bottle), grooming (animal scratching, licking, or biting any part of its anatomy), activity (including locomotion, sniffing, or rearing), inactivity (immobility when aware, or signs of sickness behavior), resting (animal curled up, resting head with eyes closed). Data were collated into 5-min period bins for display. With time spent in each of the behaviors as % of the total behavior.

2.3. Meal Pattern Analysis

On day 17 of dietary treatment, the rats were housed individually in transparent observational cages that allowed continuous recording of food intake for three days. The first two days served as the adaptation period, and the meal pattern and food intake were analyzed on the third day. The measurements were performed similar to previous studies [30]. Rats were fasted overnight for 12 h before the meal pattern analysis. Meal patterns of the nocturnal (from 8:30 p.m. to 8:30 a.m.) and diurnal (from 8:30 a.m. to 8:30 p.m.) periods were analyzed and recorded. Rats were fed respective diets ad libitum during the meal pattern analysis. The results were collected as total food intake (g), feeding rate (mg/s), meal size (g), meal duration (s), meal number, and inter-meal interval (min). A meal was defined as an intake larger than 0.3 g lasting a period longer than 13 s, and two distinct meals needed to be separated by >10 min [27]. The meal patterns for rats were recorded using monitoring equipment in a computer-based data acquisition system (Shenzhen Quick Zoom Technology Co., Ltd., N5063 960P, Shenzhen, China).

2.4. Samples Collection

On day 20 of dietary treatment, rats were fasted overnight and then given food ad libitum the following morning. Two hours after the meal presentation, the rats were anesthetized (ethylene oxide) and opened by laparotomy. Blood samples were collected by cardiac puncture and placed into tubes containing ethylene diamine tetraacetic acid (EDTA) and a peptidase inhibitor cocktail containing general protease inhibitor (Roche Diagnostics Ltd., Burgess Hill, West Sussex, UK), followed by centrifugation at 3000× *g* for 10 min at 4 °C and storage at −80 °C until GLP-1 and PYY analysis. The gut was removed to sample the contents from cecum and tissue from distal ileum. Cecal contents were stored at −80 °C until analysis of short chain fatty acids (SCFAs). Tissues from distal ileum were immersed in RNAlater (QIAGEN, Crawley, UK) for 5 days at 4 °C and then stored at −80 °C until analysis.

2.5. Chemical Analysis

Diet samples were analyzed for crude protein according to the Association of Analytical Communities (AOAC) [31]. Gross energy was determined by bomb calorimetry using a LECO Ac 300 automated calorimeter system 789-500 (Parr Instrument Co., Moline, IL, USA). Soluble dietary fiber and insoluble fiber were determined by AOAC Method 991.43 [31]. Viscosity in extracts of diets was measured as reported by Johansen et al. [32]. The water-binding capacity and swelling capacity of diets were measured as described by Serena et al. [33].

The concentrations of GLP-1 and PYY in plasma were analyzed using an ultrasensitive rat GLP-1 and PYY enzyme-linked immunosorbent assay (ELISA) kit (Biosource Inc., Sunnyvale, CA, USA) according to the instructions. The SCFAs concentration of cecal contents was analyzed by gas chromatography (Varian CP-3800, Shimadzu Co., Kyoto, Japan), as described by Bosch et al. [34]. Total SCFAs was determined as the sum of analyzed acetate, propionate, and butyrate. All procedures were performed in duplicate.

2.6. Quantitative PCR (QPCR)

QPCR technology was employed to verify changes in the mRNA levels of GLP-1 and PYY genes. Total RNA was isolated from the distal ileum tissue using TRIZOL reagent (Invitrogen, Life Technologies Co., Carlsbad, CA, USA) according to the manufacturer's recommendations. Briefly, 2.5 μg of RNA was reverse transcribed using a First-strand cDNA synthethesis kit (TOYOBO, Kyoto, Japan) and cDNAs were stored at −20 °C. After 10-fold dilution, cDNA was used for the relative quantification of gene amplification. Primer sets for all genes were designed using Primer 6.0 Software (Applied Biosystems, Foster City, CA, USA) and synthesized commercially by Sangon (Shanghai, China). The primers sequences for rat PYY were sense 5′ CCGTTATGGTCGCAATGCT 3′, antisense 5′ TCTCGCTGTCGTCTGTGAA 3′. The primers sequences for rat GLP-1 were: sense 5′ CGGAAGAAGTCGCCATAGC 3′, antisense 5′ CAGCCAGTTGATGAAGTCTCT 3′. Rat β-*actin* was selected as the internal control gene for all QPCR reactions by using the following primers sequences: 5′ CTTTCTACAATGAGCTGCGTGTG 3′, antisense 5′ GTCAGGATCTTCATGAGGTAGTCTGTC 3′. cDNA was amplified by QPCR using a Bio-Rad CFX Connect™ Real-Time PCR Detection System (Bio-Rad, Richmond, CA, USA) under the following conditions: 95 °C for 3 min for enzyme activation, followed by denaturing at 95 °C for 20 s and annealing at 59 °C for 20 s and elongation at 72 °C for 20 s, repeated for a total of 40 cycles. Gene expression levels were calculated after normalization to the standard housekeeping gene β-*actin* using the $\Delta\Delta C_t$ method. Briefly, the mean values of the triplicate cycle thresholds (CT) of the target genes (PYY and GLP-1) were normalized to the mean values of triplicate CT of the reference β-*actin* using the calculation formula "$2^{CT_{\beta\text{-}actin} - CT_{\text{target gene}}}$", which indicated a relative value as a fraction of PYY or GLP-1.

2.7. Statistical Analysis

Data were compared by repeated ANOVA measures plus Tukey's post-hoc test, using the "PROC MIXED" function of the SAS software program (SAS 9.1, SAS Institute Inc., Cary, NC, USA). Data were examined to ensure patterns of constant variance and a normal distribution. The results that did not meet these conditions were transformed to appropriate data using logarithms or square roots. Data were presented as means ± SEM, and significant differences were accepted at a probability of $p < 0.05$.

3. Results

3.1. Food Intake and Body Weight

Average daily food intake throughout the experiment was affected by the dietary treatment in the decreasing magnitude order of control > PX > PG > KF ($p < 0.05$). Accordingly, cumulative food intake was significantly lower for rats fed the KF and PG diets than their control counterparts ($p < 0.05$), but with no significant difference between control and PX groups (Figure 1B). Compared with the control group, the final body weight and body weight gain showed a lower tendency in the KF and PG groups, but was not statistically significant ($p > 0.05$) (Figure 1C,D).

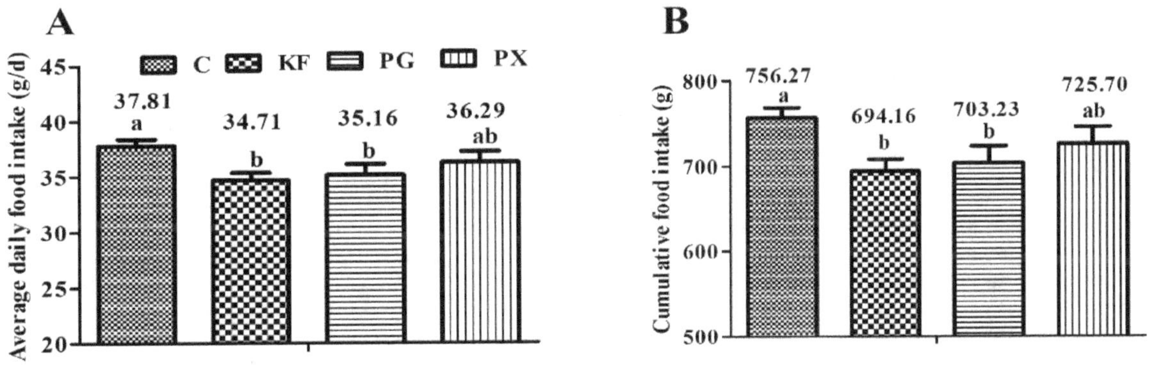

Figure 1. *Cont.*

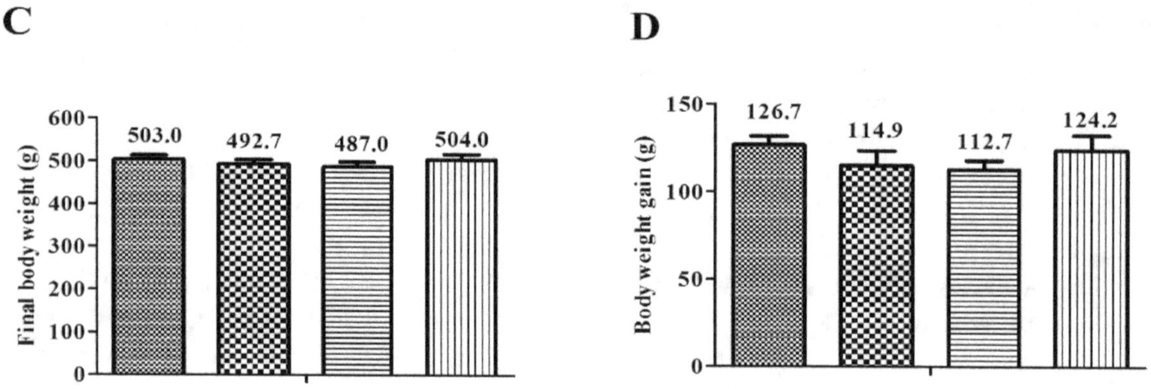

Figure 1. Food intake and body weight. (**A**) Average daily food intake; (**B**) cumulative food intake; (**C**) final body weight; and (**D**) body weight gain in rats given diets containing different dietary fibers for three weeks. Diets were control (C) or supplemented with 2% fiber of *konjac* flour (KF), pregelatinized waxy maize starch plus guar gum (PG) or pregelatinized waxy maize starch plus xanthan gum (PX); Values are mean ± SEM of $n = 8$ per group. Bars with different letters indicate a significant difference ($p < 0.05$).

3.2. Behavioral Satiety Sequence

The behavioral satiety sequence (feeding, drinking, activity, inactivity, grooming, and resting) of rats is shown in Table 2 and Figure 2. The overall pattern of behaviors was similar among all the dietary treatments. Quantification of individual behaviors indicated that the KF and PG groups spent significantly less time on feeding than the control group ($p < 0.05$; Table 2). When compared with other groups, the control group showed the feeding peak in the second time bin (control 91.88%, KF 84.38%, PG 74.38%, and PX 78.75%, respectively, $p = 0.07$; Figure 2). Furthermore, compared with bin 7 in the control group (Figure 2F–I), the KF, PG, and PX groups showed the transition from eating to resting in time bins 6, 5, and 6, respectively, which was consistent with the result that KF and PG groups had a lower food intake than the control group during the 1 h observation period ($p < 0.05$; Figure 2A).

Table 2. Behavioral satiety sequence of rats given diets containing different dietary fibers on day 15 [1].

Item	Control [2]	KF [2]	PG [2]	PX [2]	*p*-Value
Behavior (% time)					
Feeding	44.69 ± 3.45 [a]	34.53 ± 3.06 [b]	30.83 ± 3.19 [b]	35.94 ± 2.94 [a,b]	0.03
Drinking	6.04 ± 0.69	6.88 ± 0.70	5.47 ± 0.48	5.36 ± 0.80	0.38
Activity	21.15 ± 2.75	24.11 ± 3.54	21.82 ± 3.99	20.78 ± 2.12	0.88
Inactivity	10.42 ± 0.87	8.85 ± 1.52	10.73 ± 1.30	11.51 ± 2.01	0.64
Grooming	3.49 ± 0.47	4.53 ± 0.91	4.32 ± 1.09	4.11 ± 0.31	0.79
Resting	14.22 ± 4.08	21.09 ± 4.06	26.82 ± 4.28	22.29 ± 5.28	0.21

[1] After a 12-h fast, rats were given food, and their behaviors monitored for 1 h. The percentage of time spent in each behavior was calculated and represented as mean ± SEM of $n = 8$ per group. Rows with different superscript letters indicate a significant difference ($p < 0.05$); [2] Diets were control or supplemented with 2% fiber of *konjac* flour (KF), pregelatinized waxy maize starch plus guar gum (PG), or pregelatinized waxy maize starch plus xanthan gum (PX).

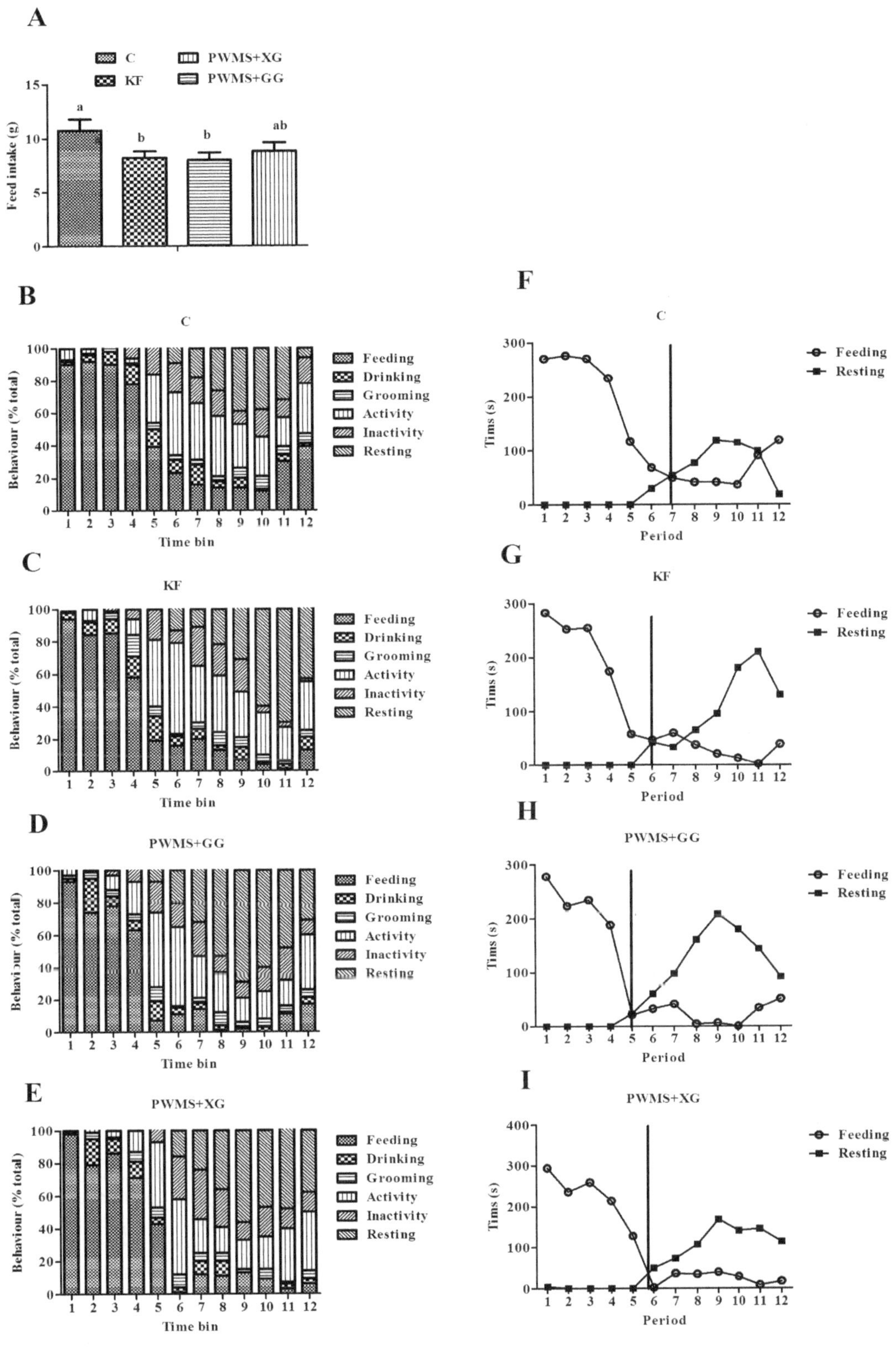

Figure 2. Food intake (**A**) in rats was calculated at 1 h and is presented as mean ± SEM for $n = 8$ per group. Bars with different letters indicate a significant difference ($p < 0.05$). Periods 1–12 correspond to the twelve 5-min time bins comprising the 60 min test session; (**B**–**E**) Frequency data within each behavioral category are expressed as a proportion of the total number of observations per time bin; (**F**–**I**) correspond to crossover graphs illustrating the point of transition from eating to resting. The perpendicular line indicates satiety point. Diets were control (C) or supplemented with 2% fiber of *konjac* flour (KF), pregelatinized waxy maize starch plus guar gum (PG), or pregelatinized waxy maize starch plus xanthan gum (PX).

3.3. Meal Pattern Parameters

Meal pattern parameters are presented in Table 3. Although the diurnal and nocturnal food intakes were similar among the four groups, the PG, KF, and PX groups were significantly lower than the control group in total food intake ($p < 0.01$). The feeding rate, meal size and meal duration (total, diurnal, and nocturnal) were similar among all the groups. However, the total and nocturnal meal numbers of the KF and PG groups were significantly lower than those of the control group ($p < 0.05$). As expected, the PG group was obviously higher than the control group in total inter-meal interval ($p < 0.05$), and the KF and PX groups were also higher, but not statistically significant.

Table 3. Meal pattern parameters of rats given diets containing different dietary fibers for three weeks [1].

Item	Control [2]	KF [2]	PG [2]	PX [2]	*p*-Value
Food intake (g/day)					
Total	51.68 ± 1.50 ^{a}	46.58 ± 0.86 ^{b}	46.01 ± 1.07 ^{b}	48.47 ± 0.79 ^{b}	<0.01
Nocturnal	23.40 ± 1.20	20.55 ± 1.04	20.79 ± 0.96	20.18 ± 1.53	0.24
Diurnal	28.29 ± 0.67	26.03 ± 1.33	25.22 ± 0.64	28.29 ± 1.62	0.16
Feeding rate (mg/s)					
Total	6.59 ± 0.93	6.54 ± 0.68	8.41 ± 1.29	5.89 ± 0.57	0.26
Nocturnal	5.67 ± 0.88	6.04 ± 0.44	7.09 ± 0.52	5.37 ± 0.62	0.26
Diurnal	6.59 ± 1.08	7.38 ± 1.25	8.47 ± 0.85	6.32 ± 0.60	0.45
Meal size (g/day)					
Total	3.12 ± 0.20	3.21 ± 0.13	3.39 ± 0.19	2.92 ± 0.19	0.33
Nocturnal	2.36 ± 0.14	2.53 ± 0.16	2.52 ± 0.15	2.20 ± 0.10	0.30
Diurnal	4.36 ± 0.41	4.22 ± 0.33	4.89 ± 0.47	3.73 ± 0.30	0.22
Meal duration (s)					
Total	507.45 ± 39.86	517.79 ± 41.60	437.35 ± 35.27	517.51 ± 41.47	0.43
Nocturnal	449.70 ± 38.00	440.70 ± 49.95	365.73 ± 28.00	437.96 ± 37.82	0.35
Diurnal	584.90 ± 49.69	620.19 ± 51.21	591.17 ± 40.64	612.64 ± 49.50	0.94
Meal number (meals/day)					
Total	16.88 ± 0.74 ^{a}	14.63 ± 0.50 ^{b}	13.88 ± 0.83 ^{b}	17.00 ± 0.89 ^{a}	0.01
Nocturnal	10.00 ± 0.38 ^{a}	8.25 ± 0.41 ^{b}	8.38 ± 0.50 ^{b}	9.25 ± 0.70 ^{a,b}	0.07
Diurnal	6.88 ± 0.61a ^{b}	6.38 ± 0.50 ^{a,b}	5.50 ± 0.53 ^{b}	7.75 ± 0.41 ^{a}	0.03
Inter-meal interval (min)					
Total	73.49 ± 4.57 ^{b}	87.72 ± 4.16 ^{a,b}	98.23 ± 9.48 ^{a}	76.53 ± 4.03 ^{b}	0.03
Nocturnal	58.34 ± 4.70	73.24 ± 6.40	70.90 ± 6.68	65.10 ± 4.74	0.27
Diurnal	106.65 ± 13.23	113.15 ± 9.48	133.19 ± 13.33	93.65 ± 5.61	0.09

[1] Values are mean ± SEM of $n = 8$, rows with different superscript letters indicate a significant difference ($p < 0.05$); [2] Diets were control or supplemented with 2% fiber of *konjac* flour (KF), pregelatinized waxy maize starch plus guar gum (PG), or pregelatinized waxy maize starch plus xanthan gum (PX).

3.4. Plasma Concentrations of GLP-1/PYY, mRNA Abundance in Distal Ileum of GLP-1/PYY, and Concentrations of SCFAs in Cecal Contents

There was no significant difference in the plasma concentrations of GLP-1 and PYY, and the mRNA abundance of GLP-1 and PYY in ileum tissue among the four dietary treatments (Figure 3). Compared with the control group, the concentrations of acetic acid and SCFAs in cecal contents were increased in the KF and PG groups ($p < 0.05$; Figure 4). Additionally, the KF, PG, and PX groups had higher concentrations of the propionic acid in cecal contents than the control group ($p < 0.05$).

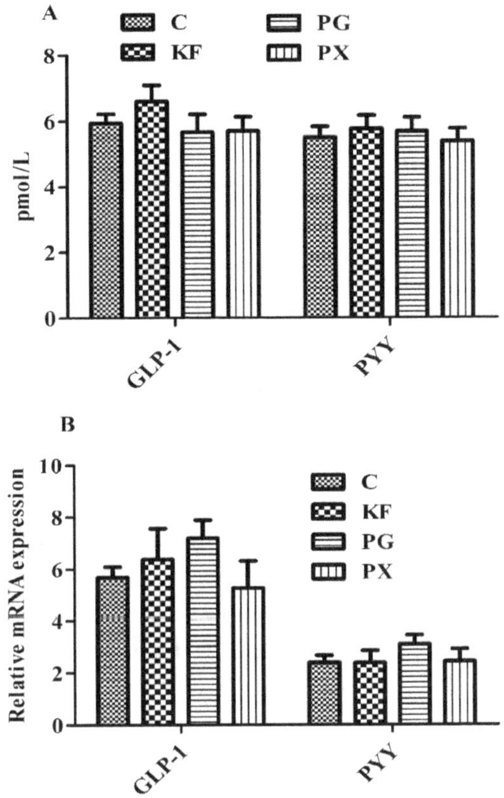

Figure 3. Plasma concentrations (**A**) and mRNA abundance in distal ileum (**B**) of GLP-1 and PYY in rats given diets containing different dietary fibers for three weeks; Diets were control (C) or supplemented with 2% fiber of *konjac* flour (KF), pregelatinized waxy maize starch plus guar gum (PG), or pregelatinized waxy maize starch plus xanthan gum (PX); Values are mean ± SEM, n = 6–8 per group. GLP-1, glucagon-like peptide-1; PYY, peptide tyrosine-tyrosine.

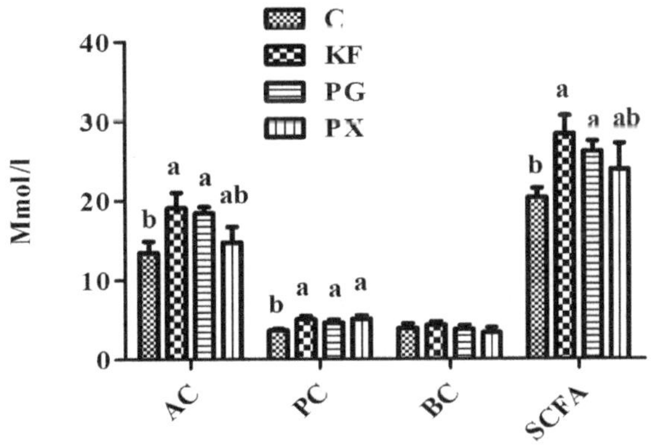

Figure 4. Concentration of SCFAs in cecal contents of rats given diets containing different dietary fibers for three weeks. Diets were control (C) or supplemented with 2% fiber of *konjac* flour (KF), pregelatinized waxy maize starch plus guar gum (PG) or pregelatinized waxy maize starch plus xanthan gum (PX); Values are mean ± SEM of n = 6–8 per group. Bars with different letters indicate a significant difference ($p < 0.05$). SCFAs, short-chain fatty acids; AC, acetate acid; PC, propionate acid; BC, butyrate acid.

4. Discussion

The present study aimed to explore whether dietary fibers regulate appetite by promoting satiety or satiation, and to this end, behavioral satiety sequence and meal pattern were monitored.

Detailed analysis of the behavioral satiety sequence revealed that the overall pattern of the behavioral response to fast-induced food intake in rats was normal. However, we observed a decrease in short-term (1 h) food intake, accompanied by reduced feeding behavior in rats fed the KF and PG diets. Furthermore, the transition from eating to resting occurred in early time bins in the PG, PX, and KF groups, indicating that satiety was induced in the three groups [35]. To our knowledge, this is probably the first report so far about a detailed analysis of the behavioral satiety sequence following dietary fiber treatments in rats.

The present results are consistent with our previous study in that supplementation of KF reduced the non-feeding oral behavior and promoted the satiety of sows [20]. In the current study, there was no significant difference in the feeding rates of rats among all the dietary treatments. Based on the association of taste and flavor aversions with a decrease in feeding rate [36], the consistent feeding rates indicated that dietary fiber supplementation did not produce a significant effect on food palatability, implying that the changes in the meal pattern observed here might be attributed to physiological factors rather than changes in diet palatability or flavor.

In the present study, dietary supplementation of KF and PG reduced the total food intake, mainly due to the increased satiety, as indicated by decreased meal numbers and increased inter-meal intervals. This is in agreement with a previous study that reported the suppression of food intake 2 h after the administration of the mixture of guar gum and fructo-oligosaccharide, due to decreased meal numbers and increased inter-meal intervals [37]. It is worth noting that the current result contrasted with a most recent study about diets supplemented with guar gum or fructo-oligosaccharide alone [30]. Although both of them reduced the food intake immediately after dietary fiber ingestion, the result was mainly attributed to a decrease of meal size and meal duration but not meal number and inter-meal intervals, indicating that the decrease in food intake is associated with increased satiation rather than satiety. In the current study, the rats consumed such a high proportion of their daily intake during the light phase, probably due to their 12-h fast overnight before the meal pattern analysis.

Pregelatinized waxy maize starch and fructo-oligosaccharide are highly fermentable fibers [38,39]' and guar gum is a viscous fiber with high water-binding capacity [3]. This suggests that the combination of fibers with different physicochemical properties may affect the physiological processes (satiation or satiety) of appetite regulation. In the present study, dietary treatments were similar in insoluble fiber and viscosity, but their soluble fiber, water-binding capacity, and swelling capacity followed the sequence of PG > KF > PX > control.

The addition of a small amount of hydrocolloids resulted in a large enhancement in water-binding capacity and swelling capacity of starch pastes, but a reduction of syneresis in starch gels, indicating that the magnitude of such changes in paste rheology and texture depends on the type of starch and gum used [40,41]. The current results (PG group with highest water-binding capacity and swelling capacity) could be explained by a previous study which showed that the most pronounced effect has been the retardation of gelation kinetics of waxy maize starch plus the guar gum, rather than the combination with other gums [42].

Gelatinized waxy maize starch was subjected to different time and temperature conditions of storage to obtain samples with different extents of amylopectin retrogradation. Increased retrogradation extents reduced the enzyme susceptibilities to pancreatic alpha amylase and amyloglucosidase at 37 °C [43]. The pregelatinized starch produced more satiety than the raw potato starch, probably because this starch was digested too slowly to increase the postprandial blood glucose concentrations to any appreciable extent [44,45].

Soluble fiber with high water-binding capacity and viscosity may slow gastric emptying and small bowel transit [46,47], and several of the aforementioned signals generated in the gastrointestinal tract cooperate to promote satiety by activating vagal afferents and/or by acting directly on the brain [48,49]. Thus, the increased satiety by dietary supplementation of KF and PG is associated with decreased food intake in rats, which may be attributed to the high water-binding capacity and swelling capacity in those diets.

In the current study, supplementation of KF and PG significantly increased the concentrations of acetic acid, propionate acid, and SCFAs in the cecal content of rats. A number of factors—including chemical structure, particle size, surface area, and solubility of the fiber—affect the fermentation in the gut and the nature of the SCFAs produced [50,51]. Carbohydrates containing glucomannan or alpha-galacturonic acid residues are generally more susceptible to fermentation [51]. A comparison of *konjac* gum, guar gum, xanthan gum, and pectin in human fecal inoculum in a 48-h static fermentation culture system showed that all the gums increased the SCFAs level, and *konjac* and guar gum had the strongest acid-reducing ability among gum dietary fibers [52]. Resistant starch is completely degraded in the large bowel, and thus long-term consumption of fermentable fiber could produce satiety benefits [53].

It has been suggested that SCFAs stimulate the production and secretion of satiety-related hormones, such as GLP-1 and PYY, possibly via G-protein coupled receptors [54]. However, in the current study, dietary treatments did not alter the GLP-1 and PYY either in plasma concentration or mRNA abundance in distal ileum two hours after feeding, which is not consistent with a previous report that dietary supplementation of fructooligosaccharide increased the plasma concentration of PYY in the fasted state of rats [37]. It can be inferred that dietary fiber effect on satiety hormones (GLP-1/PYY) is associated with fed or fasted state. PYY and GLP-1 are both synthesized and released from L-cells located in the small intestine and large intestine [55]. They showed no increased expression here in distal ileum, probably due to an overall increase in L-cell number along the enlarged intestines, which was not detectable here since the real time PCR method measures expression per mg tissue. Slowly digestible starch inclusion in pig diet decreased distal ileum SCFAs transporter mRNA abundance [56]. This is why we selected the distal ileum for anatomical analysis.

The SCFAs produced via bacterial fermentation directly suppresses appetite via central hypothalamic mechanisms in rodents [57]. Recent findings from human study suggest that propionate production may play an important role in attenuating reward-based eating behavior via striatal pathways, independent of changes in plasma PYY and GLP-1 [58]. It is well known that SCFAs serve as an additional energy source, especially at the moment when glucose absorption is decreasing (or completed) in the small intestine, which helps to stabilize glucose levels in blood [59,60]. Delayed postprandial glucose transient declines could delay the onset of the ensuing meal and induce inter-meal satiety [61].

In the current study, dietary treatments had no effect on final body weight and body weight gain in the rats. At 10 weeks of age, the tested rats were young adults. The adult rats might continue to gain body mass at a slower rate, but the juvenile rapid growth phase ceased [62]. Therefore, the similarity in the body weight gain of rats among all the dietary treatments can be explained from the analysis of short-term effects.

The slight but not significant variation in feeding behavior, meal number, and SCFAs yield in PX group may result in an overall reduction trend but not in notable changes in food intake, probably due to the reason that the PX diet did not reach the level of KF and PG diets in the physicochemical properties (water-binding capacity and swelling capacity) and fermentability (SCFAs), thus it could not produce a significant effect on the satiety and food intake in rats.

In the current study, the daily dosage of soluble fiber per kilogram of body weight in rats was 1.4 g/kg (35 g (daily food intake) × 2% (dosage)/0.5 kg (body weight) = 1.4 g/kg body weight). Based on the dose translation formula (Human equivalent doses (mg/kg) = Animal dose (mg/kg) × (Animal *Km*/Human *Km*)) from animal to human studies revisited [63,64], the corresponding soluble fiber dose for humans was estimated to be 0.23 g/kg (1.4 g/kg (Animal dose) × 6 (Animal *Km*)/37 (Human *Km*) = 0.23 g/kg), which means the soluble fiber dose for a 60 kg person is 13.8 g (0.23 g/kg × 60 kg = 13.8 g). Further work is required to translate the findings to humans.

5. Conclusions

KF and PG reduce the food intake, probably by promoting the satiety, which was supported by decreased meal numbers and increased inter-meal intervals, but without a reduction in body weight gain. Additionally, dietary soluble fibers with high levels of physicochemical properties (water-binding capacity and swelling capacity) and fermentability (SCFAs) have a more significant effect on food intake, meal pattern, and feeding behavior in rats.

Author Contributions: All authors contributed to the paper in the following ways: conception and design of the study (J.P., Y.F.Z.), acquisition of data (C.Q.T., X.C.Z., C.H.X.), analysis and interpretation of the data (J.P., C.Q.T., H.K.W.), drafting the article (C.Q.T.), and final approval (J.P., C.Q.T., Y.F.Z.).

References

1. Raghad, A.; Hala, G.; Mohamad, A.; Omar, O. Meal pattern of male rats maintained on amino acid supplemented diets: The effect of tryptophan, lysine, arginine, proline and threonine. *Nutrients* **2014**, *6*, 2509–2522.
2. Schroeder, N.; Marquart, L.F.; Gallaher, D.D. The role of viscosity and fermentability of dietary fibers on satiety- and adiposity-related hormones in rats. *Nutrients* **2013**, *5*, 2093–2113. [CrossRef] [PubMed]
3. Wanders, A.J.; Jonathan, M.C.; van den Borne, J.J.; Mars, M.; Schols, H.A.; Feskens, E.J.; de Graaf, C. The effects of bulking, viscous and gel-forming dietary fibres on satiation. *Br. J. Nutr.* **2013**, *109*, 1330–1337. [CrossRef] [PubMed]
4. Bortolotti, M.; Levorato, M.; Lugli, A.; Mazzero, G. Effect of a balanced mixture of dietary fibers on gastric emptying, intestinal transit and body weight. *Ann. Nutr. Metab.* **2008**, *52*, 221–226. [CrossRef] [PubMed]
5. Rendon-Huerta, J.A.; Juarez-Flores, B.; Pinos-Rodriguez, J.M.; Aguirre-Rivera, J.R.; Delgado-Portales, R.E. Effects of different sources of fructans on body weight, blood metabolites and fecal bacteria in normal and obese non-diabetic and diabetic rats. *Plant Foods Hum. Nutr.* **2012**, *67*, 64–70. [CrossRef] [PubMed]
6. Howarth, N.C.; Saltzman, E.; Roberts, S.B. Dietary fiber and weight regulation. *Nutr. Rev.* **2001**, *59*, 129–139. [CrossRef] [PubMed]
7. Li, J.; Zhang, N.; Hu, L.; Li, Z.; Li, R.; Li, C.; Wang, S. Improvement in chewing activity reduces energy intake in one meal and modulates plasma gut hormone concentrations in obese and lean young Chinese men. *Am. J. Clin. Nutr.* **2011**, *94*, 709–716. [CrossRef] [PubMed]
8. Zijlstra, N.; Mars, M.; de Wijk, R.A.; Westerterp-Plantenga, M.S.; de Graaf, C. The effect of viscosity on ad libitum food intake. *Int. J. Obes.* **2008**, *32*, 676–683. [CrossRef] [PubMed]
9. Dabin, B. Fibres for fertility: The inclusion of raw fibre in sow diets has many positive effects. In *Feed Mix*; Misset International: Doetinchem, The Netherlands, 2006; pp. 18–21.
10. Bergmann, J.F.; Chassany, O.; Petit, A.; Triki, R.; Caulin, C.; Segrestaa, J.M. Correlation between echographic gastric emptying and appetite: Influence of psyllium. *Gut* **1992**, *33*, 1042–1043. [CrossRef] [PubMed]
11. Phillips, R.J.; Powley, T.L. Tension and stretch receptors in gastrointestinal smooth muscle: Re-evaluating vagal mechanoreceptor electrophysiology. *Brain Res. Brain Res. Rev.* **2000**, *34*, 1–26. [CrossRef]
12. Heijboer, A.C.; Pijl, H.; van den Hoek, A.M.; Havekes, L.M.; Romijn, J.A.; Corssmit, E.P.M. Gut-brain axis: Regulation of glucose metabolism. *J. Neuroendocrinol.* **2006**, *18*, 883–894. [CrossRef] [PubMed]
13. Silva, E.; Birkenhake, M.; Scholten, E.; Sagis, L.M.C.; Linden, E.V.D. Controlling rheology and structure of sweet potato starch noodles with high broccoli powder content by hydrocolloids. *Food Hydrocoll.* **2013**, *30*, 42–52. [CrossRef]
14. Sun, H.Q.; Zhou, Y.F.; Tan, C.Q.; Zheng, L.F.; Peng, J.; Jiang, S.W. Effects of konjac flour inclusion in gestation diets on the nutrient digestibility, lactation feed intake and reproductive performance of sows. *Animal* **2014**, *8*, 1089–1094. [CrossRef] [PubMed]
15. Katsuraya, K.; Okuyama, K.; Hatanaka, K.; Oshima, R.; Sato, T.; Matsuzaki, K. Constitution of konjac glucomannan: Chemical analysis and 13 C NMR spectroscopy. *Carbohydr. Polym.* **2003**, *53*, 183–189. [CrossRef]
16. Chua, M.; Baldwin, T.C.; Hocking, T.J.; Chan, K. Traditional uses and potential health benefits of *Amorphophallus konjac* K. Koch ex NEBr. *J. Ethnopharmacol.* **2010**, *128*, 268–278. [CrossRef] [PubMed]

17. Shah, B.R.; Li, B.; Wang, L.; Liu, S.; Li, Y.; Wei, X.; Jin, W.; Li, Z. Health benefits of konjac glucomannan with special focus on diabetes. *Bioact. Carbohydr. Diet. Fibre* **2015**, *5*, 179–187. [CrossRef]
18. Tan, C.Q.; Wei, H.K.; Sun, H.Q.; Long, G.; Ao, J.T.; Jiang, S.W.; Peng, J. Effects of supplementing sow diets during two gestations with konjac flour and *Saccharomyces boulardii* on constipation in peripartal period, lactation feed intake and piglet performance. *Anim. Feed Sci. Technol.* **2015**, *210*, 254–262. [CrossRef]
19. Tan, C.Q.; Wei, H.K.; Ao, J.T.; Long, G.; Peng, J. Inclusion of konjac flour in the gestation diet changes the gut microbiota, alleviates oxidative stress, and improves insulin sensitivity in sows. *Appl. Environ. Microbiol.* **2016**, *82*, 5899–5909. [CrossRef] [PubMed]
20. Sun, H.; Tan, C.; Wei, H.; Zou, Y.; Long, G.; Ao, J.; Xue, H.; Jiang, S.; Peng, J. Effects of different amounts of konjac flour inclusion in gestation diets on physio-chemical properties of diets, postprandial satiety in pregnant sows, lactation feed intake of sows and piglet performance. *Anim. Reprod. Sci.* **2015**, *152*, 55–64. [CrossRef] [PubMed]
21. Copeland, L.; Blazek, J.; Salman, H.; Tang, M.C.M. Form and functionality of starch. *Food Hydrocoll.* **2009**, *23*, 1527–1534. [CrossRef]
22. Shimotoyodome, A.; Suzuki, J.; Kameo, Y.; Hase, T. Dietary supplementation with hydroxypropyl-distarch phosphate from waxy maize starch increases resting energy expenditure by lowering the postprandial glucose-dependent insulinotropic polypeptide response in human subjects. *Br. J. Nutr.* **2011**, *106*, 96–104. [CrossRef] [PubMed]
23. Fuongfuchat, A.; Seetapan, N.; Makmoon, T.; Pongjaruwat, W.; Methacanon, P.; Gamonpilas, C. Linear and non-linear viscoelastic behaviors of crosslinked tapioca starch/polysaccharide systems. *J. Food Eng.* **2012**, *109*, 571–578. [CrossRef]
24. Mandala, I.G.; Bayas, E. Xanthan effect on swelling, solubility and viscosity of wheat starch dispersions. *Food Hydrocoll.* **2004**, *18*, 191–201. [CrossRef]
25. Paquet, É.; Bédard, A.; Lemieux, S.; Turgeon, S.L. Effects of apple juice-based beverages enriched with dietary fibres and xanthan gum on the glycemic response and appetite sensations in healthy men. *Bioact. Carbohydr. Diet. Fibre* **2014**, *4*, 39–47. [CrossRef]
26. Tan, C.Q.; Wei, H.K.; Zhao, X.C.; Xu, C.H.; Peng, J. Effects of Water Binding Capacity and Swelling Capacity of Soluble Fibers on Physicochemical Properties of Gastrointestinal Digesta and Food Intake in Rats. *Food Nutr. Res.* **2015**, in press.
27. Glendinning, J.I.; Smith, J.C. Consistency of meal patterns in laboratory rats. *Physiol. Behav.* **1994**, *56*, 7–16. [CrossRef]
28. Halford, J.C.; Wanninayake, S.C.; Blundell, J.E. Behavioral satiety sequence (BSS) for the diagnosis of drug action on food intake. *Pharmacol. Biochem. Behav.* **1998**, *61*, 159–168. [CrossRef]
29. Lira, L.A.; Almeida, L.C.A.; Silva, A.A.M.D.; Cavalcante, T.C.F.; Melo, D.D.C.B.D.; Souza, J.A.D.; Campina, R.C.F.; Souza, S.L.D. Perinatal undernutrition increases meal size and neuronal activation of the nucleus of the solitary tract in response to feeding stimulation in adult rats. *Int. J. Dev. Neurosci.* **2014**, *38*, 23–29. [CrossRef] [PubMed]
30. Hadri, Z.; Chaumontet, C.; Fromentin, G.; Even, P.C.; Darcel, N.; Bouras, A.D.; Tome, D.; Rasoamanana, R. Long term ingestion of a preload containing fructo-oligosaccharide or guar gum decreases fat mass but not food intake in mice. *Physiol. Behav.* **2015**, *147*, 198–204. [CrossRef] [PubMed]
31. Association of Official Analytical Chemists. *Official Methods of Analysis*, 16th ed.; AOAC International: Arlington, VA, USA, 1999.
32. Johansen, H.N.; Bach Knudsen, K.E.; Wood, P.J.; Fulcher, R.G. Physico-Chemical Properties and the Degradation of Oat Bran Polysaccharides in the Gut of Pigs. *J. Sci. Food Agric.* **1997**, *73*, 81–92. [CrossRef]
33. Serena, A.; Jorgensen, H.; Knudsen, K.E.B. Digestion of carbohydrates and utilization of energy in sows fed diets with contrasting levels and physicochemical properties of dietary fiber. *J. Anim. Sci.* **2008**, *86*, 2208–2216. [CrossRef] [PubMed]
34. Bosch, G.; Pellikaan, W.F.; Rutten, P.G.P.; van der Poel, A.F.B.; Verstegen, M.W.A.; Hendriks, W.H. Comparative in vitro fermentation activity in the canine distal gastrointestinal tract and fermentation kinetics of fiber sources. *J. Anim. Sci.* **2008**, *86*, 2979–2989. [CrossRef] [PubMed]
35. Orozco-Solis, R.; Lopes-de-Souza, S.; Barbosa Matos, R.J.; Grit, I.; Le-Bloch, J.; Nguyen, P.; Manhaes-de-Castro, R.; Bolanos-Jimenez, F. Perinatal undernutrition-induced obesity is independent of the developmental programming of feeding. *Physiol. Behav.* **2009**, *96*, 481–492. [CrossRef] [PubMed]

36. Labouré, H.; Saux, S.; Nicolaidis, S. Effects of food texture change on metabolic parameters: Short- and long-term feeding patterns and body weight. *Am. J. Physiol. Regul. Integr. Comp. Physiol.* **2001**, *280*, R780–R789. [PubMed]
37. Rasoamanana, R.; Even, P.C.; Darcel, N.; Tomé, D.; Fromentin, G. Dietary fibers reduce food intake by satiation without conditioned taste aversion in mice. *Physiol. Behav.* **2013**, *17*, 13–19. [CrossRef] [PubMed]
38. Alles, M.S.; de Roos, N.M.; Bakx, J.C.; van de Lisdonk, E.; Zock, P.L.; Hautvast, G.A. Consumption of fructooligosaccharides does not favorably affect blood glucose and serum lipid concentrations in patients with type 2 diabetes. *Am. J. Clin. Nutr.* **1999**, *69*, 64–69. [PubMed]
39. Da Silva, C.S.; Bosch, G.; Bolhuis, J.E.; Stappers, L.J.N.; van Hees, H.M.J.; Gerrits, W.J.J.; Kemp, B. Effects of alginate and resistant starch on feeding patterns, behaviour and performance in ad libitum-fed growing pigs. *Animal* **2014**, *8*, 1917–1927. [CrossRef] [PubMed]
40. Eidam, D.C.D.; Kuhn, K.; Stute, R. Formation of Maize Starch Gels Selectively Regulated by the Addition of Hydrocolloids. *Starch Stärke* **1995**, *47*, 378–384. [CrossRef]
41. Sudhakar, V.; Singhal, R.S.; Kulkarni, P.R. Effect of salts on interactions of starch with guar gum. *Food Hydrocoll.* **1996**, *10*, 329–334. [CrossRef]
42. Biliaderis, C.G.; Arvanitoyannis, I.; Izydorczyk, M.S.; Prokopowich, D.J. Effect of Hydrocolloids on Gelatinization and Structure Formation in Concentrated Waxy Maize and Wheat Starch Gels. *Starch Stärke* **1997**, *49*, 278–283. [CrossRef]
43. Eerlingen, R.C.; Jacobs, H.; Delcour, J.A. Enzyme-resistant starch. V. Effect of retrogradation of waxy maize starch on enzyme susceptibility. *Cereal Chem.* **1994**, *71*, 351–355.
44. Liljeberg, H.G.; Akerberg, A.K.; Björck, I.M. Effect of the glycemic index and content of indigestible carbohydrates of cereal-based breakfast meals on glucose tolerance at lunch in healthy subjects. *Am. J. Clin. Nutr.* **1999**, *69*, 647–655. [PubMed]
45. Raben, A.; Tagliabue, A.; Christensen, N.J.; Madsen, J.; Holst, J.J.; Astrup, A. Resistant starch: The effect on postprandial glycemia, hormonal response, and satiety. *Am. J. Clin. Nutr.* **1994**, *60*, 544–551. [PubMed]
46. Burton-Freeman, B. Dietary fiber and energy regulation. *J. Nutr.* **2000**, *130*, 272S–275S. [PubMed]
47. Kristensen, M.; Jensen, M.G. Dietary fibres in the regulation of appetite and food intake. Importance of viscosity. *Appetite* **2011**, *56*, 65–70. [CrossRef] [PubMed]
48. Moran, T.H.; Ladenheim, E.E.; Schwartz, G.J. Within-meal gut feedback signaling. *Int. J. Obes. Relat. Metab. Disord.* **2001**, *25*, S39–S41. [CrossRef] [PubMed]
49. Schwartz, G. Integrative capacity of the caudal brainstem in the control of food intake. *Philos. Trans. R. Soc. B Biol. Sci.* **2006**, *361*, 1275–1280. [CrossRef] [PubMed]
50. Blackwood, A.D.; Salter, J.; Dettmar, P.W.; Chaplin, M.F. Dietary fibre, physicochemical properties and their relationship to health. *J. R. Soc. Promot. Health* **2000**, *120*, 242–247. [CrossRef] [PubMed]
51. Slavin, J.; Savarino, V.; Paredes-Diaz, A.; Fotopoulos, G. A review of the role of soluble fiber in health with specific reference to wheat dextrin. *J. Int. Med. Res.* **2009**, *37*, 1–17. [CrossRef] [PubMed]
52. Fiszman, S.; Varela, P. The role of gums in satiety/satiation. A review. *Food Hydrocoll.* **2013**, *32*, 147–154. [CrossRef]
53. Yang, H.-F.; Chen, H.-L. Utilization of Gum Dietary Fibers by the Human Fecal Inoculum in the Static Fermentation Culture System. *Taiwan J. Agric. Chem. Food Sci.* **2008**, *46*, 183–189.
54. Tilg, H.; Moschen, A.R. Microbiota and diabetes: An evolving relationship. *Gut* **2014**, *63*, 1513–1521. [CrossRef] [PubMed]
55. Del, P.A.; Iadevaia, M.; Loguercio, C. The role of gut hormones in controlling the food intake: What is their role in emerging diseases? *Endocrinol. Nutr.* **2012**, *59*, 197–206.
56. Woodward, A.D.; Regmi, P.R.; Gänzle, M.G.; van Kempen, T.A.; Zijlstra, R.T. Slowly digestible starch influences mRNA abundance of glucose and short-chain fatty acid transporters in the porcine distal intestinal tract. *J. Anim. Sci.* **2012**, *90*, 80–82. [CrossRef] [PubMed]
57. Frost, G.; Sleeth, M.L.; Sahuri-Arisoylu, M.; Lizarbe, B.; Cerdan, S.; Brody, L.; Anastasovska, J.; Ghourab, S.; Hankir, M.; Shuai, Z. The short-chain fatty acid acetate reduces appetite via a central homeostatic mechanism. *Nat. Commun.* **2014**, *5*, 3611. [CrossRef] [PubMed]
58. Byrne, C.S.; Chambers, E.S.; Alhabeeb, H.; Chhina, N.; Morrison, D.J.; Preston, T.; Tedford, C.; Fitzpatrick, J.; Irani, C.; Busza, A. Increased colonic propionate reduces anticipatory reward responses in the human striatum to high-energy foods123. *Am. J. Clin. Nutr.* **2016**, *188*, 724–732.

59. Higgins, J.A. Resistant starch: Metabolic effects and potential health benefits. *J. AOAC Int.* **2004**, *87*, 761–768. [CrossRef] [PubMed]
60. Leeuw, J.A.D.; Jongbloed, A.W.; Spoolder, H.A.M.; Verstegen, M.W.A. Effects of hindgut fermentation of non-starch polysaccharides on the stability of blood glucose and insulin levels and physical activity in empty sows. *Livest. Prod. Sci.* **2005**, *96*, 165–174. [CrossRef]
61. De Leeuw, J.A.; Jongbloed AWVerstegen, M.W. Dietary Fiber Stabilizes Blood Glucose and Insulin Levels and Reduces Physical Activity in Sows (Sus scrofa). *J. Nutr.* **2004**, *134*, 1481–1486. [PubMed]
62. Sengupta, P. The Laboratory Rat: Relating Its Age With Human's. *Int. J. Prev. Med.* **2013**, *4*, 624–630. [PubMed]
63. Food and Drug Administration. *Guidance for Industry: Estimating the Maximum Safe Starting Dose in Initial Clinical Trials for Therapeutics in Adult Healthy Volunteers*; Food and Drug Administration: Washington, DC, USA, 2005.
64. Reagan-Shaw, S.; Nihal, M.; Ahmad, N. Dose translation from animal to human studies revisited. *FASEB J.* **2008**, *22*, 659–661. [CrossRef] [PubMed]

3

The Interaction between Dietary Fiber and Fat and Risk of Colorectal Cancer in the Women's Health Initiative

Sandi L. Navarro [1,*], Marian L. Neuhouser [1,2], Ting-Yuan David Cheng [3], Lesley F. Tinker [1], James M. Shikany [4], Linda Snetselaar [5], Jessica A. Martinez [6], Ikuko Kato [7], Shirley A. A. Beresford [1,2], Robert S. Chapkin [8] and Johanna W. Lampe [1,2]

1 Division of Public Health Sciences, Fred Hutchinson Cancer Research Center, Seattle, WA 98109, USA; mneuhous@fredhutch.org (M.L.N.); ltinker@whi.org (L.F.T.); beresfrd@uw.edu (S.A.A.B.); jlampe@fredhutch.org (J.W.L.)
2 Department of Epidemiology, School of Public Health, University of Washington, Seattle, WA 98105, USA
3 Division of Cancer Prevention and Population Sciences, Roswell Park Cancer Institute, Buffalo, NY 14263, USA; david.cheng@roswellpark.org
4 Division of Preventive Medicine, University of Alabama at Birmingham, Birmingham, AL 35294, USA; jshikany@uabmc.edu
5 Department of Epidemiology, University of Iowa, Iowa City, IA 52242, USA; linda-snetselaar@uiowa.edu
6 Department of Nutritional Sciences, University of Arizona Cancer Center, Tucson, AZ 85724, USA; jam1@email.arizona.edu
7 Department of Oncology and Pathology, Wayne State University, Detroit, MI 48201, USA; katoi@karmanos.org
8 Program in Integrative Nutrition and Complex Diseases, Texas A&M University, College Station, TX 77843, USA; r-chapkin@tamu.edu
* Correspondence: snavarro@fredhutch.org;

Abstract: Combined intakes of specific dietary fiber and fat subtypes protect against colon cancer in animal models. We evaluated associations between self-reported individual and combinations of fiber (insoluble, soluble, and pectins, specifically) and fat (omega-6, omega-3, and docosahexaenoic acid (DHA) and eicosapentaenoic acid (EPA), specifically) and colorectal cancer (CRC) risk in the Women's Health Initiative prospective cohort (n = 134,017). During a mean 11.7 years (1993–2010), 1952 incident CRC cases were identified. Cox regression models computed multivariate adjusted hazard ratios to estimate the association between dietary factors and CRC risk. Assessing fiber and fat individually, there was a modest trend for lower CRC risk with increasing intakes of total and insoluble fiber (*p-trend* 0.09 and 0.08). An interaction ($p = 0.01$) was observed between soluble fiber and DHA + EPA, with protective effects of DHA + EPA with lower intakes of soluble fiber and an attenuation at higher intakes, however this association was no longer significant after correction for multiple testing. These results suggest a modest protective effect of higher fiber intake on CRC risk, but not in combination with dietary fat subtypes. Given the robust results in preclinical models and mixed results in observational studies, controlled dietary interventions with standardized intakes are needed to better understand the interaction of specific fat and fiber subtypes on colon biology and ultimately CRC susceptibility in humans.

Keywords: butyrate; colorectal cancer; DHA; EPA; fat; fiber; omega-3; pectin

---

1. Introduction

Colorectal cancer (CRC) is the third most common type of cancer in the U.S., accounting for roughly 8% of new cancer cases and 8% of all cancer deaths in 2015 [1]. Lifestyle factors such as diet, physical activity, and body weight contribute substantially to CRC, and it is generally held that risk could be greatly reduced through dietary modification [2]. Dietary fiber and fat are two of the most well-studied dietary components in this regard [3]. Although many case-control studies have found inverse associations between fiber and fat intakes and CRC [4], data from epidemiologic studies are mixed [4–25], possibly due to differences in intake assessment, the type of fiber or fat analyzed, and residual confounding by other lifestyle and dietary factors. More recent studies have attempted to control for dietary confounders such as folate, alcohol, and red meat consumption, yet the contradictions in outcomes persist [7,15,26,27]. Finally, within the Women's Health Initiative (WHI) Dietary Modification Trial, a low fat dietary pattern intervention which included a focus on increasing servings of whole grains, vegetables, and fruits, was found to have no significant benefit on CRC incidence over an average of 8.1 years [28].

There is a growing recognition that dietary exposures are complex with synergistic and antagonistic effects between different dietary components contributing to chronic disease risk. Interactions between dietary constituents and microbial metabolites may also partially explain differences in population-level study outcomes [29,30]. In contrast to the equivocal data from observational studies in humans—in which each dietary component is evaluated separately—strong evidence for a combined effect of the subtypes of fat and fiber in relation to reduced colon tumorigenesis has been demonstrated in preclinical animal models [31–35]. Gut bacteria ferment dietary fiber (e.g., pectins, a type of fermentable soluble fiber) to butyrate [36–49], a potent histone deacetylase (HDAC) inhibitor [29,30] associated with reduced CRC risk [50–52]. Omega 6 (n-6) polyunsaturated fatty acids (PUFA), commonly found in refined vegetables oils, processed and fast foods, and red meat, typical in Western diets [53], and omega 3 (n-3) PUFA in fish oils [54] are structural precursors of eicosanoids; those derived from n-6 are mainly pro-inflammatory, whereas those produced from n-3 tend to have opposing effects [55,56]. Given the strong correlation between inflammation and CRC [56], higher intakes of long-chain n-3 PUFA provide biologic validity for a chemoprotective effect [57].

Preclinical research suggests that the combined effects of n-3 PUFA in fish oils (e.g., docosahexaenoic acid (DHA) and eicosapentaenoic acid (EPA)) and butyrate from fermentable fiber (e.g., pectin) may work in concert to enhance the chemopreventive potential of either dietary component alone, primarily by increasing apoptosis [31,33,34,58–62]. While other factors, such as low dietary intakes of fiber and certain fatty acid subtypes, may contribute to the mixed results in humans, the lack of evaluation of the interaction between subtypes of dietary fat and fiber, i.e., pectins in soluble fiber and marine-derived n-3 PUFA, may also explain why the chemoprotective effects of fiber and fat have not been consistently detected in prospective cohort studies. Therefore, our objectives for this study were to determine the associations between the individual and combinations of subtypes of fiber (soluble, and pectins specifically, which leads to the production of butyrate, vs. insoluble) and fat (n-3, and DHA + EPA, specifically, vs. n-6), and risk of CRC in the WHI.

2. Materials and Methods

2.1. Study Population

The WHI is a large prospective study focused on understanding preventive strategies for major chronic diseases in postmenopausal women [63]. WHI includes both a multi-component randomized Clinical Trial (CT) and an Observational Study (OS). The CT (n = 68,132) was actually three overlapping randomized controlled trials evaluating combined hormone therapy or estrogen alone versus placebo (HRT), a low-fat dietary pattern versus comparison (Dietary Modification), and calcium and vitamin D supplementation versus placebo (CaD), on the risk of breast and colorectal cancers, coronary heart disease, and osteoporotic fractures. The OS (n = 93,676) examines a broader range of lifestyle, health, and risk factors and risk of common chronic diseases in postmenopausal women initially interested in but ineligible for one or more of the clinical trials. Postmenopausal women aged 50–79 years were recruited from the general population at 40 different Clinical Centers between

1993 and 1998, with trial follow-up information and outcome data available through 2005, and post-trial follow-up information and outcome data for these analyses available through September, 2010, the end of the first WHI Extension Study. All participants in the CT and OS were included in the present analysis except women who were randomized to the intervention arm of the Dietary Modification trial (n = 19,541). Further details on recruitment, study design, and baseline measures have been published elsewhere [63–66]. Institutional review board approval was obtained from all clinical sites, and women provided written informed consent prior to participation and for follow-up in the Extension period. The WHI ClinicalTrials.gov identifier is NCT00000611.

2.2. Data Collection and Dietary Assessment

Detailed information on demographic characteristics, medical, reproductive and familial CRC history, and lifestyle factors were collected at baseline. Weight and height were assessed with a standardized protocol using a calibrated balance beam scale and stadiometer, respectively, and body mass index (BMI) was computed as weight in kg/height in m^2. Physical activity was assessed by computing average weekly metabolic equivalents of moderate and vigorous leisure-time physical activity.

Dietary intake over the past three months was measured from the WHI food frequency questionnaire (FFQ) [67] using a standardized protocol at baseline for all women, and at year one for Dietary Modification CT participants. Follow-up FFQs were completed in years two through nine for a rotating proportion (33%) of Dietary Modification CT participants. The baseline FFQ data were used for the current study. The FFQs contained 122 food and food group items, and 19 adjustment questions, the majority of which ask about food practices pertaining to types and amounts of added fats (e.g., fat added at the table and in cooking), and three summary questions on food purchasing and preparation methods [67]. The WHI nutrient database was derived from Nutrition Data Systems for Research (NDS-R, version 2005, Nutrition Coordinating Center, University of Minnesota, Minneapolis, MN, USA). The database has over 140 nutrient values including total fat, total PUFA, n-6 and n-3 PUFA, total DHA and EPA from food sources; and total, insoluble and soluble fiber, and pectins.

2.3. Colorectal Cancer Case Ascertainment

Clinical outcomes, including cancer diagnoses, were updated annually in the OS and semi-annually in the CT until 2005 when the outcomes were thereafter reported annually using mail or telephone questionnaires. Self-reports of CRC were verified by trained physician adjudicators at the Clinical Centers who reviewed medical records and pathology reports [68]. All CRC diagnoses were then confirmed by blinded review at the WHI Clinical Coordinating Center at the Fred Hutchinson Cancer Research Center.

2.4. Statistical Analysis

Exclusions were made for women who reported history of colon or rectal cancers prior to baseline enrollment or who were missing these data (n = 946). Further exclusions were made for women with FFQs containing incomplete information, or data that suggested biologically implausible daily energy intakes of <2512 or >20,930 kJ (n = 4649), or extreme BMIs (<15 or >50 kg/m^2; n = 2069). Finally, women who were missing data for smoking, physical activity, and education variables combined (n = 9), or were lost to follow up (n = 577), were excluded, leaving a sample of 134,017 for analysis.

Cox proportional hazards models were used to estimate hazard ratios (HR) and 95% confidence intervals (95% CI) for the association of fiber (total, insoluble, soluble, and pectins) and fat (total, n-6, n-3, and DHA + EPA) intakes and CRC risk. Dietary variables were evaluated as separate main effects, as quintiles of intake, using the lowest quintile as the reference group. Quintile assignments of dietary variables from the baseline FFQ were calculated based on the distribution in non-cases. Tests for trend were performed in a separate Cox model treating quintiles 1–5 as linear. Fat variables were analyzed both as g intake/day with energy adjusted in the models, and as % energy. As the results for both were similar (data not shown) we present only fat as g intake/day. Interactions (a total of seven determined a priori: total fat × total fiber; insoluble fiber × n-6 PUFA; soluble fiber × n-3 PUFA; insoluble fiber × n-3 PUFA; soluble fiber × DHA + EPA; pectins × n-3 PUFA; pectins × DHA + EPA) were assessed by adding the multiplicative interaction term between linear quintiles of dietary fat and fiber variables to the final multivariate model. For the significant interaction of soluble fiber and DHA + EPA, post-hoc HRs and 95% CIs were computed for each quintile comparison for each of the 25 fat × fiber groups.

All models were adjusted for established or suggestive risk factors for CRC: (age (years, continuous); family history of CRC (yes/no); red and processed meat consumption (g/day, continuous); BMI (kg/m^2, continuous); leisure physical activity (total metabolic equivalent-h/week, continuous); smoking (current or past/never); alcohol use (g/day, continuous); current use of non-steroidal anti-inflammatory drugs (NSAIDs; yes/no); folate (food plus supplements; µg dietary folate equivalents/day, continuous); calcium (food plus supplements; mg/day; continuous)) [69,70], and confounders that altered point estimates for dietary outcome measures by more than 10%: total energy intake (kcal/day, continuous); history of screening colonoscopy (yes/no); education level (high school; technical school or some college; college grad or post); ever use of menopausal hormones (yes/no); and study component (OS, CT) and CT randomization assignment (HRT, Dietary Modification or CaD). We created a "missing" category for covariates with data missing for <0.5% of the participant population (NSAIDs, $n = 91$, smoking, $n = 1737$, education level, $n = 1005$, and colonoscopy screening, $n = 4736$), and imputed the median values for physical activity ($n = 5230$) to reduce the number of participants who would be dropped from the analysis. All tests for individual dietary factors were two sided and statistical significance was set at $p < 0.05$. Tests for interaction were adjusted for multiple testing using Bonferroni correction (0.05/7 tests conducted = $p < 0.007$). All analyses were conducted using Stata (v14.1; StataCorp, College Station, TX, USA).

3. Results

The distribution of baseline participant characteristics and dietary intake for CRC cases and non-cases are given in Table 1. During a mean follow up of 11.7 years (±3.5; range: 0.02–17.5 years), a total of 1952 CRC cases were reported. Women with CRC appeared less likely to have ever used hormone therapy and consumed less calcium. Intakes of all other dietary variables were very similar in cases and non-cases.

Table 1. Baseline characteristics, colorectal cancer risk factors, and dietary constituents for participants in the Women's Health Initiative 1993–2010 [1].

Characteristic	Cases (n = 1952)	Non-Cases (n = 132,065)
Age, (years)	66 (6.9)	63 (7.3)
Height (cm)	162 (6.3)	162 (6.4)
Body mass index (kg/m^2)	28 (5.7)	28 (5.5)
Race (%)		
White	85	84
Black	9	8
Other/Unknown [2]	6	8
Education (% college graduate)	38	40
Screening colonoscopy (%)	49	51
Family history of CRC (%)	19	15
NSAID (% current use)	17	19
Alcohol use at baseline (g/day)	5 (11.3)	5 (10.8)
Never smokers (%)	49	50
Physical activity (MET-h/week) [3]	12 (12.6)	13 (13.7)
Ever used post-menopausal Hormone therapy (%)	48	56
Dietary intake		
Total energy (kJ/day)	6766 (2671)	6787 (2642)
Total fiber (g/day)	16 (6.9)	16 (6.9)
Soluble fiber (g/day)	4.3 (1.8)	4.3 (1.8)
Pectins (g/day)	2.5 (1.2)	2.5 (1.2)
Insoluble fiber (g/day)	11.5 (5.1)	11.8 (5.1)

Table 1. *Cont.*

Characteristic	Cases (n = 1952)	Non-Cases (n = 132,065)
Total fat (g/day)	60 (32.7)	59 (32.0)
n-3 (g/day)	1.41 (0.8)	1.41 (0.8)
DHA + EPA (g/day)	0.12 (0.12)	0.13 (0.12)
n-6 (g/day)	10.8 (6.2)	10.7 (6.2)
Linoleic acid (g/day)	10.8 (6.2)	10.7 (6.1)
Linolenic acid (g/day)	1.3 (0.7)	1.3 (0.7)
Calcium (mg/day)	803 (439)	827 (453)
Folate (DFE, µg/day)	478 (206)	488 (207)
Red meat (g/day)	0.69 (0.57)	0.67 (0.55)

[1] Means (Standard Deviation) unless otherwise specified; [2] Includes Hispanic, American Indian, Asian/Pacific Islander, Mixed races, and Refused; [3] Total metabolic equivalent-hours/week. CRC, colorectal cancer; DFE, dietary folate equivalents; DHA, docosahexaenoic acid; EPA, eicosapentaenoic acid; NSAIDs, non-steroidal anti-inflammatory drugs.

Table 2 provides data on associations of total, insoluble, and soluble fiber, and pectins, with CRC risk. When assessing fiber as a main effect, higher versus lower total soluble and insoluble fibers were associated with modest, but non-significant lower risk of CRC. There was a suggestion of inverse linear trends for total and insoluble fiber, (*p-trend* = 0.09 for total fiber; *p-trend* = 0.08 for insoluble fiber).

Table 2. Multivariate-adjusted hazard ratios and 95% CIs for the association of fiber with colorectal cancer in the Women's Health Initiative (n = 134,017) 1993–2010.

Quintiles of Dietary Intake	No. Cases	Person-Years	Multivariate Adjusted HR (95% CI) [1]
	Total fiber (g/day)		
<10.3	420	302,828	1.00 (Reference)
10.3–13.6	426	312,546	1.00 (0.87, 1.15)
13.6–17.0	354	316,244	0.83 (0.71, 0.97)
17.0–21.5	372	318,893	0.87 (0.74, 1.03)
>21.5	380	318,844	0.90 (0.73, 1.10)
p-trend			0.09
	Soluble fiber (g/day)		
<2.8	408	304,051	1.00 (Reference)
2.8–3.7	409	312,599	0.97 (0.84, 1.12)
3.7–4.6	361	316,928	0.85 (0.73, 1.00)
4.6–5.8	410	318,628	0.96 (0.81, 1.13)
>5.8	364	317,148	0.84 (0.69, 1.03)
p-trend			0.14
	Insoluble fiber (g/day)		
<7.4	433	302,242	1.00 (Reference)
7.4–9.8	413	312,804	0.93 (0.81, 1.07)
9.8–12.3	357	316,721	0.81 (0.69, 0.94)
12.3–15.7	370	318,704	0.84 (0.72, 1.00)
>15.7	379	318,884	0.87 (0.72, 1.06)
p-trend			0.08
	Pectin (g/day)		
<1.4	399	303,832	1.00 (Reference)
1.4–2.0	397	313,746	0.97 (0.84, 1.12)
2.0–2.6	379	316,302	0.92 (0.79, 1.06)
2.6–3.5	396	318,847	0.97 (0.83, 1.13)
>3.5	381	316,626	0.94 (0.80, 1.11)
p-trend			0.56

[1] The following variables were included in both the multivariate and continuous models: total energy intake (continuous), age (continuous), body mass index (continuous), education (high school, technical school or some college, college graduate or post-graduate), family history of colorectal cancer (yes/no), history of colonoscopy (yes/no), current NSAID use (yes/no), alcohol intake (continuous), smoking history (never, former, current), physical activity (total metabolic equivalent-hours, continuous), ever use of hormone therapy (never, current/former), folate (DFE; µg/day, continuous), calcium (mg/day, continuous), and red meat intake (g/day, continuous), and study component (OS, CT) and CT randomization assignment and treatment arm. OS, observational study; CT, clinical trial; DFE, dietary folate equivalents; NSAIDs, non-steroidal anti-inflammatory drugs.

The associations of total fat, *n*-6 PUFA, *n*-3 PUFA, and EPA + DHA with CRC risk were null with most HRs near the null value of 1.0 (Table 3).

Table 3. Multivariate-adjusted hazard ratios and 95% CIs for the association of fat with colorectal cancer in the Women's Health Initiative (n = 134,017) 1993–2010.

Quintiles of Dietary Intake	No. Cases	Person-Years	Multivariate Adjusted HR (95% CI) [1]
		Total fat (g/day)	
<33.1	345	309,005	1.00 (Reference)
33.1–45.6	432	318,884	1.20 (1.04, 1.39)
45.6–59.7	394	316,808	1.05 (0.90, 1.24)
59.7–80.6	381	316,629	0.98 (0.82, 1.18)
>80.6	400	313,067	0.98 (0.76, 1.27)
p-trend			0.44
		n-6 PUFA (g/day)	
<5.9	375	309,046	1.00 (Reference)
5.9–8.1	405	314,292	1.02 (0.88, 1.18)
8.1–10.7	390	316,554	0.95 (0.81, 1.11)
10.7–14.6	394	317,021	0.92 (0.78, 1.09)
>14.6	388	312,441	0.84 (0.68, 1.05)
p-trend			0.10
		n-3 PUFA (g/day)	
<0.80	401	308,532	1.00 (Reference)
0.80–1.09	389	314,521	0.94 (0.82, 1.08)
1.09–1.41	383	316,931	0.90 (0.78, 1.05)
1.41–1.90	377	316,759	0.87 (0.75, 1.03)
>1.90	402	312,611	0.90 (0.74, 1.09)
p-trend			0.16
		DHA + EPA (g/day)	
<0.04	402	307,408	1.00 (Reference)
0.04–0.07	389	312,402	0.97 (0.84, 1.12)
0.07–0.11	393	315,998	0.98 (0.85, 1.13)
0.11–0.18	389	318,148	0.99 (0.85, 1.14)
>0.18	379	315,397	0.98 (0.84, 1.13)
p-trend			0.87

[1] The following variables were included in both the multivariate and continuous models: total energy intake (continuous), age (continuous), body mass index (continuous), education (high school, technical school or some college, college graduate or post-graduate), family history of colorectal cancer (yes/no), history of colonoscopy (yes/no), current NSAID use (yes/no), alcohol intake (continuous), smoking history (never, former, current), physical activity (total metabolic equivalent-hours, continuous), ever use of hormone therapy (never, current/former), folate (DFE μg/day, continuous), calcium (mg/day, continuous), and red meat intake (g/day, continuous), and study component (OS, CT) and CT randomization assignment and treatment arm. OS, observational study; CT, clinical trial; DFE, dietary folate equivalents; DHA, docosahexaenoic acid; EPA, eicosapentaenoic acid; NSAIDs, non-steroidal anti-inflammatory drugs. PUFA, polyunsaturated fatty acids.

We next examined the interaction of fat and fiber subtypes in relation to CRC risk. The interaction between DHA + EPA and soluble fiber was statistically significant (*p-interaction* = 0.01), with a significant decreased risk of CRC with increasing DHA + EPA intake among those in the lowest quintile of soluble fiber intake (*p-trend* = 0.02; Table 4) and a borderline increased risk of CRC with increasing DHA + EPA among those in the highest quintile of soluble fiber (*p-trend* = 0.07; Table 4). There was a marginal statistically significant association between pectins and DHA + EPA (p = 0.05), with a similar pattern of attenuation, whereby the protective effects of higher intakes of pectins were no longer apparent with higher intakes of DHA + EPA (data not shown). However, these interactions were no longer significant when adjusted for multiple comparisons. There were no other significant interactions between the various dietary fiber and fat combinations.

Table 4. Soluble fiber and DHA + EPA stratified by quintile of intake, and association with colorectal cancer in the Women's Health Initiative (n = 134,017) 1993–2010.

		DHA + EPA (g/Day)					HR (95% CI) [1]	*p*-Trend [2]
		Q1	Q2	Q3	Q4	Q5		
Soluble fiber (g/day)	Q1	1.00 (Ref) [3]	0.88 (0.68, 1.13)	0.78 (0.59, 1.04)	0.88 (0.65, 1.20)	0.59 (0.40, 0.88)	0.91 (0.84, 0.98)	0.02
	Q2	0.81 (0.62, 1.06)	0.82 (0.63, 1.07)	0.91 (0.70, 1.18)	0.80 (0.60, 1.06)	0.91 (0.69, 1.23)	1.03 (0.96, 1.11)	0.44
	Q3	0.71 (0.53, 0.96)	0.84 (0.63, 1.11)	0.73 (0.55, 0.97)	0.65 (0.48, 0.87)	0.79 (0.59, 1.06)	0.99 (0.91, 1.06)	0.70
	Q4	0.76 (0.56, 1.05)	0.86 (0.65, 1.15)	0.87 (0.66, 1.15)	0.90 (0.68, 1.18)	0.77 (0.57, 1.02)	1.00 (0.93, 1.07)	0.96
	Q5	0.70 (0.49, 1.01)	0.53 (0.37, 0.78)	0.73 (0.53, 1.00)	0.81 (0.60, 1.08)	0.80 (0.60, 1.08)	1.08 (1.00, 1.17)	0.07
HR (95% CI) [1]		0.97 (0.89, 1.08)	0.90 (0.81, 1.00)	1.02 (0.92, 1.13)	0.99 (0.89, 1.09)	1.00 (0.89, 1.11)		
p-trend [2]		0.62	0.05	0.72	0.80	0.95		

[1] HR and 95% CI across quintiles of soluble fiber and DHA + EPA; [2] *p*-trend values from linear interactions across each row and column. The following variables were included in the model: total energy intake (continuous), age (continuous), body mass index (continuous), education (high school, technical school or some college, college graduate or post-graduate), family history of colorectal cancer (yes/no), history of colonoscopy (yes/no), current NSAID use (yes/no), alcohol intake (continuous), smoking history (never, former, current), physical activity (total metabolic equivalent-hours, continuous), ever use of hormone therapy (never, current/former), folate (μg/day, continuous), calcium (mg/day, continuous), and red meat intake (g/day, continuous), and study component (OS, CT) and CT randomization assignment and treatment arm; [3] the combination of the first quintiles for soluble fiber and DHA + EPA is the reference group for all comparisons within quintiles. OS, observational study; CT, clinical trial; DFE, dietary folate equivalents; DHA, docosahexaenoic acid; EPA, eicosapentaenoic acid; NSAIDs, non-steroidal anti-inflammatory drugs. PUFA, polyunsaturated fatty acids.

4. Discussion

The results of the present analysis in a large, prospective cohort of postmenopausal women do not support the results obtained in preclinical studies demonstrating that combinations of higher fiber and fat subtypes are associated with reduced risk of CRC. While there was a modest additional protective effect of either dietary component when intake of the other was low, this protective effect was attenuated with greater consumption in our study population. Intakes and ranges were very low such that only women in the highest quintile of fiber were consuming adequate intakes for this age group (21 g/day for women ages 51–70 years), with a very small percentage consuming high intakes [71]. Further, intakes of n-3 PUFA, and DHA and EPA, specifically, were substantially lower than the levels used in experimental diets. These factors may have prevented detection of an association.

It is generally thought that CRC risk could be reduced through dietary modification, including increased dietary fiber intake and reduced fat intake [3]. Dietary fiber mainly includes remnants of plant foods resistant to digestion by human enzymes and therefore arrives in the colon relatively intact, where it undergoes metabolism by gut microbiota. In the 2011 Colorectal Cancer Report, part of the Continuous Update Project, the World Cancer Research Fund/American Institute for Cancer Research Expert Panel classified evidence supporting consumption of fiber-containing foods and CRC protection as 'convincing' [72], noting that for every 10 g/day increase in fiber, there was a 10% decrease in CRC risk. Mechanisms hypothesized to explain how dietary fiber may reduce CRC include increased stool bulk and reduced intestinal transit time, resulting in reduced exposure to potential carcinogens; decreased secondary bile acids and subsequent generation of reactive oxygen species; and fiber fermentation by gut microbiota to short-chain fatty acids, particularly butyrate [73–75]. It is now well-documented that butyrate induces apoptosis in tumor cells through inhibition of HDAC and subsequent activation of the Fas receptor-mediated extrinsic death pathway [31,76–79]. Given the potential importance of fiber fermentation on CRC risk, consideration of fiber subtypes may be important; however, few studies have examined fiber subtype (i.e., soluble and insoluble, or more and less fermentable), and associations are similar, with both null [9,10] and inverse associations [80–83] reported.

When evaluating total fiber and subtypes in the present study, CRC risk was reduced for all quintiles of increased consumption and a marginal linear trend was observed; however, most quintiles did not reach statistical significance. Inconsistencies across epidemiologic studies may be attributed in part to lower overall fiber intakes and narrow ranges of fiber intakes in Western populations which reduce statistical power [13]. Mean fiber intake in the U.S. is ~15 g/day [4]. Intakes at or above current recommended intakes (25 g/day for women and 38 g/day for men) [71] show robust protection against CRC with relative risks ranging from 0.72 to 0.90 [4,6,26]. Only 10% of our study population reported intakes of dietary fiber >25 g/day, thus our ability to detect a protective effect was compromised.

Overlaying the conflicting data observed with dietary fiber and CRC is a similar body of inconsistent literature on the association between subtypes of fat, particularly *n*-3 PUFA, and CRC risk. In addition to the anti-inflammatory effects promulgated by changes in the eicosanoid milieu, other putative actions of *n*-3 PUFA have been proposed. These include alterations in membrane fluidity and lipid raft composition, which may affect receptor signaling involved in proliferation and apoptosis [84], and modulation of oxidative stress [57,85]. As with dietary fiber, laboratory data consistently show reduced CRC risk with marine *n*-3 PUFA [58], while epidemiologic data are less convincing. Whereas two meta-analyses reported reduced CRC risk with *n*-3 PUFA from fish intake [86,87], two systematic reviews concluded that there is insufficient [15] or limited [7] evidence to suggest an association between long-chain *n*-3 PUFA intake and CRC risk. A more recent publication reported no overall association between *n*-3 PUFA and CRC risk among 123,529 individuals; however, among women in the same cohort, *n*-3 PUFA intake after CRC diagnosis had a protective effect on survival [88].

In the WHI population, we did not observe an association between any dietary fat subtypes and CRC risk. As with fiber, intakes of *n*-3 PUFA were very low; mean intakes were 1.4 g/day (range 0.1–10.4) for *n*-3, and 0.04 and 0.08 g/day (range 0–1.4 and 0–3.1, respectively) for EPA and DHA. While specific recommendations for *n*-3 PUFA intake have not been determined, the Food and Nutrition Board of the Institute of Medicine established adequate intake levels for alpha-linolenic acid (ALA), the precursor of long-chain *n*-3 PUFA, of 1.1 g/day for women over the age of 19 [71]. Only about half of our study population had intakes at that level. Furthermore, the Academy of Nutrition and Dietetics recommends a minimum intake of 0.5 g/day of combined EPA and DHA [89]. Less than 2% of the women in our study cohort reached an intake level above 0.5 g/day.

Despite the inconsistent epidemiologic data for dietary fiber and fat, studies in preclinical animal models have shown that combinations of fiber and fat work synergistically to protect against colon cancer [58–62]. In a series of experiments, the effects of different types of fat (fish oil or corn oil; 15 g/100 g) and fiber (pectin or cellulose; 6 g/100 g) diets were tested on tumorigenesis and various other aspects of colonocyte physiology [58,90]. Both fish oil and pectin alone, relative to corn oil and cellulose feeding, resulted in a significantly lower proportion of animals with adenocarcinomas; however, the combination of fish oil and pectin led to an even greater reduction [58]. Additional work showed changes to the re-dox environment within rat colonocytes with a concomitant reduction in DNA damage [35,59,91]. Serving as the primary energy source for colonic epithelial cells, butyrate induces cellular reactive oxygen species (ROS) generation, creating a pro-oxidant environment [31]. At the same time, long chain *n*-3 PUFA from fish oil (e.g., DHA) incorporated into cell membranes, are susceptible to oxidation due to their high degree of unsaturation [33]. These physiological attributes of butyrate and DHA are relevant as lipid peroxidation can directly trigger the release of pro-apoptotic factors from mitochondria into the cytosol, through a p53-independent, calcium-mediated cell death pathway [33]. Given that butyrate independently induces apoptosis through an extrinsic, HDAC inhibition-mediated pathway, the combination of dietary constituents, and subsequent effects on intrinsic apoptotic pathways, would be expected to exponentially increase apoptosis.

Dietary fiber and fatty acids, in combination, and risk of CRC in humans has only recently begun to be evaluated. In a large cohort study (n = 96,354) of Seventh Day Adventists, risk of CRC was reduced by 22% among all vegetarians combined compared to non-vegetarians, but protection was greatest among pescovegetarians who consume high amounts of both fiber and n-3 PUFA-containing fish (HR: 0.57; 95% CI: 0.40, 0.82) [92]. Furthermore, striking reciprocal changes in gut mucosal cancer risk biomarkers, the microbiome, and the metabolome were reported after African Americans were given a high-fiber (primarily in the form of resistant starch, including pectin), low-fat diet and rural Africans were given a high-fat, low-fiber Western-style diet [93]. Significantly increased butyrate production and suppressed secondary bile acid synthesis were also noted after the diet exchange to high-fiber, low-fat intake in African Americans [93].

An analysis in the Rotterdam prospective cohort (n = 4967) lends support to the hypothesis that higher intakes of fat and fiber are an important factor mediating the relationship between these dietary variables. An increased risk of CRC was observed with n-3 PUFA intake and dietary fiber intakes below the median, but not when fiber intakes were above [22]. It is noteworthy that the levels of fiber intakes were markedly lower (mean 26 g/day) relative to the intakes among pescovegetarians in the Seventh Day Adventist population (mean 40 g/day) and the African American intervention participants (mean 55 g/day), but higher than the intakes in our population (mean 16 g/day). Adding to the complexity of the relationship, when evaluated by food sources of n-3 PUFA in the Rotterdam study, increased CRC risk was restricted to intake from non-marine sources which contain ALA; there was no association when n-3 PUFA from marine-derived (e.g., EPA and DHA) sources were evaluated [22]. Contrary to these results, evaluation by n-3 PUFA source in a case-control study did not show any difference between non-marine and marine sources and interaction with dietary fiber. In this instance, greater protection of n-3 PUFA was found among individuals with lower dietary fiber intakes although overall intake was low (median 18.6 g/day) [94], consistent with our observation of the significant reduced risk of CRC among women with the lowest soluble fiber and highest DHA + EPA intakes. The authors speculated that high fiber intake may interfere with lipid absorption, offsetting potential beneficial effects of certain fatty acids [94].

While intakes in animal models do not directly translate to human intakes, the amount of fiber and fat used in preclinical experiments is comparable, as a proportion of intake, to what is currently recommended for humans. For example, the amount of fiber in the rat diets was 6% by weight, which is approximately equivalent to 30 g/day for humans [58]. This level of intake was only approached in the highest quintile of total fiber intake (>21.5 g/day). Similarly, all rat diets contained fat at 15% by weight and 30% of energy, with fish oil comprising approximately 1%–5% [58]. Women in WHI consumed 33% of their calories from fat on average, but less than 1% from n-3 PUFA and even less from combined DHA and EPA from fish oil (highest quintile >0.18 g/day). In the VITamins And Lifestyle (VITAL) cohort (n = 68,109), individuals using fish oil supplements on 4+ days/week for 3+ years experienced 49% lower CRC risk than non-users (HR = 0.51, 95% CI = 0.26–1.00; *p-trend* = 0.06) [17]. An average serving of oily fish (e.g., salmon or mackerel) provides 1.5–3 g of marine fish oil [95]. Thus, it may be difficult to achieve the levels of n-3 PUFA needed for a chemoprotective effect through diet alone.

Strengths of this study include the large, well-characterized prospective cohort. As CRC was one of the primary outcomes of WHI, incident cases were expertly adjudicated and confirmed. Additionally, detailed information was collected on a wide range of exposures, including diet, with reliability subsequently assessed [65]. Finally, this is the largest prospective cohort to evaluate the interactions of subtypes of fiber and fat on CRC to date.

As with all observational studies, there are limitations. First, we relied on self-report via FFQ to capture usual dietary intake, therefore we cannot rule out measurement error. FFQs are subject to lack of precision and inaccurate recall of dietary intake [96]. As dietary intakes were only assessed at baseline, it is possible that diets changed over time. However, we performed a sensitivity analysis using FFQ from women in the Dietary Modification comparison arm (the only group for which FFQ data from multiple time-points were collected) between years 0, 1, 3, 6, and 9, and found that correlations were 0.62 for fiber intake and 0.44 for total fat intake, suggesting that intake remained relatively stable during the follow-up. The WHI FFQ has been shown to yield nutrient estimates that are similar to those obtained from short-term dietary recall and recording methods, and test-retest reliability for most nutrients was high (e.g., FFQ estimates for total, saturated, and polyunsaturated fat variables were all within 10% of those from food records and 24-h recalls, although dietary fiber was slightly higher ~17%, and information on fat and fiber subtypes was not evaluated) [67]. Our fiber exposure also did not include the integration of dietary fiber supplement use, which is known to be higher with age and among women [97]. Lastly, measurement of the level of EPA/DHA incorporation in plasma or the tissue level was not conducted. It is widely known that the biological activities of these compounds depend on their bioavailability [98] and FFQ estimates only provide a surrogate for exposure.

Finally, while we adjusted for several potential confounders, we did not directly evaluate antioxidant content of the diet. Because the combination of butyrate and n-3 PUFA drive apoptosis via an oxidative-dependent mechanism, higher antioxidant intakes might antagonize this protective effect. In addition, there is some evidence that high antioxidants promote CRC in both preclinical [59,91] and epidemiologic [99–101] studies. Although mean intakes for several individual nutrients with antioxidant capacity (e.g., vitamins C, E, and beta-carotene) were very similar between cases and controls at baseline (<1% difference), total antioxidant capacity of dietary intakes was not considered.

5. Conclusions

In summary, at the levels of dietary intake consumed by women in WHI, we did not find evidence of a protective association between increased subtypes of fiber and fat intakes in combination, and reduced risk of CRC. Our results for fat and fiber separately are in agreement with what has been reported previously, namely modest inverse associations with fiber, but no consistent trends across intakes. Given the biologic plausibility of a protective effect for fiber and n-3 PUFA, the robust results from preclinical models, and the mixed results in observational studies, controlled feeding trials with standardized intakes and consideration of the potential impact of the gut microbiome are urgently needed.

Acknowledgments: We acknowledge the WHI Investigator Group, short list: Program Office: (National Heart, Lung, and Blood Institute, Bethesda, Maryland); Jacques Rossouw, Shari Ludlam, Dale Burwen, Joan McGowan, Leslie Ford, and Nancy Geller; Clinical Coordinating Center: (Fred Hutchinson Cancer Research Center, Seattle, WA, USA) Garnet Anderson, Ross Prentice, Andrea LaCroix, and Charles Kooperberg; Investigators and Academic Centers: (Brigham and Women's Hospital, Harvard Medical School, Boston, MA, USA) JoAnn E. Manson; (MedStar Health Research Institute/Howard University, Washington, DC, USA) Barbara V. Howard; (Stanford Prevention Research Center, Stanford, CA, USA) Marcia L. Stefanick; (The Ohio State University, Columbus, OH, USA) Rebecca Jackson; (University of Arizona, Tucson/Phoenix, AZ, USA) Cynthia A. Thomson; (University at Buffalo, Buffalo, NY, USA) Jean Wactawski-Wende; (University of Florida, Gainesville/Jacksonville, FL, USA) Marian Limacher; (University of Iowa, Iowa City/Davenport, IA, USA) Robert Wallace; (University of Pittsburgh, Pittsburgh, PA, USA) Lewis Kuller; (Wake Forest University School of Medicine, Winston-Salem, NC, USA) Sally Shumaker. Women's Health Initiative Memory Study: (Wake Forest University School of Medicine, Winston-Salem, NC, USA) Sally Shumaker; WHI is supported by National Heart, Lung, and Blood Institute, National Institutes of Health, U.S. Department of Health and Human Services through contracts, HHSN268201100046C (Fred Hutch), HHSN268201100001C (SUNY Buffalo), HHSN268201100002C (The Ohio State University), HHSN268201100003C (Stanford), HHSN268201100004C (Wake Forest), and HHSN271201100004C (WHI Memory Study), and grants P30 CA015704, R35 CA197707, and T32 CA09168.

Author Contributions: Author contributions: S.L.N., J.W.L., M.L.N., S.A.A.B., T.-Y.D.C., L.F.T. and R.S.C. conceived the study; S.L.N., T.-Y.D.C. and M.L.N. conducted the data analysis; S.L.N., M.L.N., T.-Y.D.C., R.S.C. and J.W.L. interpreted the results; S.L.N. wrote the manuscript; M.L.N., J.W.L., R.S.C., T.-Y.D.C., L.F.T., J.M.S., L.S., J.A.M., I.K. and S.A.A.B. critically revised the manuscript.

References

1. American Cancer Society. *Cancer Facts & Figures 2016*; American Cancer Society: Atlanta, GA, USA, 2016.
2. World Cancer Research Fund. *Food, Nutrition, Physical Activity, and the Prevention of Cancer: A Global Perspective*; American Institute for Cancer Research: Washington, DC, USA, 2007.

3. Perez-Cueto, F.J.; Verbeke, W. Consumer implications of the WCRF's permanent update on colorectal cancer. *Meat. Sci.* **2012**, *90*, 977–978. [CrossRef] [PubMed]
4. Ben, Q.; Sun, Y.; Chai, R.; Qian, A.; Xu, B.; Yuan, Y. Dietary fiber intake reduces risk for colorectal adenoma: A meta-analysis. *Gastroenterology* **2014**, *146*, 689–699. [CrossRef] [PubMed]
5. Michels, K.B.; Fuchs, C.S.; Giovannucci, E.; Colditz, G.A.; Hunter, D.J.; Stampfer, M.J.; Willett, W.C. Fiber intake and incidence of colorectal cancer among 76,947 women and 47,279 men. *Cancer Epidemiol. Biomark. Prev.* **2005**, *14*, 842–849. [CrossRef] [PubMed]
6. Murphy, N.; Norat, T.; Ferrari, P.; Jenab, M.; Bueno-de-Mesquita, B.; Skeie, G.; Dahm, C.C.; Overvad, K.; Olsen, A.; Tjonneland, A.; et al. Dietary fibre intake and risks of cancers of the colon and rectum in the european prospective investigation into cancer and nutrition (epic). *PLoS ONE* **2012**, *7*, e39361. [CrossRef] [PubMed]
7. Gerber, M. Omega-3 fatty acids and cancers: A systematic update review of epidemiological studies. *Br. J. Nutr.* **2012**, *107*, S228–S239. [CrossRef] [PubMed]
8. Kunzmann, A.T.; Coleman, H.G.; Huang, W.Y.; Kitahara, C.M.; Cantwell, M.M.; Berndt, S.I. Dietary fiber intake and risk of colorectal cancer and incident and recurrent adenoma in the prostate, lung, colorectal, and ovarian cancer screening trial. *Am. J. Clin. Nutr.* **2015**, *102*, 881–890. [CrossRef] [PubMed]
9. Wakai, K.; Date, C.; Fukui, M.; Tamakoshi, K.; Watanabe, Y.; Hayakawa, N.; Kojima, M.; Kawado, M.; Suzuki, K.; Hashimoto, S.; et al. Dietary fiber and risk of colorectal cancer in the japan collaborative cohort study. *Cancer Epidemiol. Biomark. Prev.* **2007**, *16*, 668–675. [CrossRef] [PubMed]
10. Uchida, K.; Kono, S.; Yin, G.; Toyomura, K.; Nagano, J.; Mizoue, T.; Mibu, R.; Tanaka, M.; Kakeji, Y.; Maehara, Y.; et al. Dietary fiber, source foods and colorectal cancer risk: The fukuoka colorectal cancer study. *Scand. J. Gastroenterol.* **2010**, *45*, 1223–1231. [CrossRef] [PubMed]
11. Park, Y.; Hunter, D.J.; Spiegelman, D.; Bergkvist, L.; Berrino, F.; van den Brandt, P.A.; Buring, J.E.; Colditz, G.A.; Freudenheim, J.L.; Fuchs, C.S.; et al. Dietary fiber intake and risk of colorectal cancer: A pooled analysis of prospective cohort studies. *JAMA* **2005**, *294*, 2849–2857. [CrossRef] [PubMed]
12. Willett, W.C.; Stampfer, M.J.; Colditz, G.A.; Rosner, B.A.; Speizer, F.E. Relation of meat, fat, and fiber intake to the risk of colon cancer in a prospective-study among women. *N. Engl. J. Med.* **1990**, *323*, 1664–1672. [CrossRef] [PubMed]
13. Schatzkin, A.; Mouw, T.; Park, Y.; Subar, A.F.; Kipnis, V.; Hollenbeck, A.; Leitzmann, M.F.; Thompson, F.E. Dietary fiber and whole-grain consumption in relation to colorectal cancer in the nih-aarp diet and health study. *Am. J. Clin. Nutr.* **2007**, *85*, 1353–1360. [PubMed]
14. Fuchs, C.S.; Giovannucci, E.L.; Colditz, G.A.; Hunter, D.J.; Stampfer, M.J.; Rosner, B.; Speizer, F.E.; Willett, W.C. Dietary fiber and the risk of colorectal cancer and adenoma in women. *N. Engl. J. Med.* **1999**, *340*, 169–176. [CrossRef] [PubMed]
15. MacLean, C.H.; Newberry, S.J.; Mojica, W.A.; Khanna, P.; Issa, A.M.; Suttorp, M.J.; Lim, Y.W.; Traina, S.B.; Hilton, L.; Garland, R.; et al. Effects of omega-3 fatty acids on cancer risk: A systematic review. *JAMA* **2006**, *295*, 403–415. [CrossRef] [PubMed]
16. Daniel, C.R.; McCullough, M.L.; Patel, R.C.; Jacobs, E.J.; Flanders, W.D.; Thun, M.J.; Calle, E.E. Dietary intake of omega-6 and omega-3 fatty acids and risk of colorectal cancer in a prospective cohort of US men and women. *Cancer Epidemiol. Biomark. Prev.* **2009**, *18*, 516–525. [CrossRef] [PubMed]
17. Kantor, E.D.; Lampe, J.W.; Peters, U.; Vaughan, T.L.; White, E. Long-chain omega-3 polyunsaturated fatty acid intake and risk of colorectal cancer. *Nutr. Cancer* **2014**, *66*, 716–727. [CrossRef] [PubMed]
18. Ward, H.A.; Norat, T.; Overvad, K.; Dahm, C.C.; Bueno-de-Mesquita, H.B.; Jenab, M.; Fedirko, V.; van Duijnhoven, F.J.; Skeie, G.; Romaguera-Bosch, D.; et al. Pre-diagnostic meat and fibre intakes in relation to colorectal cancer survival in the european prospective investigation into cancer and nutrition. *Br. J. Nutr.* **2016**, *116*, 316–325. [CrossRef] [PubMed]
19. Liu, L.; Wang, S.; Liu, J. Fiber consumption and all-cause, cardiovascular, and cancer mortalities: A systematic review and meta-analysis of cohort studies. *Mol. Nutr. Food Res.* **2015**, *59*, 139–146. [CrossRef] [PubMed]
20. Hajishafiee, M.; Saneei, P.; Benisi-Kohansal, S.; Esmaillzadeh, A. Cereal fibre intake and risk of mortality from all causes, cvd, cancer and inflammatory diseases: A systematic review and meta-analysis of prospective cohort studies. *Br. J. Nutr.* **2016**, *116*, 343–352. [CrossRef] [PubMed]

21. Song, M.; Chan, A.T.; Fuchs, C.S.; Ogino, S.; Hu, F.B.; Mozaffarian, D.; Ma, J.; Willett, W.C.; Giovannucci, E.L.; Wu, K. Dietary intake of fish, omega-3 and omega-6 fatty acids and risk of colorectal cancer: A prospective study in U.S. Men and women. *Int. J. Cancer* **2014**, *135*, 2413–2423. [CrossRef] [PubMed]
22. Kraja, B.; Muka, T.; Ruiter, R.; de Keyser, C.E.; Hofman, A.; Franco, O.H.; Stricker, B.H.; Kiefte-de Jong, J.C. Dietary fiber intake modifies the positive association between *n*-3 pufa intake and colorectal cancer risk in a Caucasian population. *J. Nutr.* **2015**, *145*, 1709–1716. [CrossRef] [PubMed]
23. Trock, B.; Lanza, E.; Greenwald, P. Dietary fiber, vegetables, and colon cancer: Critical review and meta-analyses of the epidemiologic evidence. *J. Natl. Cancer Inst.* **1990**, *82*, 650–661. [CrossRef] [PubMed]
24. Vargas, A.J.; Neuhouser, M.L.; George, S.M.; Thomson, C.A.; Ho, G.Y.; Rohan, T.E.; Kato, I.; Nassir, R.; Hou, L.; Manson, J.E. Diet quality and colorectal cancer risk in the women's health initiative observational study. *Am. J. Epidemiol.* **2016**, *184*, 23–32. [CrossRef] [PubMed]
25. Makarem, N.; Nicholson, J.M.; Bandera, E.V.; McKeown, N.M.; Parekh, N. Consumption of whole grains and cereal fiber in relation to cancer risk: A systematic review of longitudinal studies. *Nutr. Rev.* **2016**, *74*, 353–373. [CrossRef] [PubMed]
26. Aune, D.; Chan, D.S.; Lau, R.; Vieira, R.; Greenwood, D.C.; Kampman, E.; Norat, T. Dietary fibre, whole grains, and risk of colorectal cancer: Systematic review and dose-response meta-analysis of prospective studies. *BMJ* **2011**, *343*, d6617. [CrossRef] [PubMed]
27. Aune, D.; Lau, R.; Chan, D.S.; Vieira, R.; Greenwood, D.C.; Kampman, E.; Norat, T. Nonlinear reduction in risk for colorectal cancer by fruit and vegetable intake based on meta-analysis of prospective studies. *Gastroenterology* **2011**, *141*, 106–118. [CrossRef] [PubMed]
28. Beresford, S.A.; Johnson, K.C.; Ritenbaugh, C.; Lasser, N.L.; Snetselaar, L.G.; Black, H.R.; Anderson, G.L.; Assaf, A.R.; Bassford, T.; Bowen, D.; et al. Low-fat dietary pattern and risk of colorectal cancer: The women's health initiative randomized controlled dietary modification trial. *JAMA* **2006**, *295*, 643–654. [CrossRef] [PubMed]
29. Donohoe, D.R.; Bultman, S.J. Metaboloepigenetics: Interrelationships between energy metabolism and epigenetic control of gene expression. *J. Cell. Physiol.* **2012**, *227*, 3169–3177. [CrossRef] [PubMed]
30. Donohoe, D.R.; Garge, N.; Zhang, X.X.; Sun, W.; O'Connell, T.M.; Bunger, M.K.; Bultman, S.J. The microbiome and butyrate regulate energy metabolism and autophagy in the mammalian colon. *Cell Metab.* **2011**, *13*, 517–526. [CrossRef] [PubMed]
31. Kolar, S.; Barhoumi, R.; Jones, C.K.; Wesley, J.; Lupton, J.R.; Fan, Y.Y.; Chapkin, R.S. Interactive effects of fatty acid and butyrate-induced mitochondrial Ca(2)(+) loading and apoptosis in colonocytes. *Cancer* **2011**, *117*, 5294–5303. [CrossRef] [PubMed]
32. Kansal, S.; Negi, A.K.; Bhatnagar, A.; Agnihotri, N. Ras signaling pathway in the chemopreventive action of different ratios of fish oil and corn oil in experimentally induced colon carcinogenesis. *Nutr. Cancer* **2012**, *64*, 559–568. [CrossRef] [PubMed]
33. Kolar, S.S.; Barhoumi, R.; Callaway, E.S.; Fan, Y.Y.; Wang, N.; Lupton, J.R.; Chapkin, R.S. Synergy between docosahexaenoic acid and butyrate elicits p53-independent apoptosis via mitochondrial Ca(2+) accumulation in colonocytes. *Am. J. Physiol. Gastrointest. Liver Physiol.* **2007**, *293*, G935–G943. [CrossRef] [PubMed]
34. Kolar, S.S.; Barhoumi, R.; Lupton, J.R.; Chapkin, R.S. Docosahexaenoic acid and butyrate synergistically induce colonocyte apoptosis by enhancing mitochondrial Ca2+ accumulation. *Cancer Res.* **2007**, *67*, 5561–5568. [CrossRef] [PubMed]
35. Ng, Y.; Barhoumi, R.; Tjalkens, R.B.; Fan, Y.Y.; Kolar, S.; Wang, N.; Lupton, J.R.; Chapkin, R.S. The role of docosahexaenoic acid in mediating mitochondrial membrane lipid oxidation and apoptosis in colonocytes. *Carcinogenesis* **2005**, *26*, 1914–1921. [CrossRef] [PubMed]
36. Hooda, S.; Boler, B.M.; Serao, M.C.; Brulc, J.M.; Staeger, M.A.; Boileau, T.W.; Dowd, S.E.; Fahey, G.C., Jr.; Swanson, K.S. 454 pyrosequencing reveals a shift in fecal microbiota of healthy adult men consuming polydextrose or soluble corn fiber. *J. Nutr.* **2012**, *142*, 1259–1265. [CrossRef] [PubMed]
37. Ross, A.B.; Bruce, S.J.; Blondel-Lubrano, A.; Oguey-Araymon, S.; Beaumont, M.; Bourgeois, A.; Nielsen-Moennoz, C.; Vigo, M.; Fay, L.B.; Kochhar, S.; et al. A whole-grain cereal-rich diet increases plasma betaine, and tends to decrease total and ldl-cholesterol compared with a refined-grain diet in healthy subjects. *Br. J. Nutr.* **2011**, *105*, 1492–1502. [CrossRef] [PubMed]

38. Costabile, A.; Klinder, A.; Fava, F.; Napolitano, A.; Fogliano, V.; Leonard, C.; Gibson, G.R.; Tuohy, K.M. Whole-grain wheat breakfast cereal has a prebiotic effect on the human gut microbiota: A double-blind, placebo-controlled, crossover study. *Br. J. Nutr.* **2008**, *99*, 110–120. [CrossRef] [PubMed]
39. Finley, J.W.; Burrell, J.B.; Reeves, P.G. Pinto bean consumption changes scfa profiles in fecal fermentations, bacterial populations of the lower bowel, and lipid profiles in blood of humans. *J. Nutr.* **2007**, *137*, 2391–2398. [PubMed]
40. Smith, S.C.; Choy, R.; Johnson, S.K.; Hall, R.S.; Wildeboer-Veloo, A.C.; Welling, G.W. Lupin kernel fiber consumption modifies fecal microbiota in healthy men as determined by rrna gene fluorescent in situ hybridization. *Eur. J. Nutr.* **2006**, *45*, 335–341. [CrossRef] [PubMed]
41. Johnson, S.K.; Chua, V.; Hall, R.S.; Baxter, A.L. Lupin kernel fibre foods improve bowel function and beneficially modify some putative faecal risk factors for colon cancer in men. *Br. J. Nutr.* **2006**, *95*, 372–378. [CrossRef] [PubMed]
42. Tuohy, K.M.; Kolida, S.; Lustenberger, A.M.; Gibson, G.R. The prebiotic effects of biscuits containing partially hydrolysed guar gum and fructo-oligosaccharides—A human volunteer study. *Br. J. Nutr.* **2001**, *86*, 341–348. [CrossRef] [PubMed]
43. Hylla, S.; Gostner, A.; Dusel, G.; Anger, H.; Bartram, H.P.; Christl, S.U.; Kasper, H.; Scheppach, W. Effects of resistant starch on the colon in healthy volunteers: Possible implications for cancer prevention. *Am. J. Clin. Nutr.* **1998**, *67*, 136–142. [PubMed]
44. Arumugam, M.; Raes, J.; Pelletier, E.; Le Paslier, D.; Yamada, T.; Mende, D.R.; Fernandes, G.R.; Tap, J.; Bruls, T.; Batto, J.M.; et al. Enterotypes of the human gut microbiome. *Nature* **2011**, *473*, 174–180. [CrossRef] [PubMed]
45. Faust, K.; Raes, J. Microbial interactions: From networks to models. *Nat. Rev. Microbiol.* **2012**, *10*, 538–550. [CrossRef] [PubMed]
46. Faust, K.; Sathirapongsasuti, J.F.; Izard, J.; Segata, N.; Gevers, D.; Raes, J.; Huttenhower, C. Microbial co-occurrence relationships in the human microbiome. *PLoS Comput. Biol.* **2012**, *8*, e1002606. [CrossRef] [PubMed]
47. Lozupone, C.; Faust, K.; Raes, J.; Faith, J.J.; Frank, D.N.; Zaneveld, J.; Gordon, J.I.; Knight, R. Identifying genomic and metabolic features that can underline early successional and opportunistic lifestyles of human gut symbionts. *Genome Res.* **2012**, *22*, 1974–1984. [CrossRef] [PubMed]
48. Bolca, S.; van de Wiele, T.; Possemiers, S. Gut metabotypes govern health effects of dietary polyphenols. *Curr. Opin. Biotechnol.* **2013**, *24*, 220–225. [CrossRef] [PubMed]
49. Heinzmann, S.S.; Merrifield, C.A.; Rezzi, S.; Kochhar, S.; Lindon, J.C.; Holmes, E.; Nicholson, J.K. Stability and robustness of human metabolic phenotypes in response to sequential food challenges. *J. Proteome Res.* **2012**, *11*, 643–655. [CrossRef] [PubMed]
50. Wang, T.; Cai, G.; Qiu, Y.; Fei, N.; Zhang, M.; Pang, X.; Jia, W.; Cai, S.; Zhao, L. Structural segregation of gut microbiota between colorectal cancer patients and healthy volunteers. *ISME J.* **2012**, *6*, 320–329. [CrossRef] [PubMed]
51. Weir, T.L.; Manter, D.K.; Sheflin, A.M.; Barnett, B.A.; Heuberger, A.L.; Ryan, E.P. Stool microbiome and metabolome differences between colorectal cancer patients and healthy adults. *PLoS ONE* **2013**, *8*, e70803. [CrossRef] [PubMed]
52. Wu, N.; Yang, X.; Zhang, R.; Li, J.; Xiao, X.; Hu, Y.; Chen, Y.; Yang, F.; Lu, N.; Wang, Z.; et al. Dysbiosis signature of fecal microbiota in colorectal cancer patients. *Microb. Ecol.* **2013**, *66*, 462–470. [CrossRef] [PubMed]
53. Simopoulos, A.P. Importance of the omega-6/omega-3 balance in health and disease: Evolutionary aspects of diet. *World Rev. Nutr. Diet.* **2011**, *102*, 10–21. [PubMed]
54. Strobel, C.; Jahreis, G.; Kuhnt, K. Survey of *n*-3 and *n*-6 polyunsaturated fatty acids in fish and fish products. *Lipids Health Dis.* **2012**, *11*, 144. [CrossRef] [PubMed]
55. Skender, B.; Hyrslova Vaculova, A.; Hofmanova, J. Docosahexaenoic fatty acid (dha) in the regulation of colon cell growth and cell death: A review. *Biomed. Pap. Med. Fac. Univ. Palacky Olomouc Czech. Repub.* **2012**, *156*, 186–199. [CrossRef] [PubMed]
56. Azer, S.A. Overview of molecular pathways in inflammatory bowel disease associated with colorectal cancer development. *Eur. J. Gastroenterol. Hepatol.* **2012**, *25*, 271–281. [CrossRef] [PubMed]

57. Cockbain, A.J.; Toogood, G.J.; Hull, M.A. Omega-3 polyunsaturated fatty acids for the treatment and prevention of colorectal cancer. *Gut* **2012**, *61*, 135–149. [CrossRef] [PubMed]
58. Chang, W.C.; Chapkin, R.S.; Lupton, J.R. Predictive value of proliferation, differentiation and apoptosis as intermediate markers for colon tumorigenesis. *Carcinogenesis* **1997**, *18*, 721–730. [CrossRef] [PubMed]
59. Sanders, L.M.; Henderson, C.E.; Hong, M.Y.; Barhoumi, R.; Burghardt, R.C.; Wang, N.; Spinka, C.M.; Carroll, R.J.; Turner, N.D.; Chapkin, R.S.; et al. An increase in reactive oxygen species by dietary fish oil coupled with the attenuation of antioxidant defenses by dietary pectin enhances rat colonocyte apoptosis. *J. Nutr.* **2004**, *134*, 3233–3238. [PubMed]
60. Vanamala, J.; Glagolenko, A.; Yang, P.; Carroll, R.J.; Murphy, M.E.; Newman, R.A.; Ford, J.R.; Braby, L.A.; Chapkin, R.S.; Turner, N.D.; et al. Dietary fish oil and pectin enhance colonocyte apoptosis in part through suppression of ppardelta/pge2 and elevation of pge3. *Carcinogenesis* **2008**, *29*, 790–796. [CrossRef] [PubMed]
61. Crim, K.C.; Sanders, L.M.; Hong, M.Y.; Taddeo, S.S.; Turner, N.D.; Chapkin, R.S.; Lupton, J.R. Upregulation of p21waf1/cip1 expression in vivo by butyrate administration can be chemoprotective or chemopromotive depending on the lipid component of the diet. *Carcinogenesis* **2008**, *29*, 1415–1420. [CrossRef] [PubMed]
62. Cho, Y.; Kim, H.; Turner, N.D.; Mann, J.C.; Wei, J.; Taddeo, S.S.; Davidson, L.A.; Wang, N.; Vannucci, M.; Carroll, R.J.; et al. A chemoprotective fish oil- and pectin-containing diet temporally alters gene expression profiles in exfoliated rat colonocytes throughout oncogenesis. *J. Nutr.* **2011**, *141*, 1029–1035. [CrossRef] [PubMed]
63. The Women's Health Initiative Study Group. Design of the women's health initiative clinical trial and observational study. *Control. Clin. Trials* **1998**, *19*, 61–109.
64. Anderson, G.L.; Manson, J.; Wallace, R.; Lund, B.; Hall, D.; Davis, S.; Shumaker, S.; Wang, C.Y.; Stein, E.; Prentice, R.L. Implementation of the women's health initiative study design. *Ann. Epidemiol.* **2003**, *13*, S5–S17. [CrossRef]
65. Langer, R.D.; White, E.; Lewis, C.E.; Kotchen, J.M.; Hendrix, S.L.; Trevisan, M. The women's health initiative observational study: Baseline characteristics of participants and reliability of baseline measures. *Ann. Epidemiol.* **2003**, *13*, S107–S121. [CrossRef]
66. Hays, J.; Hunt, J.R.; Hubbell, F.A.; Anderson, G.L.; Limacher, M.; Allen, C.; Rossouw, J.E. The women's health initiative recruitment methods and results. *Ann. Epidemiol.* **2003**, *13*, S18–S77. [CrossRef]
67. Patterson, R.E.; Kristal, A.R.; Tinker, L.F.; Carter, R.A.; Bolton, M.P.; Agurs-Collins, T. Measurement characteristics of the women's health initiative food frequency questionnaire. *Ann. Epidemiol.* **1999**, *9*, 178–187. [CrossRef]
68. Curb, J.D.; McTiernan, A.; Heckbert, S.R.; Kooperberg, C.; Stanford, J.; Nevitt, M.; Johnson, K.C.; Proulx-Burns, L.; Pastore, L.; Criqui, M.; et al. Outcomes ascertainment and adjudication methods in the women's health initiative. *Ann. Epidemiol.* **2003**, *13*, S122–S128. [CrossRef]
69. Haggar, F.A.; Boushey, R.P. Colorectal cancer epidemiology: Incidence, mortality, survival, and risk factors. *Clin. Colon Rectal Surg.* **2009**, *22*, 191–197. [CrossRef] [PubMed]
70. Edwards, B.K.; Ward, E.; Kohler, B.A.; Eheman, C.; Zauber, A.G.; Anderson, R.N.; Jemal, A.; Schymura, M.J.; Lansdorp-Vogelaar, I.; Seeff, L.C.; et al. Annual report to the nation on the status of cancer, 1975–2006, featuring colorectal cancer trends and impact of interventions (risk factors, screening, and treatment) to reduce future rates. *Cancer* **2010**, *116*, 544–573. [CrossRef] [PubMed]
71. National Academy of Sciences-Institute of Medicine. Food and Nutrition Board. *Dietary Reference Intakes for Energy, Carbohydrate, Fiber, Fat, Fatty Acids, Cholesterol, Protein, and Amino Acids*; National Academy Press: Washington, DC, USA, 2005.
72. American Institute For Cancer Research. Available online: http://www.Aicr.Org/continuous-update-project/colorectal-cancer.Html (accessed on 4 November 2016).
73. Bingham, S.A. Diet and large bowel cancer. *J. R. Soc. Med.* **1990**, *83*, 420–422. [PubMed]
74. Young, G.P.; Hu, Y.; Le Leu, R.K.; Nyskohus, L. Dietary fibre and colorectal cancer: A model for environment–gene interactions. *Mol. Nutr. Food Res.* **2005**, *49*, 571–584. [CrossRef] [PubMed]
75. Slavin, J.L. Dietary fiber and body weight. *Nutrition* **2005**, *21*, 411–418. [CrossRef] [PubMed]
76. Donohoe, D.R.; Collins, L.B.; Wali, A.; Bigler, R.; Sun, W.; Bultman, S.J. The warburg effect dictates the mechanism of butyrate-mediated histone acetylation and cell proliferation. *Mol. Cell* **2012**, *48*, 612–626. [CrossRef] [PubMed]

77. Bultman, S.J. Molecular pathways: Gene-environment interactions regulating dietary fiber induction of proliferation and apoptosis via butyrate for cancer prevention. *Clin. Cancer Res.* **2014**, *20*, 799–803. [CrossRef] [PubMed]
78. Triff, K.; Kim, E.; Chapkin, R.S. Chemoprotective epigenetic mechanisms in a colorectal cancer model: Modulation by *n*-3 pufa in combination with fermentable fiber. *Curr. Pharmacol. Rep.* **2015**, *1*, 11–20. [CrossRef] [PubMed]
79. Chapkin, R.S.; Seo, J.; McMurray, D.N.; Lupton, J.R. Mechanisms by which docosahexaenoic acid and related fatty acids reduce colon cancer risk and inflammatory disorders of the intestine. *Chem. Phys. Lipids* **2008**, *153*, 14–23. [CrossRef] [PubMed]
80. Levi, F.; Pasche, C.; Lucchini, F.; la Vecchia, C. Dietary fibre and the risk of colorectal cancer. *Eur. J. Cancer* **2001**, *37*, 2091–2096. [CrossRef]
81. Freudenheim, J.L.; Graham, S.; Horvath, P.J.; Marshall, J.R.; Haughey, B.P.; Wilkinson, G. Risks associated with source of fiber and fiber components in cancer of the colon and rectum. *Cancer Res.* **1990**, *50*, 3295–3300. [PubMed]
82. Le Marchand, L.; Hankin, J.H.; Wilkens, L.R.; Kolonel, L.N.; Englyst, H.N.; Lyu, L.C. Dietary fiber and colorectal cancer risk. *Epidemiology* **1997**, *8*, 658–665. [CrossRef] [PubMed]
83. Negri, E.; Franceschi, S.; Parpinel, M.; La Vecchia, C. Fiber intake and risk of colorectal cancer. *Cancer Epidemiol. Biomark. Prev.* **1998**, *7*, 667–671.
84. Turk, H.F.; Monk, J.M.; Fan, Y.Y.; Callaway, E.S.; Weeks, B.; Chapkin, R.S. Inhibitory effects of omega-3 fatty acids on injury-induced epidermal growth factor receptor transactivation contribute to delayed wound healing. *Am. J. Physiol. Cell Physiol.* **2013**, *304*, C905–C917. [CrossRef] [PubMed]
85. Larsson, S.C.; Kumlin, M.; Ingelman-Sundberg, M.; Wolk, A. Dietary long-chain *n*-3 fatty acids for the prevention of cancer: A review of potential mechanisms. *Am. J. Clin. Nutr.* **2004**, *79*, 935–945. [PubMed]
86. Wu, S.; Feng, B.; Li, K.; Zhu, X.; Liang, S.; Liu, X.; Han, S.; Wang, B.; Wu, K.; Miao, D.; et al. Fish consumption and colorectal cancer risk in humans: A systematic review and meta-analysis. *Am. J. Med.* **2012**, *125*, 551–559. [CrossRef] [PubMed]
87. Geelen, A.; Schouten, J.M.; Kamphuis, C.; Stam, B.E.; Burema, J.; Renkema, J.M.; Bakker, E.J.; van't Veer, P.; Kampman, E. Fish consumption, *n*-3 fatty acids, and colorectal cancer: A meta-analysis of prospective cohort studies. *Am. J. Epidemiol.* **2007**, *166*, 1116–1125. [CrossRef] [PubMed]
88. Song, M.; Zhang, X.; Meyerhardt, J.A.; Giovannucci, E.L.; Ogino, S.; Fuchs, C.S.; Chan, A.T. Marine omega-3 polyunsaturated fatty acid intake and survival after colorectal cancer diagnosis. *Gut* **2016**. [CrossRef] [PubMed]
89. Vannice, G.; Rasmussen, H. Position of the academy of nutrition and dietetics: Dietary fatty acids for healthy adults. *J. Acad. Nutr. Diet.* **2014**, *114*, 136–153. [CrossRef] [PubMed]
90. Jiang, Y.H.; Lupton, J.R.; Chapkin, R.S. Dietary fat and fiber modulate the effect of carcinogen on colonic protein kinase c lambda expression in rats. *J. Nutr.* **1997**, *127*, 1938–1943. [PubMed]
91. Fan, Y.Y.; Ran, Q.; Toyokuni, S.; Okazaki, Y.; Callaway, E.S.; Lupton, J.R.; Chapkin, R.S. Dietary fish oil promotes colonic apoptosis and mitochondrial proton leak in oxidatively stressed mice. *Cancer Prev. Res.* **2011**, *4*, 1267–1274. [CrossRef] [PubMed]
92. Orlich, M.J.; Singh, P.N.; Sabate, J.; Fan, J.; Sveen, L.; Bennett, H.; Knutsen, S.F.; Beeson, W.L.; Jaceldo-Siegl, K.; Butler, T.L.; et al. Vegetarian dietary patterns and the risk of colorectal cancers. *JAMA Intern. Med.* **2015**, *175*, 767–776. [CrossRef] [PubMed]
93. O'Keefe, S.J.; Li, J.V.; Lahti, L.; Ou, J.; Carbonero, F.; Mohammed, K.; Posma, J.M.; Kinross, J.; Wahl, E.; Ruder, E.; et al. Fat, fibre and cancer risk in African americans and rural Africans. *Nat. Commun.* **2015**, *6*, 6342. [CrossRef] [PubMed]
94. Kato, I.; Majumdar, A.P.; Land, S.J.; Barnholtz-Sloan, J.S.; Severson, R.K. Dietary fatty acids, luminal modifiers, and risk of colorectal cancer. *Int. J. Cancer* **2010**, *127*, 942–951. [CrossRef] [PubMed]
95. US Department of Agriculture, Agriculture Research Services. Nutrient Intakes from Food: Mean Amounts Consumed per Individual, by Gender and Age. Available online: http://www.ars.usda.gov/ba/bhnrc/fsrg (accessed on 4 November 2016).
96. Kristal, A.R.; Shattuck, A.L.; Williams, A.E. Food Frequency Questionnaires for Diet Intervention Research. In Proceedings of the 17th National Nutrient Databank Conference, Baltimore, MD, USA, 7–10 June 1992.

97. Satia-Abouta, J.; Kristal, A.R.; Patterson, R.E.; Littman, A.J.; Stratton, K.L.; White, E. Dietary supplement use and medical conditions: The vital study. *Am. J. Prev. Med.* **2003**, *24*, 43–51. [CrossRef]
98. Fasano, E.; Serini, S.; Cittadini, A.; Calviello, G. Long-chain *n*-3 pufa against breast and prostate cancer: Which are the appropriate doses for intervention studies in animals and humans? *Crit. Rev. Food Sci. Nutr.* **2015**. [CrossRef] [PubMed]
99. Vece, M.M.; Agnoli, C.; Grioni, S.; Sieri, S.; Pala, V.; Pellegrini, N.; Frasca, G.; Tumino, R.; Mattiello, A.; Panico, S.; et al. Dietary total antioxidant capacity and colorectal cancer in the italian epic cohort. *PLoS ONE* **2015**, *10*, e0142995. [CrossRef] [PubMed]
100. La Vecchia, C.; Decarli, A.; Serafini, M.; Parpinel, M.; Bellocco, R.; Galeone, C.; Bosetti, C.; Zucchetto, A.; Polesel, J.; Lagiou, P.; et al. Dietary total antioxidant capacity and colorectal cancer: A large case-control study in italy. *Int. J. Cancer* **2013**, *133*, 1447–1451. [CrossRef] [PubMed]
101. Bjelakovic, G.; Nikolova, D.; Simonetti, R.G.; Gluud, C. Antioxidant supplements for prevention of gastrointestinal cancers: A systematic review and meta-analysis. *Lancet* **2004**, *364*, 1219–1228. [CrossRef]

4

Consumption of Fruit or Fiber-Fruit Decreases the Risk of Cardiovascular Disease in a Mediterranean Young Cohort

Pilar Buil-Cosiales [1,2,3], Miguel Angel Martinez-Gonzalez [2,3,4,5], Miguel Ruiz-Canela [2,3,4], Javier Díez-Espino [1,2,3], Ana García-Arellano [6] and Estefania Toledo [2,3,4,*]

1 Atención Primaria, Servicio Navarro de Salud-Osasunbidea, 08010 Navarra, Spain; pilarbuil@ono.com (P.B.-C.); javierdiezesp@ono.com (J.D.-E.)
2 Centro de Investigación Biomédica en Red Fisiopatología de la Obesidad y Nutrición (CIBERobn), Instituto de Salud Carlos III, 28029 Madrid, Spain; mamartinez@unav.es (M.A.M.-G.); mcanela@unav.es (M.R.C.)
3 IdiSNA, Navarra Institute for Health Research, 31008 Pamplona, Navarra, Spain
4 Department of Preventive Medicine and Public Health, University of Navarra, 31008 Pamplona, Navarra, Spain
5 Department of Nutrition, Harvard School of Public Health, Boston, MA 02115, USA
6 Department of Emergency, Complejo Hospitalario de Navarra Servicio Navarro de Salud-Osasunbidea, 31008 Pamplona, Navarra, Spain; agarare@gmail.com
* Correspondence: etoledo@unav.es or etoledo@unav.com;

Abstract: Fiber and fiber-rich foods have been inversely associated with cardiovascular disease (CVD), but the evidence is scarce in young and Mediterranean cohorts. We used Cox regression models to assess the association between quintiles of total fiber and fiber from different sources, and the risk of CVD adjusted for the principal confounding factors in a Mediterranean cohort of young adults, the SUN (Seguimiento Universidad de Navarra, Follow-up) cohort. After a median follow-up of 10.3 years, we observed 112 cases of CVD among 17,007 participants (61% female, mean age 38 years). We observed an inverse association between fiber intake and CVD events (p for trend = 0.024) and also between the highest quintile of fruit consumption (hazard ratio (HR) 0.51, 95% confidence interval (CI) 0.27–0.95) or whole grains consumption (HR 0.43 95% CI 0.20–0.93) and CVD compared to the lowest quintile, and also a HR of 0.58 (95% CI 0.37–0.90) for the participants who ate at least 175 g/day of fruit. Only the participants in the highest quintile of fruit-derived fiber intake had a significantly lower risk of CVD (HR 0.52, 95% CI 0.28–0.97). The participants who ate at least one serving per week of cruciferous vegetables had a lower risk than those who did not (HR 0.52, 95% CI 0.30–0.89). In conclusion, high fruit consumption, whole grain consumption, or consumption of at least one serving/week of cruciferous vegetables may be protective against CVD in young Mediterranean populations.

Keywords: fiber; fruit; vegetables; cardiovascular disease; legumes; whole grains

---

1. Introduction

Cardiovascular disease (CVD) is the leading cause of morbidity and mortality in developed countries [1,2] and its prevalence is increasing in developing countries. Lifestyles are the most important determinants of CVD, among which nutritional habits play an important role.

Higher dietary fiber intake has been recognized to be inversely associated with coronary heart disease (CHD) [3] and stroke [4]. Nevertheless, studies that have assessed the association between fiber intake and CVD in Mediterranean countries are scarce. It is also noteworthy that the foods that mainly contribute to the high intake of fiber—namely fruits, vegetables, legumes, and whole grains—have other micronutrients that have been postulated to be even more important for the prevention of CVD [5,6].

Fruits and vegetables are a heterogeneous food group with different contents of vitamins, minerals, and other bioactive phytochemicals [7]. There are not many studies that have evaluated the association between specific fruits or vegetables or groups of them, and it is unclear which fruit or vegetable subgroup may be the most protective against CVD. Also, fruits and vegetables consumed in different regions differ, and this could explain the differences observed in their reported effects [8].

Epidemiologic studies that have analyzed the relationship between fruit and vegetable consumption, which represent the principal source of fiber in Mediterranean countries, and CHD found inconsistent results. A meta-analysis published in 2015 [8], that analyzed 23 studies assessing this relationship, found an inverse association but showed heterogeneity with geographical differences. Concretely, an inverse association between fruit and vegetable consumption and CHD was observed only in Western countries. In addition, only one of the included studies had been conducted in a Mediterranean country [9] and this latter study found no significant association of fruit and vegetable consumption with the risk of CHD. More recently, two studies [10,11] conducted within the PREDIMED trial (PREvención con DIeta MEDiterránea) that recruited older participants in the Mediterranean area found an inverse association between fruit consumption and cardiovascular mortality, but not with non-fatal CVD. Albeit there are cohort studies and even a meta-analysis [12] that have observed an inverse association between fruits and vegetables and stroke, none of the included studies had been conducted in Mediterranean countries.

On the other hand, legumes and whole grains are also good sources of dietary fiber, and both have been suggested to be protective against CVD [13–15]. There is a wide body of evidence regarding the inverse association between whole grains and the risk of cardiovascular risk factors, such as type 2 diabetes [16,17], dyslipidaemia [18,19], high blood pressure [20], and obesity [17], but the research on their association with CVD clinical hard end-points is not large. A meta-analysis [21] included only nine publications that assessed the relationship between whole grains and CVD and found an inverse association. Six out of the nine studies had been conducted in the US, and only one in a Mediterranean country, and this latter study only reported on cardiovascular mortality. Even less are the studies which have assessed the relationship between legume consumption and the risk of CVD events [19,22,23].

Additionally, most of the studies have been conducted in aged adults and older people, and none in young adults. Therefore, we analyzed the association between fiber-rich foods and CVD in a Mediterranean cohort of young adults in order to advance in the knowledge of this relationship.

2. Materials and Methods

The SUN (Seguimiento Universidad de Navarra, Follow-up) project is a prospective, multipurpose, dynamic cohort of university graduates conducted in Spain. As a dynamic cohort, the recruitment of the participants is permanently open. Methodological aspects of this cohort have been published in detail previously [24]. Briefly, the cohort began in December 1999 and the recruitment of participants is permanently open. Information is gathered biennially by mailed questionnaires. Several validation studies of this self-reported information have been conducted, including anthropometric data [25], physical activity [26], the diagnosis of hypertension [27] and the specific criteria used for metabolic syndrome definition [28], all of them supporting the quality of the collected information.

For the present study, we included 22,476 subjects recruited before March 2013, so that they could have at least one follow-up questionnaire by the time of the last update of the dataset (December 2015). For the current analysis, we excluded 2113 participants with an energy intake out of sex specific predefined limits (>4000 kcal/day and <800 kcal/day for men and >3500 kcal/day and <500 kcal/day for women) [29]. We also excluded 947 participants who had prevalent cardiovascular disease at baseline and 2409 subjects with no follow-up information. After exclusions, the final sample population included a total of 17,007 participants. The retention in the cohort was 88%.

The study was approved by the Institutional Review Board of the University of Navarra on 30 August 2001. Voluntary completion of the first questionnaire was considered to imply informed consent.

Dietary intake was assessed through a validated 136-item semi-quantitative food-frequency questionnaire [30,31], which showed an intra-class correlation coefficient of 0.71 for fruits and 0.82 for vegetables.

Each item in the questionnaire included a typical portion size. Daily food consumption was estimated by multiplying the portion size by the consumption frequency for each item (nine options ranging from never or almost never to six times per day). Nutrient intake was estimated using Spanish food composition tables. We defined moderate alcohol consumption between 5 and 25 g/day for women and between 10 and 50 g/day for men. Based on the dietary information collected with the food-frequency questionnaire we calculated a score of adherence to the traditional Mediterranean diet [13].

Incidence of cardiovascular events, defined as non-fatal myocardial infarction, non-fatal stroke reported by participants on a follow-up questionnaire, or deaths due to cardiovascular disease, was the primary endpoint. An expert panel of physicians, blinded to the information on diet, anthropometric indexes, and risk factors, reviewed medical records of participants and adjudicated events applying universal criteria for myocardial infarction and clinical criteria for the other outcomes. A non-fatal stroke was defined as a focal neurological deficit of sudden onset and vascular mechanism lasting >24 h. Cases of fatal stroke were documented if there was evidence of a cerebrovascular mechanism. Deaths were reported to our research team by the participants' next of kin, work associates, and postal authorities. For participants lost to follow-up, we consulted the National Death Index every six months to identify deceased cohort members and to obtain their cause of death. Cases of fatal CHD or stroke reported by families or postal authorities were confirmed by a review of medical records with permission of the next of kin.

Statistical Analysis

Participants were categorized in quintiles of fiber, fruits, vegetables, legumes, or whole grain consumption. We used the residuals method to adjust the assessed foods for total energy intake.

Baseline characteristics are presented according to quintiles of baseline consumption of fruit and vegetables, as mean (SD) for quantitative traits, and percentage for categorical variables.

We used Cox regression models to assess the relationship between quintiles of baseline fiber, fruit, vegetables, legumes, or whole grains consumption and the subsequent incidence of CVD during follow-up. Hazard ratios (HRs) and their 95% confidence intervals (95% CIs) were calculated using the first quintile as the reference category. We used age as the underlying time variable. Entry time was defined as the date of completion of the first questionnaire and exit time as the date of CVD, the date of the completion of the last questionnaire, or date of death, whichever occurred first.

In addition, we analyzed specific subgroups of fruit and vegetables. The definition of composite groups was based on a report by Joshipura et al. [32] which we adapted to our Food Frequency Questionnaire (FFQ) and to the usual habits of the Spanish population. The fruits and vegetables included in each subgroup are presented in Table 1.

Three multivariable models were constructed to adjust for the known or suspected predictors of CVD. First, we adjusted only for sex. In the second model, we adjusted additionally for marital status (married, single, widowed, separated, others), highest attained educational level (five categories), family history of CHD (dichotomous), type 2 diabetes (dichotomous), high blood pressure (dichotomous), dyslipidemia (dichotomous), smoking status (four categories), total energy intake (kcal/day), body mass index (kg/m^2), alcohol intake (three categories), and use of cholesterol-lowering drugs. We also fitted a third model with additional adjustments for nutritional variables: olive oil (g/day) for all the groups and vegetables (g/day), legumes (g/day), and whole grains (g/day) in the analysis of fruit consumption; fruits (g/day), legumes (g/day), and whole grains (g/day) in an analysis that assessed vegetable consumption; fruits (g/day), vegetables (g/day), and whole grains (g/day) consumption in the analysis of legumes and fruits (g/day), vegetables (g/day), and legumes (g/day) consumption in the analysis that assessed whole grains consumption. All the models were also stratified by age in decades.

Table 1. Definitions for various fruit and vegetable subgroups.

Subgroups	Individual Foods
Orange group	Orange, tangerine, grapefruit
Apple/pear group	Apple/pear
Green leafy vegetables	Spinach, lettuce, chard greens
Cruciferous vegetables	Broccoli, cabbage, cauliflower, Brussels sprouts
β-carotene-rich fruits and vegetables	Carrots, spinach, pumpkin, chard greens
Lutein-rich fruits and vegetables	Spinach, chard greens
Lycopene-rich fruits and vegetables	Tomatoes, tomato sauce, "gazpacho" *
Vitamin C-rich fruits and vegetables	Orange, tangerine, grapefruit, peppers

* Cold tomato-based soup with pepper, cucumber, garlic, and onion.

Tests for linear trend were conducted by assigning the quintile specific median value of consumption of each food item or nutrient and regressing the risk of CVD on the resulting variable, which was treated as a continuous variable.

For some foods for which the point estimates obtained with the quintiles suggested a threshold effect, we generated a new dichotomous variable and assessed the relationship between this new variable and CVD with the same multivariable models.

Statistical tests were two-sided, and p values of less than 0.05 were considered to indicate statistical significance.

3. Results

The final sample comprised 17,007 participants, of whom 61% were women and the mean age was 38 years. The median follow-up was 10.3 years (mean = 9.6 years). We observed 112 confirmed cases of CVD during this follow-up period (56 myocardial infarctions, 32 strokes, and 33 cardiovascular deaths). The mean consumption of fruits, vegetables, legumes, and whole grains was 343 g/day, 525 g/day, 23 g/day, and 12 g/day, respectively. The most consumed fruit was oranges and the most consumed vegetables were tomatoes and lettuce. The main sources of fiber were mostly vegetables (10.4 g/day) and fruits (6 g/day).

Table 2 presents the baseline characteristics of the study participants according to quintiles of baseline fiber consumption. Participants in the highest quintile were older, and more likely to be diagnosed with dyslipidemia, type 2 diabetes, and high blood pressure. As expected, participants in the higher quintiles consumed more fruits, vegetables, legumes, and whole grains, and of all the items of the fruits and vegetables groups. Also, participants with the highest fiber intake showed a higher adherence to the traditional Mediterranean diet.

When we compared the highest quintile of fruit or whole grains consumption with the lowest quintile, we observed an inverse association between them and CVD in the fully adjusted model, and also a significant inverse trend for fiber intake. Table 3 shows the association of fiber intake, fruits, vegetables, legumes, or whole grains consumption at baseline with the incidence of CVD. When we compared the participants who consumed at least 160 g/day of fruit (two servings) with those with a lower consumption we found a HR of CVD of 0.62 (95% CI 0.39–0.99, $p = 0.045$) and HR of 0.58 (95% CI 0.37–0.90; $p = 0.015$) for the participants who consumed at least 175 g/day compared with those with a lower consumption. We observed no threshold for vegetables consumption.

Table 2. Baseline characteristics * of the study participants according to baseline quintiles of fiber intake, SUN (Seguimiento Universidad de Navarra, Follow-up) Project 1999–2013.

	Quintiles of Fiber Intake				
	Q1	Q2	Q3	Q4	Q5
Age (years)	34 (10)	36 (11)	38 (12)	40 (12)	42 (13)
Sex (% women)	60.6	60.6	60.6	60.6	60.6
Marital Status, %					
Single	55.3	47.4	42.9	40.6	37.9
Married	41.8	48.9	52.6	53.8	55.6
Others	2.9	3.8	4.6	5.6	6.5
Highest attained educational level					
Degree or licenciate degree, %	56	53	53	52	53
Master's degree, %	7	8	8	8	8
Doctoral degree, %	7	9	11	11	11
Family history of CHD, %	11	12	14	14	16
Use of lipid-lowering drugs, %	1.2	1.5	3.0	3.1	4.0
Type 2 diabetes, %	0.7	0.9	1.7	2.2	3.0
Body mass index (Kg/m^2)	23 (11)	23 (3.3)	24 (3.5)	24 (3.5)	24 (3.5)
Hypertension, %	3.7	4.9	6.7	7.9	9.3
Dyslipidemia, %	11.7	14.9	16.9	16.2	20.1
Smoking status, %					
Current smoker	28.5	23.4	21.6	18.6	16.1
Former smoker	22.5	26.5	28.0	32.6	33.3
Carbohydrate intake (% of total energy)	40 (7)	42 (7)	43 (7)	44 (7)	48 (7)
Protein intake (% of total energy)	17 (4)	18 (3)	18 (3)	19 (3)	19 (3)
Fat intake (% of total energy)	40 (7)	38 (6)	37 (6)	36 (6)	32 (6)
Olive oil consumption (g/day) **	18 (14)	18 (14)	19 (13)	19 (13)	18 (13)
Fiber intake (g/day) **	16 (3.4)	22 (1.5)	26 (1.6)	31 (2.1)	44 (10.0)
Fruit consumption (g/day) **	144 (116)	246 (143)	312 (159)	407 (219)	604 (419)
Vegetable consumption (g/day) **	271 (138)	397 (151)	493 (176)	601 (218)	863 (458)
Legume consumption (g/day) **	16 (9)	20 (10)	22 (12)	24 (14)	31 (29)
Whole grains (g/day) **	2 (10)	6 (15)	10 (21)	16 (29)	32 (52)
Orange group (portions/week) **	1.8 (2.7)	3.3 (3.5)	4.5 (4.4)	5.7 (5.3)	8.2 (7.7)
Apples/pear (portions/week) **	1.1 (1.5)	1.9 (2.0)	2.5 (2.6)	3.3 (3.4)	5.2 (5.8)
Lutein-rich fruits and vegetables (portions/week) **	0.4 (0.4)	0.6 (0.6)	0.8 (0.7)	1.0 (1.0)	1.7 (1.9)
Cruciferous (portions/week) **	0.3 (0.4)	0.5 (0.5)	0.6 (0.6)	0.8 (0.9)	1.2 (1.6)
Green-leafy vegetables (portions/week) **	2.5 (1.9)	3.6 (2.3)	4.5 (2.5)	5.5 (3.1)	7.8 (5.6)
Lycopene-rich fruits and vegetables (portions/week) **	2.0 (2.1)	3.7 (2.3)	3.7 (2.8)	4.5 (3.1)	6.2 (5.5)
Carotene-rich fruits and vegetables (portions/week) **	1.0 (1.0)	1.7 (1.2)	2.3 (1.5)	3.0 (1.9)	5.1 (4.1)
Vitamin C-rich fruits and vegetables (portions/week) **	3.1 (3.0)	5.0 (3.8)	6.5 (4.6)	8.1 (5.6)	11.5 (8.7)
Alcohol consumption (g/day) **	6.1 (11.7)	5.0 (7.8)	4.3 (6.8)	4.2 (12.9)	3.5 (6.0)
Moderate alcohol consumption (%) **	24.6	22.38	19.43	18.32	15.08
Physical activity (METs-h/week) **	21.6 (19.0)	21.6 (19.0)	22.4 (19.4)	23.3 (20.0)	24.3 (20.0)
Total energy intake (Kcal/day) **	2525 (616)	2283 (591)	2223 (595)	2237 (610)	2420 (610)
MDS (0–9 items) ***	2.7 (1.4)	3.5 (1.5)	4.1 (1.4)	4.8 (1.4)	5.6 (1.4)

* Mean (SD) unless otherwise stated; ** Adjusted for total energy intake by the residual method; *** MDS, Mediterranean diet score [13]; CHD, coronary heart disease; METs, metabolic equivalent of task.

Table 3. Hazard ratios (HRs) (95% confidence intervals) of cardiovascular disease (CVD) according to baseline quintiles (Q) of fiber, fruit, vegetables, pulses, or whole-grain consumption.

	Quintiles of Fiber Intake					
	Q1	Q2	Q3	Q4	Q5	*p* for Trend
N	3402	3401	3402	3401	3401	
Time at risk	33,643	33,107	32,496	32,132	31,381	
# of cases	18	24	22	22	26	
Median g/day	16.76	22.06	26.09	31.12	40.88	
Sex adjusted	1 (ref)	1.24 (0.66–2.30)	0.77 (0.41–1.45)	0.67 (0.36–1.28)	0.57 (0.31–1.06)	0.015
Multivariable adjusted 1	1 (ref)	1.31 (0.70–2.49)	0.81 (0.42–1.57)	0.70 (0.37–1.35)	0.61 (0.32–1.16)	0.025
Multivariable adjusted 2	1 (ref)	1.32 (0.70–2.49)	0.81 (0.42–1.56)	0.70 (0.36–1.35)	0.60 (0.32–1.15)	0.024
	Quintiles of Fruit Consumption					
	Q1	Q2	Q3	Q4	Q5	*p* for Trend
N	3402	3401	3402	3401	3401	
Time at risk	33,824	32,929	32,684	31,714	31,608	
# of cases	23	19	17	25	28	
Median g/day	90	192	280	398	653	
Sex adjusted	1 (ref)	0.60 (0.32–1.11)	0.45 (0.24–0.85)	0.49 (0.28–0.88)	0.45 (0.25–0.81)	0.036
Multivariable adjusted 1	1 (ref)	0.61 (0.32–1.17)	0.48 (0.24–0.94)	0.51 (0.27–0.94)	0.48 (0.26–0.87)	0.057
Multivariable adjusted 3	1 (ref)	0.62 (0.32–1.18)	0.50 (0.26–0.98)	0.54 (0.29–1.00)	0.51 (0.27–0.95)	0.114
	Quintiles of Vegetable Consumption					
	Q1	Q2	Q3	Q4	Q5	*p* for Trend
N	3402	3401	3402	3401	3401	
Time at risk	33,695	32,816	32,870	32,100	31,278	
# of cases	20	24	25	18	25	
Median g/day	209	348	468	609	884	
Sex adjusted	1 (ref)	1.18 (0.65–2.15)	1.06 (0.58–1.92)	0.71 (0.37–1.35)	0.80 (0.44–1.47)	0.191
Multivariable adjusted 1	1 (ref)	1.29 (0.70–2.38)	1.07 (0.58–1.96)	0.77 (0.40–1.48)	0.81 (0.44–1.49)	0.180
Multivariable adjusted 4	1 (ref)	1.37 (0.74–2.54)	1.14 (0.62–2.11)	0.86 (0.44–1.67)	0.96 (0.51–1.82)	0.458

Table 3. *Cont.*

	Q1	Q2	Q3	Q4	Q5	*p* for Trend
Quintiles of Legumes Consumption						
N	3402	3401	3402	3401	3401	
Time at risk	32,311	32,682	32,726	33,244	31,796	
# of cases	26	24	20	15	27	
Median g/day	8.4	15.2	20	25	36	
Sex adjusted	1 (ref)	0.91 (0.52–1.60)	0.78 (0.43–1.40)	0.58 (0.30–1.10)	0.96 (0.59–1.65)	0.674
Multivariable adjusted 1	1 (ref)	0.92 (0.52–1.62)	0.80 (0.44–1.45)	0.58 (0.30–1.11)	0.92 (0.53–1.59)	0.559
Multivariable adjusted 5	1 (ref)	0.95 (0.54–1.68)	0.83 (0.46–1.52)	0.59 (0.31–1.15)	0.95 (0.54–1.66)	0.622
Quintiles of Whole Grains Consumption						
	Q1	Q2	Q3	Q4	Q5	*p* for Trend
N	3402	3401	3402	3401	3401	
Time at risk	34,089	34,090	33,207	32,620	31,255	
# of cases	26	17	25	28	16	
Median g/day	0	0	1.9	5.7	54.7	
Sex adjusted	1 (ref)	0.59 (0.31–1.10)	0.79 (0.45–1.37)	0.71 (0.41–1.22)	0.51 (0.27–0.95)	0.110
Multivariable adjusted 1	1 (ref)	0.49 (0.24–0.99)	0.62 (0.29–1.31)	0.48 (0.20–1.15)	0.40 (0.19–0.86)	0.102
Multivariable adjusted 6	1 (ref)	0.51 (0.25–1.02)	0.64 (0.30–1.36)	0.49 (0.20–1.18)	0.43 (0.20–0.93)	0.149

Note: Multivariable adjusted 1: sex, marital status (five categories), highest attained educational level (five categories), family history of CHD (yes/no), type 2 diabetes (yes/no), high blood pressure (yes/no), dyslipidaemia (yes/no), smoking status (four categories), total energy intake (kcal/day), body mass index, physical activity (METs-h/day), alcohol intake (three categories) and use of lipid-lowering drugs, and stratified by age in decades. Age as underlying time variable. Multivariable adjusted 2: additionally adjusted for and olive oil consumption (g/day). Multivariable adjusted 3: additionally adjusted for olive oil (g/day), vegetables, legumes (g/day), and whole-grains (g/day) consumption. Multivariable adjusted 4: additionally adjusted for olive oil (g/day), fruits (g/day), legumes (g/day), and whole-grains (g/day) consumption. Multivariable adjusted 5: additionally adjusted for olive oil (g/day), fruits (g/day), vegetables (g/day), and whole-grains (g/day) consumption. Multivariable adjusted 6: additionally adjusted for olive oil (g/day), fruits (g/day), vegetables (g/day), and legumes (g/day) consumption.

When we analyzed fiber intake according to its source as exposure, participants in the highest quintile of fruit fiber consumption had the lowest risk of CVD, which was significantly lower than the risk of those in the first quintile (HR 0.52, 95% CI 0.28–0.97). No statistically significant differences were found for other fiber sources.

We found no significant association between legume consumption and CVD.

When we analyzed specific groups of fruits and vegetables, only higher intakes of cruciferous vegetables were associated with CVD with a HR of 0.52 (95% CI 0.30–0.89, $p = 0.16$) for the participants who ate at least one serving/week in comparison with those who did not. We also observed an inverse significant trend in the association between cruciferous vegetable consumption and CVD (Table 4).

Table 4. Hazard ratios (HRs) of CVD according to baseline quintiles (Q) of specific groups of fruits and vegetables consumption. (HR and 95% confidence intervals).

	Q1	Q2	Q3	Q4	Q5	*p* for Trend
Orange Group						
N	3402	3401	3402	3401	3401	
Time at risk	32,607	32,155	32,253	32,686	33,057	
# of cases	21	22	21	21	27	
Median (servings/week)	0.23	1.58	3.09	5.64	15.34	
Sex adjusted	1 (ref)	0.80 (0.43–1.46)	0.73 (0.40–1.34)	0.53 (0.29–0.98)	0.60 (0.34–1.08)	0.166
Multivariable adjusted 1	1 (ref)	0.81 (0.43–1.55)	0.79 (0.42–1.50)	0.56 (0.30–1.05)	0.65 (0.35–1.19)	0.234
Multivariable adjusted 2	1 (ref)	0.81 (0.43–1.56)	0.80 (0.42–1.52)	0.56 (0.30–1.07)	0.65 (0.35–1.20)	0.267
Apple/Pear Group						
	Q1	Q2	Q3	Q4	Q5	*p* for Trend
N	3402	3401	3402	3401	3401	
Time at risk	33,274	32,993	32,058	31,793	32,641	
# of cases	24	16	17	25	30	
Median (servings/week)	0.16	0.79	1.55	3.12	6.68	
Sex adjusted	1 (ref)	0.51 (0.27–0.97)	0.47 (0.25–0.89)	0.75 (0.42–1.32)	0.61 (0.35–1.06)	0.715
Multivariable adjusted 1	1 (ref)	0.46 (0.23–0.92)	0.44 (0.22–0.88)	0.74 (0.41–1.35)	0.61 (0.34–1.08)	0.816
Multivariable adjusted 2	1 (ref)	0.47 (0.24–0.93)	0.45 (0.23–0.91)	0.79 (0.44–1.44)	0.65 (0.37–1.16)	0.997

Table 4. *Cont.*

	Q1	Q2	Q3	Q4	Q5	*p* for Trend
Green Leafy Group						
N	3402	3401	3402	3401	3401	
Time at risk	32,830	32,494	32,226	32,498	32,711	
# of cases	19	23	25	22	23	
Median (servings/week)	1.14	2.81	3.99	6.16	8.21	
Sex adjusted	1 (ref)	1.47 (0.79–2.72)	1.42 (0.77–2.59)	0.90 (0.48–1.66)	0.92 (0.50–1.71)	0.268
Multivariable adjusted 1	1 (ref)	1.48 (0.79–2.77)	1.57 (0.85–2.91)	0.90 (0.48–1.68)	0.97 (0.52–1.80)	0.298
Multivariable adjusted 2	1 (ref)	1.54 (0.82–2.89)	1.61 (0.87–2.99)	0.93 (0.49–1.75)	1.05 (0.56–1.96)	0.431
Cruciferous Group						
	Q1	Q2	Q3	Q4	Q5	*p* for Trend
N	3402	3401	3402	3401	3401	
Time at risk	32,604	32,972	32,488	32,817	31,878	
# of cases	19	26	27	21	19	
Median (servings/week)	0	0.37	0.48	0.93	1.07	
Sex adjusted	1 (ref)	1.03 (0.56–1.88)	1.25 (0.69–2.27)	0.81 (0.43–1.51)	0.56 (0.30–1.08)	0.035
Multivariable adjusted 1	1 (ref)	0.97 (0.52–1.79)	1.35 (0.73–2.47)	0.82 (0.43–1.55)	0.54 (0.28–1.04)	0.033
Multivariable adjusted 2	1 (ref)	0.98 (0.53–1.81)	1.37 (0.75–2.52)	0.83 (0.44–1.58)	0.56 (0.29–1.09)	0.046
Carotene-Rich Fruits and Vegetables						
	Q1	Q2	Q3	Q4	Q5	*p* for Trend
N	3402	3401	3402	3401	3401	
Time at risk	33,385	33,226	32,328	32,002	31,817	
# of cases	25	19	24	20	24	
Median (servings/week)	0.44	1.16	1.78	3–28	5.92	
Sex adjusted	1 (ref)	0.69 (0.38–1.26)	0.82 (0.47–1.45)	0.62 (0.34–1.14)	0.60 (0.33–1.06)	0.111
Multivariable adjusted 1	1 (ref)	0.74 (0.40–1.38)	0.90 (0.50–1.62)	0.67 (0.36–1.24)	0.64 (0.35–1.14)	0.142
Multivariable adjusted 2	1 (ref)	0.77 (0.41–1.43)	0.92 (0.51–1.67)	0.71 (0.38–1.31)	0.68 (0.38–1.23)	0.218
Lutein-Rich Fruits and Vegetables						
	Q1	Q2	Q3	Q4	Q5	*p* for Trend
N	3402	3401	3402	3401	3401	
Time at risk	32,106	32,994	32,316	32,995	32,408	
# of cases	21	23	22	18	27	
Median (servings/week)	0	0.4	0.58	0.98	2.88	
Sex adjusted	1 (ref)	0.90 (0.49–1.65)	0.90 (0.49–1.65)	0.76 (0.40–1.43)	0.76 (0.43–1.36)	0.381
Multivariable adjusted 1	1 (ref)	1.07 (0.58–1.99)	1.0 (0.54–1.87)	0.82 (0.43–1.56)	0.81 (0.45–1.48)	0.354
Multivariable adjusted 2	1 (ref)	1.10 (0.59–2.05)	1.03 (0.56–1.93)	0.84 (0.44–1.60)	0.86 (0.47–1.55)	0.439
Lycopene-Rich Fruits and Vegetables						
	Q1	Q2	Q3	Q4	Q5	*p* for Trend
N	3402	3401	3402	3401	3401	
Time at risk	34,332	33,347	32,602	31,537	31,041	
# of cases	23	26	19	23	21	
Median (servings/week)	0.44	1.91	3.24	4.87	7.23	
Sex adjusted	1 (ref)	1.04 (0.59–1.84)	0.81 (0.44–1.50)	0.78 (0.43–1.39)	0.70 (0.38–1.27)	0.137
Multivariable adjusted 1	1 (ref)	0.98 (0.54–1.76)	0.80 (0.43–1.49)	0.81 (0.44–1.47)	0.69 (0.38–1.28)	0.181
Multivariable adjusted 2	1 (ref)	1.0 (0.55–1.79)	0.8 (0.43–1.49)	0.84 (0.46–1.53)	0.73 (0.40–1.35)	0.249
Vitamin C-rich fruits and vegetables						
	Q1	Q2	Q3	Q3	Q5	*p* for Trend
N	3402	3401	3402	3401	3401	
Time at risk	32,746	32,672	32,371	32,628	32,341	
# of cases	20	21	25	19	27	
Median (servings/week)	1.46	3.4	5.33	7.84	16.41	
Sex adjusted	1 (ref)	0.78 (0.42–1.46)	0.91 (0.50–1.65)	0.55 (0.29–1.03)	0.61 (0.33–1.11)	0.103
Multivariable adjusted 1	1 (ref)	0.79 (0.42–1.53)	0.99 (0.54–1.84)	0.56 (0.29–1.07)	0.66 (0.38–1.22)	0.171
Multivariable adjusted 2	1 (ref)	0.83 (0.43–1.61)	1.00 (0.54–1.86)	0.58 (0.30–1.11)	0.68 (0.37–1.27)	0.191

Note: Multivariable adjusted 1: sex, marital status (five categories), studies (five categories), family history of CHD (yes/no), type 2 diabetes (yes/no), high blood pressure (yes/no), dyslipidemia (yes/no), smoking status (four categories), total energy intake (kc/day), body mass index, physical activity (METs-h/day), alcohol intake (three categories), stratified by age in decades. Age as underlying time variable. Multivariable adjusted 2: additionally adjusted for legumes (g/day), whole-grains (g/day), and olive oil consumption (g/day).

4. Discussion

In this young, highly educated, Mediterranean cohort, we found an inverse association between fiber intake and CVD. This observed association was consistent with previous studies [3,33,34], but the results for fruit and vegetables subtypes, for the different fiber sources, or for rich-fiber foods remain unclear.

We also found an inverse association between fruit consumption and fruit fiber and CVD. Our findings are consistent with various meta-analyses [12,33–37], even though the individual studies seldom reached statistical significance. In a previous work with participants of an old Mediterranean cohort [11], our results suggested that higher fruit consumption was likely to be inversely associated with the future occurrence of CVD, but the results were no longer statistically significant in the multivariable analysis. The EPIC study (European Prospective Investigation into Cancer and Nutrition) that included participants from several Mediterranean countries did not find an association between fruit consumption and cardiovascular mortality either [38]. A meta-analysis [33] found a marginally significant inverse association for each 4 g/day greater intake of fiber fruit with CVD (HR 0.96 (95% CI 0.93–1.00)), but another meta-analysis that included one further publication [3] found a clearly decreased risk of 8% (95% CI 2%–14%) for CHD. None of these meta-analyses included studies with Mediterranean populations. In our work, we also found that consumptions of at least two portions a day of fruit (160 g/day) could be protective against CVD, and higher consumptions did not appear to provide additional protection.

We found no significant association with vegetable consumption nor with fiber from vegetables. Similarly, a recent meta-analysis [3] did not find a statistically significant association between vegetable fiber and CVD. It is also noteworthy that in our study vegetable consumption was very high (mean 525 g/day) and the median of the first quintile was already 209 g/day. Lack of variability in a lower range of vegetable consumption may have precluded us from finding significant associations. In addition, the number of observed cases was low, as expected in this educated, slim, and young Mediterranean cohort. The statistical power of our study would be sufficient only to detect relative risks between extreme quintiles in the range of 0.40–0.55, but not other relative risks closer to the null. However, we expected to find strong associations, on the basis of a previous case-control study conducted by our group [39].

Fruit and vegetables are rich sources of fiber, but they also provide antioxidants, vitamin K, folate, and other phytochemicals—some of them have other micronutrients, thus leading to heterogeneity between the different types. Therefore, some classifications have been suggested according these differences. Nevertheless, studies that have assessed the association between a food or group and CVD are scarce. Oude Griep et al. [40] found no significant association between different varieties of fruits and vegetables and CHD or stroke, but found a strong correlation between the different fruit varieties and total fruit intake (0.72), and a less strong correlation between the different vegetables varieties and total vegetable consumption (0.53). Their results suggest that the quantity of fruit and vegetable consumption may be more relevant than their variety for the prevention of CVD. In a different classification according to the color of vegetables, the same authors [41,42] found a significant protective association with stroke only for white fruits and vegetables; no significant association was observed for CHD. In our analysis, we found an inverse association between cruciferous vegetable consumption and CVD, where eating at least one serving of cruciferous vegetables per week could reduce the risk of CVD by 48%. Our results differ from other studies that found no association between cruciferous vegetables and stroke [12] or CHD [32,43], but are consistent with our results from a previous study on an old Mediterranean cohort [11]. Bendinelli [9] analyzed the association between fruit and vegetable consumption and CHD in a Mediterranean cohort of women, and found an inverse association with green leafy vegetables, which was consistent with other studies [32,44,45], but did not report the results for cruciferous vegetables alone. Cruciferous vegetables contain sulforaphane [7], the most widely studied and best characterized isothiocyanate [46] which is a long-acting antioxidant, but also has anti-inflammatory activity by inhibition of cytokine production. The relationship between sulforaphane and the atherosclerosis process seems to be clear [46]. In animal models, sulforaphane has shown an inverse association with hypertension, diabetes, and diabetes complications [47,48].

A higher consumption of legumes did not have any association with the risk of CVD in our cohort. Legumes are high in vegetable proteins and dietary fiber, and have a low glycemic index. To our knowledge, only Bazzano et al. [49] and Wang et al. [50] reported an inverse association between the consumption of legumes and CVD, with tangible benefits observed for the consumption of legumes at least four times per week. A recently published meta-analysis [51] found an inverse association between legume consumption and CHD (HR 0.90 CI 95% 0.84–0.97). Additionally, the authors of this latter meta-analysis also found a marginally significant association between legume consumption and CVD (HR 0.94 CI 95% 0.89–1.00). Our participants had a high legume consumption (median in the fifth quintile: 36 g/day) and a priori we expected to find a risk reduction. Legumes are an important food in the Mediterranean diet and Trichopoulou et al. [13] found that the observed inverse association between adherence to the Mediterranean diet and cardiovascular mortality was toned down when legumes were taken out from their score. Another meta-analysis [52] conducted with 20 studies that analyzed the association between adherence to the Mediterranean diet or its individual components and CVD also found an inverse association between legume consumption and CVD (HR 0.90 CI 95% 0.83–0.98). Our results are similar in the magnitude and the direction of the association, but we did not achieve statistical significance. Again, the low number of cases could explain this result. Moreover, there are important differences in composition across legumes in macronutrients [53] (specifically in their protein content), fiber content, micronutrients, and phytochemicals, which could also explain the differences across different cohorts. Additionally, there are differences in the way they are cooked in the different Mediterranean countries, which could also contribute to the diverse results in the different studies.

We found an inverse association between whole grain consumption and risk of CVD (HR for the fifth vs. first quintile of 0.43 (95% CI 0.20–0.93)). Our study is consistent with a meta-analysis of ten cohort studies [21] that found an inverse association between whole grain consumption and risk of CHD, stroke, and CVD, with no evidence of linearity and with a stronger risk reduction from no consumption up to 50 g/day than with higher intakes. Most of the studies included in the last meta-analysis were from USA, only one of the included cohorts originating from a Mediterranean setting, and even then, only cardiovascular mortality was assessed. We found no association between whole grain consumption and CVD in a cohort with older Mediterranean participants [11].

Different plant foods, including fruits, vegetables, and whole grains among others, have their distinctive phytochemical contents. These distinctive phytochemicals have different biochemical properties, such as molecular size and solubility [5]. All these properties will affect the interactions between the various biochemicals and thus their antioxidant or anti-inflammatory effect. Also, different plant-based foods contain different fiber types. Eating a wide variety of fruits, vegetables, whole grains, and other plant foods and following a health dietary pattern—like the Mediterranean diet—has been postulated as being more important for CVD prevention than eating isolated food items [54]. A recent meta-analysis has shed light on this association [52], finding that some of the individual components did not achieve significance, but that the overall diet decreased CVD disease rates.

We acknowledge that our study may have some limitations. First, our participants have a high educational level, and are young and predominantly females, potentially limiting the generalizability of our results. However, the high educational level of our participants enhances the quality of their self-reported information and increases the internal validity of our results. In addition, lack of representativeness does not preclude from finding associations valid for other populations [55]. In fact, there are no biological mechanisms that suggest that our observed associations may no longer hold for other populations. Finally, literature on the covered topic in middle-aged cohort was previously absent. Second, the use of a validated FFQ does not rule out the existence of an information bias, but it has good or reasonable correlation coefficients for the considered exposures. Since the possible measurement error in the assessment of diet is expected to be non-differential, it would presumably bias our results towards the null value. Third, the absence of repeated measurements may have also led to a misclassification bias, because our participants may have experienced changes in their consumption along the follow-up. Fourth, we might have missed some CVD events. Nevertheless, all of our participants are university graduates, who are highly educated and highly motivated, and more than half of them are health professionals, thereby reducing the risk of underreporting. Additionally, we regularly consulted the National Death Index. Fifth, the incidence of CVD was low in our cohort. Thus, we may have low statistical power to assess associations, especially in adjusted models. Nevertheless, it is noteworthy that the point estimates hardly changed with successive adjustment and that the point estimates point towards the a priori expected association based on the available literature. Finally, observing significant associations may have been hindered by a considerably high consumption of healthy foods in the lowest quintiles, compared to other available studies. High consumption of the considered food items may show protective effects when compared to really low consumptions, but may show no additional protection beyond moderate consumptions.

The major strengths of the current study include its prospective design, its relatively large sample and long-term follow-up, and its high retention rate. Another potential strength is the use of a validated FFQ, with good correlations with the analyzed foods. Moreover, we adjusted the models for a wide array of potential confounders, in an attempt to control for potential confounders.

In conclusion, consumptions of at least two servings/day of fruit, and one serving/week of cruciferous vegetables or whole grains may be protective against CVD in young Mediterranean populations.

Acknowledgments: The authors are indebted to the participants of the SUN study for their continued cooperation and participation. We are also grateful to the members of the Department of Nutrition of the Harvard School of Public Health (Willett WC, Hu FB, and Ascherio A) who helped us to design the SUN study. We also thank the other members of the SUN Group: Alonso A, Barrio López MT, Basterra-Gortari FJ, Benito Corchón S, Bes-Rastrollo M, Beunza JJ, Carlos Chillerón S, Carmona L, Cervantes S, de Irala Estévez J, de la Rosa PA, Delgado Rodríguez M, Donat Vargas CL, Donázar M, Fernández Montero A, Galbete Ciáurriz C, García López M, Gea A, Goñi Ochandorena E, Guillén Grima F, Hernández A, Lahortiga F, Llorca J, López del Burgo C, Marí Sanchís A, Martí del Moral A, Martín Calvo N, Martínez JA, Núñez-Córdoba JM, Pimenta AM, Ramallal R, Ruiz Zambrana A, Sánchez Adán D, Sayón Orea C, Toledo Atucha J, Vázquez Ruiz Z, and Zazpe García I. The SUN Project has received funding from the Spanish Government-Instituto de Salud Carlos III, and the European Regional Development Fund (FEDER) (RD 06/0045, CIBER-OBN, Grants PI10/02658, PI10/02293, PI13/00615, PI14/01668, PI14/01798, PI14/01764, and G03/140), the Navarra Regional Government (45/2011, 122/2014), and the University of Navarra.

Author Contributions: M.A.M.-G. and M.R.-C. conceived and designed the experiments; J.D.-E. and A.G.-A. contributed to data collection; P.B.-C. and E.T. analyzed the data and wrote the paper. All authors have revised the manuscript critically for important intellectual content and have given final approval of the version to be published.

References

1. Mozaffarian, D.; Benjamin, E.J.; Go, A.S.; Arnett, D.K.; Blaha, M.J.; Cushman, M.; Das, S.H.; De Ferranti, S.; Despres, J.D.; Fullerton, H.J.; et al. Heart Disease and Stroke Statistics—2016 Update. *Circulation* **2016**, *133*, e38–e360. [CrossRef] [PubMed]
2. World Health Organization. Global Health Observatory (GHO) data. *World Health Statistics 2016: Monitoring health for the SDGs*. Available online: http://www.who.int/gho/publications/world_health_statistics/2016/en/ (accessed on 16 March 2017).
3. Wu, Y.; Qian, Y.; Pan, Y.; Li, P.; Yang, J.; Ye, X.; Xu, G. Association between dietary fiber intake and risk of coronary heart disease: A meta-analysis. *Clin. Nutr.* **2015**, *34*, 603–611. [CrossRef] [PubMed]
4. Wang, S.; Moustaid-Moussa, N.; Chen, L.; Mo, H.; Shastri, A.; Su, R.; Bapak, P.; KWun, J.; Shen, C.L. Novel insights of dietary polyphenols and obesity. *J. Nutr. Biochem.* **2014**, *25*, 1–18. [CrossRef] [PubMed]
5. Liu, R.H. Health-promoting components of fruits and vegetables in the Diet. *Adv. Nutr.* **2013**, *4*, 384S–392S. [CrossRef] [PubMed]
6. Liu, R.H. Potential synergy of phytochemicals in cancer prevention: Mechanism of action. *J. Nutr.* **2004**, *134*, 3479S–3485S. [PubMed]
7. Rodriguez-Casado, A. The health potential of fruits and vegetables phytochemicals: Notable examples. *Crit. Rev. Food Sci. Nutr.* **2014**. [CrossRef] [PubMed]
8. Gan, Y.; Tong, X.; Li, L.; Cao, S.; Yin, X.; Gao, C.; Merath, C.; Li, W.; Jin, Z.; Chen, Y.; et al. Consumption of fruit and vegetable and risk of coronary heart disease: A meta-analysis of prospective cohort studies. *Int. J. Cardiol.* **2015**, *183*, 129–137. [CrossRef] [PubMed]

9. Bendinelli, B.; Masala, G.; Saieva, C.; Salvini, S.; Calonico, C.; Sacerdote, C.; Agnoli, C.; Grioni, S.; Frasca, G.; Mattiello, A.; et al. Fruit, vegetables, and olive oil and risk of coronary heart disease in Italian women: The EPICOR Study. *Am. J. Clin. Nutr.* **2011**, *93*, 275–283. [CrossRef] [PubMed]
10. Buil-Cosiales, P.; Zazpe, I.; Toledo, E.E.; Corella, D.; Salas-Salvadó, J.; Diez-Espino, J.; Ros, E.; Fernandez-Creuet Navajas, J.; Santos-Lozano, J.M.; Aros, F.; et al. Dietary Fiber intake and all-cause mortality in the Prevencio (PREDIMED) study Mediterra. *Am. J. Clin. Nutr.* **2014**, *100*, 1498–1507. [CrossRef] [PubMed]
11. Buil-Cosiales, P.; Toledo, E.; Salas-Salvadó, J.; Zazpe, I.; Farràs, M.; Basterra-Gortari, F.J.; Diez-Espino, J.; Estruch, R.; Corella, D.; Ros, E.; et al. Association between dietary fibre intake and fruit, vegetable or whole-grain consumption and the risk of CVD: Results from the PREvención con DIeta MEDiterránea (PREDIMED) trial. *Br. J. Nutr.* **2016**, *1*, 1–13. [CrossRef] [PubMed]
12. Hu, D.; Huang, J.; Wang, Y.; Zhang, D.; Qu, Y. Fruits and vegetables consumption and risk of stroke: A meta-analysis of prospective cohort studies. *Stroke* **2014**, *45*, 1613–1619. [CrossRef] [PubMed]
13. Trichopoulou, A.; Bamia, C.; Trichopoulos, D. Anatomy of health effects of Mediterranean diet: Greek EPIC prospective cohort study. *BMJ* **2009**, *338*, b2337. [CrossRef] [PubMed]
14. Nagura, J.; Iso, H.; Watanabe, Y.; Maruyama, K.; Date, C.; Toyoshima, H.; Yamamoto, A.; Kikuchi, S.; Koizumi, A.; Kondal, T.; et al. Fruit, vegetable and bean intake and mortality from cardiovascular disease among Japanese men and women: The JACC Study. *Br. J. Nutr.* **2009**, *102*, 285–292. [CrossRef] [PubMed]
15. Flight, I.; Clifton, P. Cereal grains and legumes in the prevention of coronary heart disease and stroke: A review of the literature. *Eur. J. Clin. Nutr.* **2006**, *60*, 1145–1159. [CrossRef] [PubMed]
16. De Munter, J.S.L.; Hu, F.B.; Spiegelman, D.; Franz, M.; Van Dam, R.M. Whole grain, bran, and germ intake and risk of type 2 diabetes: A prospective cohort study and systematic review. *PLoS Med.* **2007**, *4*, 1385–1395. [CrossRef] [PubMed]
17. Ye, E.; Chacko, S.; Chou, E.; Kugizaki, M.; Liu, S. Greater whole-grain intake is associated with lower risk of type 2 diabetes, cardiovascular disease, and weight gain. *J. Nutr.* **2012**, *142*, 1304–1313. [CrossRef] [PubMed]
18. Leinonen, K.S.; Poutanen, K.S.; Mykkänen, H.M. Rye bread decreases serum total and LDL cholesterol in men with moderately elevated serum cholesterol. *J. Nutr.* **2000**, *130*, 164–170. [PubMed]
19. Ha, V.; Sievenpiper, J.L.; de Souza, R.J.; Jayalath, V.H.; Mirrahimi, A.; Agarwal, A.; Chiavaroli, L.; Mejia, S.B.; Sacks, F.H.; Di Buono, M.; et al. Effect of dietary pulse intake on established therapeutic review and meta-analysis of randomized controlled trials. *Can. Med. Assoc. J.* **2014**, *186*, 252–262. [CrossRef] [PubMed]
20. Kirwan, J.P.; Malin, S.K.; Scelsi, A.R.; Kullman, E.L.; Navaneethan, S.D.; Haus, J.M.; Fillion, J.; Godin, J.P.; Kochher, S.; Ross, A.B. A whole grain diet reduces cardiovascular risk factors in overweight and obese adults: A randomized controlled trial. *J. Nutr.* **2016**, *146*, 2244–2251. [CrossRef] [PubMed]
21. Aune, D.; Keum, N.; Giovannucci, E.; Fadnes, L.T.; Boffetta, P.; Greenwood, D.C.; Tonstad, S.; Vatten, L.J.; Riboli, E.; Narat, T. Whole grain consumption and risk of cardiovascular disease, cancer, and all cause and cause specific mortality: Systematic review and dose-response meta-analysis of prospective studies. *BMJ* **2016**, *353*, i2716. [CrossRef] [PubMed]
22. Bouchenak, M.; Lamri-Senhadji, M. Nutritional quality of legumes, and their role in cardiometabolic risk prevention: A review. *J. Med. Food* **2013**, *16*, 1–14. [CrossRef] [PubMed]
23. Hosseinpour-Niazi, S.; Mirmiran, P.; Amiri, Z.; Hosseini-Esfahani, F.; Shakeri, N.; Azizi, F. Legume intake is inversely associated with metabolic syndrome in adults. *Arch. Iran. Med.* **2012**, *15*, 538–544. [PubMed]
24. Seguí-Gómez, M.; de la Fuente, C.; Vázquez, Z.; de Irala, J.; Martínez-González, M.A. Cohort profile: The "Seguimiento Universidad de Navarra" (SUN) study. *Int. J. Epidemiol.* **2006**, *35*, 1417–1422. [CrossRef] [PubMed]
25. The British Geriatrics Society. Fit for Frailty-Consensus Best Practice Guidance for the Care of Older People Living in Community and Outpatient Settings-a Report from the British Geriatrics Society 2014. Available online: http://www.bgs.org.uk/campaigns/fff/fff_full.pdf (accessed on 15 March 2017).
26. Eguaras, S.; Toledo, E.; Hernández-Hernández, A.; Cervantes, S.; Martínez-González, M.A. Better adherence to the mediterranean diet could mitigate the adverse consequences of obesity on cardiovascular disease: The SUN prospective cohort. *Nutrients* **2015**, *7*, 9154–9162. [CrossRef] [PubMed]
27. Alonso, A.; Beunza, J.J.; Delgado-Rodríguez, M.; Martínez-González, M.A. Validation of self reported diagnosis of hypertension in a cohort of university graduates in Spain. *BMC Public Health* **2005**, *5*, 94. [CrossRef] [PubMed]

28. Fernandez-Montero, A.; Beunza, J.J.; Bes-Rastrollo, M.; Barrio, M.T.; de la Fuente-Arrillaga, C.; Moreno-Galarraga, L.; Martinez-Gonzalez, M.A. Validacion de los componentes del sindrome metabolico autodeclarados en un estudio de cohortes. *Gac. Sanit.* **2011**, *25*, 303–307. (In Spanish) [CrossRef] [PubMed]
29. Willett, W.C. Implications of total energy intake for epidemiologic analyses. In *Nutritional Epidemiology*, 3rd ed.; Willett, W.C., Ed.; Oxford University Press: New York, NY, USA, 2013.
30. Martin-Moreno, J.M.; Boyle, P.; Gorgojo, L.; Maisonneuve, P.; Fernandez-Rodriguez, J.C.; Salvini, S.; Willet, W.C. Development and validation of a food frequency questionnaire in Spain. *Int. J. Epidemiol.* **1993**, *22*, 512–519. [CrossRef] [PubMed]
31. Fernández-Ballart, J.D.; Piñol, J.L.; Zazpe, I.; Corella, D.; Carrasco, P.; Toledo, E.; Perez-Bauer, M.; Fernandez-Gonzalez, M.A.; Salas-Salvado, J.; Martin-Moreno, J.M. Relative validity of a semi-quantitative food-frequency questionnaire in an elderly Mediterranean population of Spain. *Br. J. Nutr.* **2010**, *103*, 1808–1816. [CrossRef] [PubMed]
32. Joshipura, K.J.; Hu, F.B.; Manson, J.E.; Stampfer, M.J.; Rimm, E.B.; Speizer, F.E.; Colditz, G.; Ascherio, A.; Rossner, B.; Spiegelman, D.; et al. The effect of fruit and vegetable intake on risk for coronary heart disease. *Ann. Intern. Med.* **2001**, *134*, 1106–1114. [CrossRef] [PubMed]
33. Threapleton, D.E.; Greenwood, D.C.; Evans, C.E.L.; Cleghorn, C.L.; Nykjaer, C.; Woodhead, C.; Cade, J.E.; Gale, C.P.; Burley, V.J. Dietary fibre intake and risk of cardiovascular disease: Systematic review and meta-analysis. *BMJ* **2013**, *347*, f6879. [CrossRef] [PubMed]
34. Dauchet, L.; Amouyel, P.; Hercberg, S.; Dallongeville, J. Fruit and vegetable consumption and risk of coronary heart disease: A meta-analysis of cohort studies. *J. Nutr.* **2006**, *136*, 2588–2593. [PubMed]
35. Chen, G.-C.C.; Lv, D.-B.B.; Pang, Z.; Dong, J.-Y.Y.; Liu, Q.-F.F. Dietary fiber intake and stroke risk: A meta-analysis of prospective cohort studies. *Eur. J. Clin. Nutr.* **2013**, *67*, 96–100. [CrossRef] [PubMed]
36. He, F.J.; Nowson, C.A.; MacGregor, G.A. Fruit and vegetable consumption and stroke: Meta-analysis of cohort studies. *Lancet* **2006**, *367*, 320–326. [CrossRef]
37. Dauchet, L.; Amouyel, P.; Dallongeville, J. Fruit and vegetable consumption and risk of stroke: A meta-analysis of cohort studies. *Neurology* **2005**, *65*, 1193–1197. [CrossRef] [PubMed]
38. Leenders, M.; Sluijs, I.; Ros, M.M.; Boshuizen, H.C.; Siersema, P.D.; Ferrari, P.; Weikert, C.; Tjonneland, A.; Olsen, D.; Boutron-Ruault, M.C. Fruit and vegetable consumption and mortality European prospective investigation into cancer and nutrition. *Am. J. Epidemiol.* **2013**. [CrossRef] [PubMed]
39. Martínez-González, M.A.; Fernández-Jarne, E.; Martínez-Losa, E.; Prado-Santamaría, M.; Brugarolas-Brufau, C.; Serrano-Martinez, M. Role of fibre and fruit in the Mediterranean diet to protect against myocardial infarction: A case-control study in Spain. *Eur. J. Clin. Nutr.* **2002**, *56*, 715–722. [CrossRef] [PubMed]
40. Oude Griep, L.M.; Verschuren, W.M.; Kromhout, D.; Ocké, M.C.; Geleijnse, J.M. Variety in fruit and vegetable consumption and 10-year incidence of CHD and stroke. *Public Health Nutr.* **2012**, 1–7. [CrossRef] [PubMed]
41. Oude Griep, L.M.; Verschuren, W.M.M.; Kromhout, D.; Ocké, M.C.; Geleijnse, J.M. Colors of fruit and vegetables and 10-year incidence of stroke. *Stroke* **2011**, *42*, 3190–3195. [CrossRef] [PubMed]
42. Oude Griep, L.M.; Monique Verschuren, W.M.; Kromhout, D.; Ocké, M.C.; Geleijnse, J.M. Colours of fruit and vegetables and 10-year incidence of CHD. *Br. J. Nutr.* **2011**, *106*, 1562–1569. [CrossRef] [PubMed]
43. Bhupathiraju, S.N.; Wedick, N.M.; Pan, A.; Manson, J.E.; Rexrode, K.M.; Willett, W.C.; Rimm, E.B.; Hu, F.B. Quantity and variety in fruit and vegetable intake and risk of coronary heart disease. *Am. J. Clin. Nutr.* **2013**. [CrossRef] [PubMed]
44. Joshipura, K.J.; Ascherio, A.; Manson, J.E.; Stampfer, M.J.; Rimm, E.B.; Speizer, F.E.; Mennkens, C.H.; Spiegelmam, D.; Willet, W.C. Fruit and vegetable intake in relation to risk of ischemic stroke. *JAMA* **1999**, *282*, 1233–1239. [CrossRef] [PubMed]
45. Pollock, R.L. The effect of green leafy and cruciferous vegetable intake on the incidence of cardiovascular disease: A meta-analysis. *JRSM Cardiovasc. Dis.* **2016**, *5*, 1–9. [CrossRef] [PubMed]
46. Bai, Y.; Wang, X.; Zhao, S.; Ma, C.; Cui, J.; Zheng, Y. Sulforaphane Protects against Cardiovascular Disease via Nrf2 Activation. *Oxid. Med. Cell. Longev.* **2015**. [CrossRef] [PubMed]
47. Bahadoran, Z.; Mirmiran, P.; Hosseinpanah, F.; Rajab, A.; Asghari, G.; Azizi, F. Broccoli sprouts powder could improve serum triglyceride and oxidized LDL/LDL-cholesterol ratio in type 2 diabetic patients: A randomized double-blind placebo-controlled clinical trial. *Diabetes Res. Clin. Pract.* **2012**, *96*, 348–354. [CrossRef] [PubMed]

48. Bahadoran, Z.; Tohidi, M.; Nazeri, P.; Mehran, M.; Azizi, F.; Mirmiran, P. Effect of broccoli sprouts on insulin resistance in type 2 diabetic patients: A randomized double-blind clinical trial. *Int. J. Food Sci. Nutr.* **2012**, *63*, 767–771. [CrossRef] [PubMed]
49. Bazzano, L.A.; He, J.; Ogden, L.G.; Loria, C.; Vupputuri, S.; Myers, L.; Whelton, P.K. Legume Consumption and Risk of Coronary Heart Disease in US Men and Women. *Arch. Intern. Med.* **2001**, *161*, 2573. [CrossRef] [PubMed]
50. Wang, J.-B.; Fan, J.-H.; Dawsey, S.M.; Sinha, R.; Freedman, N.D.; Taylor, P.R.; Qiao, Y.-L.; Abnet, C.C. Dietary components and risk of total, cancer and cardiovascular disease mortality in the Linxian Nutrition Intervention Trials cohort in China. *Sci. Rep.* **2016**, *6*, 22619. [CrossRef] [PubMed]
51. Marventano, S.; Izquierdo Pulido, M.; Sánchez-González, C.; Godos, J.; Speciani, A.; Galvano, F.; Grosso, G. Legume consumption and CVD risk: A systematic review and meta-analysis. *Public Health Nutr.* **2017**, *20*, 245–254. [CrossRef] [PubMed]
52. Grosso, G.; Marventano, S.; Yang, J.; Micek, A.; Pajak, A.; Scalfi, L.; Galvano, F.; Kales, S.N. A comprehensive meta-analysis on evidence of Mediterranean diet and cardiovascular disease: Are individual components equal? *Crit. Rev. Food Sci. Nutr.* **2015**. [CrossRef] [PubMed]
53. Ros, E.; Hu, F.B. Consumption of plant seeds and cardiovascular health: Epidemiological and clinical trial evidence. *Circulation* **2013**, *128*, 553–565. [CrossRef] [PubMed]
54. Martínez-González, M.A.; Gea, A. Mediterranean diet: The whole is more than the sum of its parts. *Br. J. Nutr.* **2012**, *108*, 577–578. [CrossRef] [PubMed]
55. Rothman, K.J. Six persistent research misconceptions. *J. Gen. Intern. Med.* **2014**, *29*, 1060–1064. [CrossRef] [PubMed]

5

Toward a Personalized Approach in Prebiotics Research

Moul Dey

Department of Health and Nutritional Sciences, Box 2203, South Dakota State University, Brookings, SD 57007, USA; Moul.Dey@sdstate.edu;

Abstract: Recent characterization of the human microbiome and its influences on health have led to dramatic conceptual shifts in dietary bioactives research. Prebiotic foods that include many dietary fibers and resistant starches are perceived as beneficial for maintaining a healthy gut microbiota. This article brings forward some current perspectives in prebiotic research to discuss why reporting of individual variations in response to interventions will be important to discern suitability of prebiotics as a disease prevention tool.

Keywords: prebiotics; disease prevention; dietary bioactives; resistant starch type 4; intervention response variability

---

The ancient Greek physician Hippocrates perceived food as the key player in the maintenance of health, not just as a fuel to run the human body. Since then, scientists have probed deeper into the role of diet in nutrient absorption and bodily function. In the late 1800s, scientists began isolating microorganisms from different parts of the human body including from the digestive tract. Some of these organisms were considered harmful and others beneficial. However, the concept of the human microbiome and its critical role in human health and diseases is more recent, emerging in the 21st century after the advent of next generation sequencing. Mapping microbiome diversity has unlocked many mysteries—but also triggered new questions. The answers to many such questions still elude us, including a very basic but pressing question, "what diet is ideal for a healthy gut microbiome?" It remains unknown if there is an ideal gut microbiome that can be considered "healthy", nor do we know of one ideal diet that can positively manipulate the microbiome of people of all ages across the globe. Furthermore, a plethora of contradictory research findings on what dietary component may or may not be healthy frequently confuse the public. Not too long ago, dietary fat used to be our worst enemy. With time, that spot was taken over by dietary sugars. Another example is soy, with its many known health benefits and a host of negative side effects [1]. While the reasons behind contradictory nutritional research are multi-faceted, one contributing factor may be researchers designing studies like modern medical research that predominantly aims for disease-specific diagnostic and therapeutic avenues. Scientists prioritize collective outcomes with high statistical significance. While these benchmarks are a sign of a successful clinical trial, individual responses to the dietary treatment are often ignored. For example, recently Zeevi et al. reported widespread and high interpersonal variability in post-prandial glucose response among healthy participants to common dietary components [2]. It is possible that researchers in dietary intervention studies frequently encounter similar variations, but they are under-reported.

Prebiotics are selectively fermented dietary ingredients such as resistant starches and some dietary fibers that change the composition and/or activity of the gastrointestinal microbiota, thus conferring benefits to the host's health [3]. While this newer type of functional food is increasingly popular, a recent systematic review of six prebiotic trials published before 6 November 2015 suggests that more randomized controlled trials are needed to support their clinical use [4]. More recently our group reported a microbiome signature in response to a resistant starch type 4 (RS4)-enriched diet in individuals with metabolic syndrome (NCT01887964, [5]). It was concluded that RS4 has prebiotic effects with a potential for metabolic disease prevention. This double-blind and placebo-controlled study is among a small number of prebiotic intervention studies conducted under a free-living setting reporting statistically significant changes across microbial composition and abundance, fecal short chain fatty acid levels, and host immunometabolic functions in response to RS4 consumption. More frequently, intervention studies end up being inconclusive or lack statistical power due to wide variability in responses among participants, particularly when conducted within natural living conditions [6]. Interestingly in our study, although statistical significance across most endpoints was observed, response variability was commonplace for bacterial abundance and metabolites as well as clinical endpoints in the host. Relative to average Americans, the study population (Hutterites living in eastern South Dakota) was more genetically homogeneous and had fewer differences in daily lifestyle due to their communal style of living. Their variability in microbiome response, however, came as little surprise. In earlier reports, microbiota varied both in steady state conditions and in response to diet, aging, and other lifestyle changes [7–9]. Quite possibly, a deeper mechanistic investigation on how RS4 functions at the molecular level may shed some light on such response variations in the future. However, here the author focusses on one other question that emerges from all of this: will it benefit the scientific community in the long run if such side observations of response variability are routinely reported? Is it possible that we are missing out on information that may hold the key to unlocking some of the mysteries of diet and the microbiome interactions by not reporting individual responses to dietary interventions? Currently, there is little enthusiasm from both scientists and publishers to report such information, as data without statistical significance would rarely contribute to the conclusions drawn from the work. The viewpoint is illustrated in Figure 1. We observed increases in *Ruminococcus lactaris* and *Eubacterium oxidoreducens* in the RS4 group compared to baseline and post-CF (control group, CF) [5]. The most common format for reporting such data is mean % change or fold change along with the *p*-value. Less frequently, individual data points with column means and associated descriptive statistical information are shown (Figure 1B,C). Collective data presentation formats, such as the one shown in Figure 1A, are less helpful in revealing the distinct nature of the two datasets.

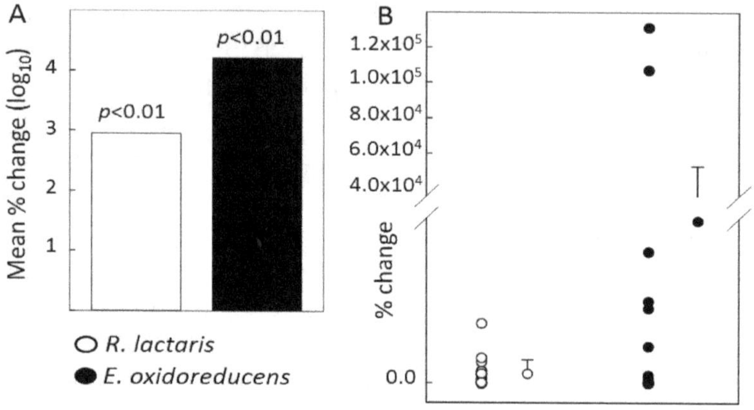

C

	R. lactaris	*E. oxidoreducens*
Sample size	19.0	19.0
Mean % change from baseline	901.5	15736.7
Std deviation	1378.9	37234.9
Std error	316.4	8542.3
C.I. of mean	664.6	17946.7
Range of change	5858.8	131,000.0
Maximum effect	5800.0	131,000.0
Minimum effect	-58.8 (decreased)	0.0
Median	437.5	135.7

Figure 1. Data presentation formats. (**A**) Relative abundance of two bacterial species before and after RS4 treatment shown as mean % change (log_{10}) with corresponding *p* values; (**B**) Percent change from before intervention of the same two bacterial species shown as individual data points with means and standard deviations on the side; (**C**) Descriptive statistical information from the two data sets presented in A and B. The information presented in the last four rows are less frequently reported in clinical trial publications.

Assessing disease risk in susceptible populations remains one major objective of personalized or precision nutrition, allowing for stratifications of subpopulations in a manner that improves the accuracy and cost-effectiveness of interventions and follow-ups. In addition, early prognosis and/or diagnosis may facilitate prophylactic treatment that would otherwise be unsuitable for a larger population. In this context, Zeevi et al. has proposed a machine-learning algorithm approach that integrates multiple features based on a preexisting large cohort data set to predict, for example, glycemic response to real-life meals [2]. While they have reported feasibility, cost-effectiveness of such an approach has not been determined. It must be taken into consideration that no one outcome alone, such as glycemic response, determines the overall health outcome of an individual. For example, being able to predict glycemic response may attenuate the risk of type 2 diabetes, but will not help with the prognosis of hyperlipidemia, heart disease, or cancer. Therefore, many large-scale endeavors, such as those reported by Zeevi et al., will be necessary to predict multiple clinical end-points or intermediate biomarkers before personalized overall health risk determination followed by preventive intervention is possible. For similar reasons, personalized microbiome profiling, while deemed promising as a tool for disease risk stratification, is not ready for translation to a clinical setting. It is only proposed that a predictive microbiome modeling system with more sophisticated readouts integrating multiple aspects of gut microbiota (composition, abundance, metagenomics, meta-transcriptomic, metabolomics, etc.) should be incorporated [10]. In addition, microbiome-based biomarkers for personalized prognostic, diagnostic, and treatment may vary by geographic locations, lifestyle, and many other factors. Therefore, while personalized microbiome profiling may be useful for predicting and mitigating disease, it will take a huge scientific undertaking before it is ready for the clinical setting.

In the past few decades, there has been a surge in metabolic diseases that affect quality of life and pose a substantial medical and economic burden on society. There is a growing interest in preventive measures to modify the risk of metabolic diseases, with diet proposed as a major player in public health promotion. Decades of generalized nutritional recommendations do not seem to be mitigating the metabolic health crisis, although at present there is no alternate to an overall healthy diet and regular physical activity recommendation for long-term health maintenance. Mounting evidence suggests a more personalized approach is required for health promotion through disease prevention and that such personalization cannot entirely rely on human genomic variations in case of complex metabolic diseases. Even taking into account the huge undertaking discussed above, current knowledge about the microbiome suggests that integrating microbiome profiling into patient care will likely allow for a faster, more accurate, and less invasive clinical decision-making processes. In this context, prebiotics will be critical components of personally tailored dietary interventions aimed at altering the microbiome to a more beneficial configuration for disease prevention. While the benefits of dietary fibers, many of which have prebiotic properties, are well-known, their mechanisms of action mostly remain a mystery. Without the knowledge of structure-function relationships between various prebiotics and microbial species as well as further consideration of the bilateral relationship of the microbiome and the host, personalized and effective use of prebiotics for disease prevention will be difficult. Large-scale characterization of the nutrition-microbiome-host metabolism axis will help delineate the integration of prebiotics in personalized diets for prevention of multi-factorial metabolic diseases. One caveat toward such effort is that disease prevention trials typically focus on intermediate outcomes because long-term follow-up of a large enough population, that will both adhere to the intervention as well as provide sufficient statistical power to detect differences, is technically difficult and prohibitively expensive. Regrettably, intermediate outcome measures do not always reflect the true preventive potential of an intervention as reported from the Look AHEAD (Action for Health in Diabetes) trial [11].

Looking to the future, it will be critical to consider the collective effects that are statistically significant, as well as individual response variations, for harnessing the many potential health benefits of prebiotics. Encouraging the scientific community to report variations observed in clinical trials, even if such observations may not meaningfully contribute to the main conclusions of the current study, will be important. Such data may be presented in formats that allow more holistic visualization of study results, including but not limited to, effect sizes, percentile ranking, minimum and maximum values, outliers, means, and medians. A recent commentary in Nature Methods discussed similar data presentation approaches in lieu of sample-to-sample variability and irreproducibility of scientific data, particularly in biomedical disciplines [12]. In addition to that, the author believes, this may also provide an opportunity to build on the vast repertoire of individual response variations that may not otherwise be possible for any one research study to capture. How such data may precisely inform clinical study designs and/or results in the future will depend on effective systematic reviews and meta-analysis outcome from the growing body of such data sets. Nevertheless, the author is hopeful that the information generated will facilitate better predictability of microbial and/or host-physiological response behavior in the direction of early prognosis and prevention.

Acknowledgments: The author's laboratory is currently supported by USDA National Institute of Food and Agriculture Hatch grant [1004817] as well as state and industry grants. No funding was directly utilized toward preparation of this manuscript.

References

1. Messina, M. Soy and Health Update: Evaluation of the Clinical and Epidemiologic Literature. *Nutrients* **2016**, *8*, 754. [CrossRef] [PubMed]
2. Zeevi, D.; Korem, T.; Zmora, N.; Israeli, D.; Rothschild, D.; Weinberger, A.; Ben-Yacov, O.; Lador, D.; Avnit-Sagi, T.; Lotan-Pompan, M.; et al. Personalized Nutrition by Prediction of Glycemic Responses. *Cell* **2015**, *163*, 1079–1094. [CrossRef] [PubMed]
3. Roberfroid, M.; Gibson, G.R.; Hoyles, L.; McCartney, A.L.; Rastall, R.; Rowland, I.; Wolvers, D.; Watzl, B.; Szajewska, H.; Stahl, B.; et al. Prebiotic effects: Metabolic and health benefits. *Br. J. Nutr.* **2010**, *104*, S1–S63. [CrossRef] [PubMed]
4. Fernandes, R.; do Rosario, V.A.; Mocellin, M.C.; Kuntz, M.G.; Trindade, E.B. Effects of inulin-type fructans, galacto-oligosaccharides and related synbiotics on inflammatory markers in adult patients with overweight or obesity: A systematic review. *Clin. Nutr.* **2016**. [CrossRef] [PubMed]
5. Upadhyaya, B.; McCormack, L.; Fardin-Kia, A.R.; Juenemann, R.; Clapper, J.; Specker, B.; Dey, M. Impact of dietary resistant starch type 4 on human gut microbiota and immunometabolic functions. *Sci. Rep.* **2016**, *6*, 28797. [CrossRef] [PubMed]
6. Satija, A.; Yu, E.; Willett, W.C.; Hu, F.B. Understanding nutritional epidemiology and its role in policy. *Adv. Nutr.* **2015**, *6*, 5–18. [CrossRef] [PubMed]
7. Eckburg, P.B.; Bik, E.M.; Bernstein, C.N.; Purdom, E.; Dethlefsen, L.; Sargent, M.; Gill, S.R.; Nelson, K.E.; Relman, D.A. Diversity of the Human Intestinal Microbial Flora. *Science* **2005**, *308*, 1635–1638. [CrossRef] [PubMed]
8. Claesson, M.J.; Jeffery, I.B.; Conde, S.; Power, S.E.; O'Connor, E.M.; Cusack, S.; Harris, H.M.; Coakley, M.; Lakshminarayanan, B.; O'Sullivan, O.; et al. Gut microbiota composition correlates with diet and health in the elderly. *Nature* **2012**, *488*, 178–184. [CrossRef] [PubMed]
9. Carmody, R.N.; Gerber, G.K.; Luevano, J.M., Jr.; Gatti, D.M.; Somes, L.; Svenson, K.L.; Turnbaugh, P.J. Diet dominates host genotype in shaping the murine gut microbiota. *Cell Host Microbe* **2015**, *17*, 72–84. [CrossRef] [PubMed]
10. Zmora, N.; Zeevi, D.; Korem, T.; Segal, E.; Elinav, E. Taking it Personally: Personalized Utilization of the Human Microbiome in Health and Disease. *Cell Host Microbe* **2016**, *19*, 12–20. [CrossRef] [PubMed]
11. Look, A.R.G.; Wing, R.R.; Bolin, P.; Brancati, F.L.; Bray, G.A.; Clark, J.M.; Coday, M.; Crow, R.S.; Curtis, J.M.; Egan, C.M.; et al. Cardiovascular effects of intensive lifestyle intervention in type 2 diabetes. *N. Engl. J. Med.* **2013**, *369*, 145–154.
12. Halsey, L.G.; Curran-Everett, D.; Vowler, S.L.; Drummond, G.B. The fickle *p* value generates irreproducible results. *Nat. Methods* **2015**, *12*, 179–185. [CrossRef] [PubMed]

6

The Effects of Moderate Whole Grain Consumption on Fasting Glucose and Lipids, Gastrointestinal Symptoms, and Microbiota

Danielle N. Cooper [1], Mary E. Kable [2], Maria L. Marco [3], Angela De Leon [1], Bret Rust [1,2], Julita E. Baker [1], William Horn [2], Dustin Burnett [2] and Nancy L. Keim [1,2,*]

1 Department of Nutrition, University of California at Davis, 1 Shields Ave, Davis, CA 95616, USA; dncooper@ucdavis.edu (D.N.C.); adeleon@ucdavis.edu (A.D.L.); brust@ucdavis.edu (B.R.); jemadejska@ucdavis.edu (J.E.B.)

2 Western Human Nutrition Research Center, USDA-ARS, 430 West Health Sciences Drive, Davis, CA 95616, USA; Mary.Kable@ars.usda.gov (M.E.K.); William.Horn@ars.usda.gov (W.H.); Dustin.Burnett@ars.usda.gov (D.B.)

3 Food Science and Technology, University of California at Davis, 1 Shields Ave, Davis, CA 95616, USA; mmarco@ucdavis.edu

* Correspondence: Nancy.Keim@ars.usda.gov;

Abstract: This study was designed to determine if providing wheat, corn, and rice as whole (WG) or refined grains (RG) under free-living conditions will change parameters of health over a six-week intervention in healthy, habitual non-WG consumers. Measurements of body composition, fecal microbiota, fasting blood glucose, total cholesterol, high density lipoprotein (HDL), low density lipoprotein (LDL), and triglycerides were made at baseline and post intervention. Subjects were given adequate servings of either WG or RG products based on their caloric need and asked to keep records of grain consumption, bowel movements, and GI symptoms weekly. After six weeks, subjects repeated baseline testing. Significant decreases in total, LDL, and non-HDL cholesterol were seen after the WG treatments but were not observed in the RG treatment. During Week 6, bowel movement frequency increased with increased WG consumption. No significant differences in microbiota were seen between baseline and post intervention, although, abundance of order *Erysipelotrichales* increased in RG subjects who ate more than 50% of the RG market basket products. Increasing consumption of WGs can alter parameters of health, but more research is needed to better elucidate the relationship between the amount consumed and the health-related outcome.

Keywords: whole grains; maize; brown rice; whole wheat; fasting glucose; fasting blood lipids; microbiota; bowel movement frequency; gastrointestinal symptoms

1. Introduction

Grains are a staple of the average American diet and therefore changes to grain products, especially the level of refinement, can have a notable effect on Americans' consumption of fiber, minerals, and vitamins [1]. The topic of whole grains has come to wider public attention since the publication of the 2005 Dietary Guidelines for Americans, which recommends half of one's daily grain intake (3–5 servings or 48–80 g for adults) should be in the form of whole grains [2]. However, there is still a huge disparity between the recommended level of whole grain consumption and the actual amount of consumption in the US with most adults only consuming on average 9.76 g of whole grains daily, as reported by the 2009–2010 National Health and Nutrition Examination Survey (NHANES) [3].

Botanically, grains are defined as the caryopsis or dried fruit (also called corn) of a cereal plant [4]. True cereals include wheat (*Triticum* spp.), corn/maize (*Zea mays*), rice (*Oryza* spp.), oats (*Avena* spp.), and barley (*Hordeum* spp.), whereas the pseudocereals include foods such as amaranth (*Amaranthus* spp.), buckwheat (*Fagopyrum esculentum*) and quinoa (*Chenopodium quinoa*) [5]. Grains are made up of three distinct components: the fibrous bran, the starchy endosperm, and the lipid containing germ. In addition to these three components, some grains, such as oats, grow within an inedible husk which is removed prior to human consumption. Whole grains are defined as the intact edible portion of the fruit of the cereal plant or the ground, cracked, flaked, or rolled fruit so long as the original proportions of the bran, endosperm, and germ are present in nearly the same proportions in the processed grain as were found in the intact grain [5,6].

Refined grains are grains that have been altered so that they are devoid of some, or all, of their naturally occurring germ and/or bran. In removing the germ, the shelf life of the grain is generally improved due to the absence of the lipid component of the germ that can become rancid [5]. Removal of the bran is often done to remove fibrous and potentially bitter components of the grain to improve the hedonic experience of the consumer and lighten the color of the resulting grain product [7]. Unfortunately, the removal of the bran and germ removes many bioactive components including vitamins, minerals, antioxidants, phenolics, flavonoids, carotenoids and critically fiber, particularly insoluble fiber [4,8]. To ameliorate some of the losses in the refining process and increase consumption of vitamins and minerals, enrichment or fortification is done with riboflavin, niacin, thiamin, folate, iron, and calcium, however nothing is done to increase the fiber level of refined grains [9].

In addition to not consuming enough whole grains, Americans are also not consuming enough fiber. The 2009–2010 NHANES data reported adults were only consuming on average 17 g of fiber per day despite the recommendation to consume 25 to 38 g per day [3]. Consumption of more whole grains has been suggested as an excellent way for Americans to bridge the fiber gap because many palatability studies have shown that in moderate proportions substituting whole grains for refined grains does not change the "liking" of grain based foods [3,10].

Consumption of whole grains is associated with decreased risk of type 2 diabetes and major chronic diseases, such as cardiovascular disease, and may even decrease the risk for some types of cancers, such as colorectal cancer [4,11,12]. Alteration of glucose homeostasis [13–16] and reduction of total cholesterol and low density lipoprotein (LDL) have been somewhat inconsistently reported in connection with increased whole grain consumption [12,13,17,18]. Beneficial alteration of the gut microbiota is often cited as a possible reason for health improvements seen with increased whole grain consumption, although a relationship between the two is not always observed [8,13,14,19]. Fiber can be mechanistically linked to all these health improvements and the content of fiber varies from grain to grain, which might explain some of the mixed reports. Another potential confounding variable is how much fiber subjects are consuming either prior to the dietary interventions or as part of their background diet [20,21].

Our study was conducted to document biological changes that occur with increased whole grain consumption. We hypothesized that compared to the subjects consuming refined grains the whole grain consumers would have lower concentrations of fasting blood glucose, total cholesterol and LDL, increased bowel movement frequency, a shift to midrange fecal firmness, and increased abundance of *Bacteroidetes*. The three grains most commonly consumed in the United States, wheat, maize, and rice [1] were used in the grain interventions, which were provided in weekly "market baskets" containing an array of either whole or refined grain foods. The number of servings per day provided to each subject was intended to be ~100% of the total grain recommendations for their maintenance calorie level.

We found that measures of fasting blood cholesterol significantly improved with the whole grain intervention. We also found that bowel movement frequency was significantly improved relative to percent consumption of the whole grains, and blood glucose tended to decrease as well with increased percent consumption of whole grains. Additionally, we observed increased abundance of order *Erysipelotrichales*, with greater amounts of refined grain consumption.

2. Materials and Methods

Prior to initiating the study, the study plan and consent form were reviewed by the Institutional Review Board (IRB) of the University of California-Davis and approved (IRB ID 235561). The study is registered with clinicaltrials.gov (NCT01403857).

2.1. Subjects and Study Design

This study was a six-week intervention trial that was preceded by a screening period to determine eligibility and a pre-intervention baseline test visit (Table 1).

Table 1. Study design and procedures.

Screening	Baseline Test Day	Six Week Intervention (Each Event Occurred Weekly)	Post-Intervention Test Day

• Consent to participate
• Determine eligibility
	• Fasted blood draw
	• Fecal sample collected
	• Body composition testing
		• Pick up the market basket and dropping off the last week's unconsumed food
		• Complete and return logs of:
		  • market basket consumption
		  • bowel movements
		  • gastrointestinal symptoms
			• Fasted blood draw
			• Fecal sample collected
			• Body composition testing

Subjects were consented and went through a screening process to determine if they were eligible to participate based on inclusion and exclusion criteria. To be included, subjects needed to be healthy adults, between the ages of 19 to 46 years with body mass index (BMI) 20 to 28 kg/m^2. They had to be "low whole grain consumers" consuming not more than 1 serving of whole grains/whole grain products per day, on average. This was evaluated using a screener that probed 81 different grain products including food items like breads, pastas, cereals, and snack bars. Subjects were asked to report how often they consumed these products by circling the option most appropriate to their consumption habits from consuming a serving of the product "never or less than once per month", "1–3 per month" then one through seven times per week, to the greatest frequency queried "2 per day". Subjects were disqualified for the study if they reported consuming seven or more servings of whole grain products per week. They also reported that their body weight had remained stable (within ±3 kg) for the past 6 months and they were not currently dieting to lose weight. It was also necessary that subjects be able to prepare and eat the majority of their meals at home.

Potential subjects were excluded if they reported having a diagnosis of type 1 or 2 diabetes mellitus, gastrointestinal diseases including malabsorption syndromes, chronic inflammatory bowel disease, colorectal cancer, celiac disease (gluten sensitivity), diverticulitis, Crohn's disease; regular use of colonics and/or laxatives; recent (within 3 months) use of antibiotics, appetite suppressants, mood altering medications, and/or regular use of tobacco/tobacco products. Females were excluded if they were currently pregnant or were pregnant within the last six months. Eating habits were also queried, and subjects were excluded if the majority of meals were eaten away from home, in restaurants, or from fast food establishments. If qualified based on these criteria, a fasting blood sample was sent to a certified clinical chemistry lab at the University of California at Davis for a comprehensive clinical chemistry panel and a complete blood count to rule-out existing health problems, of which the subject may be unaware.

Eligible subjects were randomly assigned in blocks to the control (refined grain market basket) or treatment (whole grain market basket) groups to achieve a 1:2 ratio of those receiving refined grain to whole grain. Overall 46 subjects enrolled in the study. Results from the analysis of fasting blood samples are based on 45 subjects due to a missing post intervention sample; body composition data were available for only for 43 subjects due to equipment malfunction; gastrointestinal (GI) symptoms were assessed for 37 subjects due to incomplete record keeping by subjects, microbial analysis was performed on 28 subjects due to fecal sample loss or poor reading depth resulting from sequencing. Table 2 contains information about the subjects.

Table 2. Demographic information of subjects who received refined grain (RG) or whole grain (WG) market baskets [1].

Subjects	Sex F = Female M = Male	Age (Years)	BMI (kg/m^2)	Calculated Daily Calorie Needs (kcal/day)	Percent of Market Basket Consumed
			All Subjects in Sample		
Total (n = 46)	25 F, 21 M	25.8 ± 0.9	23.4 ± 0.6	2247.8 ± 48.2	47.1 ± 2.9
RG (n = 11)	3 F, 8 M	24.6 ± 1.6	25.5 ± 2.1	2363.6 ± 96.6	44.7 ± 7.8
WG (n = 35)	22 F, 13 M	26.2 ± 1	22.8 ± 0.5	2211.4 ± 55	47.9 ± 3

[1] Values are means ± standard error of the mean (SEM).

2.2. Market Baskets and Consumption Log

The market baskets consisted of foods made of either refined or whole wheat (representing ~75% of the products), corn (~15%), or rice (~10%). Three grain products were developed for the study: cookies, muffins and baking mixes; the others were commercially prepared items: bread, ready to eat cereals, couscous, crackers, pastas, rice, and tortillas (Table 3).

Table 3. Products contained in the market baskets. For reference the 2000 kcal portions are provided. All products were packaged by the metabolic kitchen, and no original labels or brand names were attached to the products given to the subjects.

Consumable	Refined Grain Products		Whole Grain Products		Servings/Week
Food Item	Description	Brand	Description	Brand	At 2000 kcal
Wheat bread	White, slices	Sysco Classic	100% whole wheat, slices	Hi Vibe	7 slices
Cereal	Cornflakes	Kellogg's	Wheaties	General Mills	5 cups
Cookie	Chocolate chip with white enriched flour	Recipe developed for study	Chocolate chip with whole wheat flour	Recipe developed for study	2 cookies, 2 $\frac{1}{2}$ inch diameter
Couscous	Refined Wheat	Giusto	Whole Wheat	Woodland Farms	$\frac{1}{2}$ cup prepared + 3 oz. dry
Crackers	Goldfish, cheddar, original	Pepperidge Farms	Goldfish, cheddar, whole wheat	Pepperidge Farms	26 crackers
Corn Muffin	Made with finely ground cornmeal	Recipe developed for study	Made with whole kernel cornmeal	Recipe developed for study	2 muffins
Penne Pasta	Semolina Wheat	La Bella	Semolina Whole Wheat	La Bella	$\frac{1}{2}$ cup prepared + 2 oz. dry
Rice	Long-rain, white	Sysco Classic	Long-grain, brown	Sysco Classic	$\frac{1}{2}$ cup prepared + 4 oz. dry
Spaghetti	Semolina Wheat	La Bella	Semolina, Whole Wheat	La Bella	$\frac{1}{2}$ cup prepared + 2 oz. dry
Tortilla	Wheat	Mi Rancho	Whole Wheat	Mi Rancho	1 tortilla (12-inch diameter)
Baking Mix	Based on enriched white flour	Formula developed for study	Based on whole wheat flour	Formula developed for study	1 cup

The contents of the market baskets (number of grain servings per week) were determined based on the caloric needs of the subjects, determined using the Harris-Benedict equation [22]. The calorie prescriptions were made in 200-kcal intervals. For example, a subject with an estimated energy expenditure of 1960 kcals would be provided a 2000 kcal per day basket and would receive six servings of grains per day, and a total of 42 servings of grains in their weekly market basket. All grain products were weighed prior to being given to the subjects. At the 2000 kcal level the whole grain market basket supplied 96 g of fiber, an average of 13.7 g per day whereas the refined grain market basket supplied 29.7 g of fiber, an average of 4.2 g per day. Subjects were asked to maintain their typical diet during the market basket intervention. We had planned to monitor dietary intake using unannounced multi-pass 24-h recalls collected by phone interview. However, we were unable to obtain a sufficient number of recalls, and between-interviewer variation was problematic. Thus, we have deemed the 24-h recall data of poor quality and have chosen not to present those data.

Subjects were asked to record the type, amount, preparation, as well as date and time of the grains used from the market basket. The grain products were pre-portioned for the subjects to increase convenience and help with record keeping in the log books (Figure A1). Subjects were not required to consume all grain products but where encouraged to replace what they would normally consume with products from the provided market baskets whenever possible. The log data were compared with the disappearance data generated by weighing back the returned market basket containing the prepared or unprepared unused grain products. If there was a discrepancy between the log data and what was returned in the market basket, in absence of a note from the subject explaining the discrepancy, the weigh back data was deemed preferred and used in the consumption calculation. After the initial basket was picked up subjects returned once weekly to return their past week's unused food, return their log books, and pick up materials for the following week. The intervention period was six weeks. The post-intervention test day was scheduled during the sixth week.

2.3. Body Composition

Subject's body composition was determined using air displacement plethysmometry (BodPod, COSMED, USA, Inc., Concord, CA, USA) in conjunction with a calibrated digital scale (Scale-tronic model 6002, Wheaton, IL, USA). Height was determined by a wall-mounted stadiometer (Ayrton Stadiometer model S100, Prior Lake, MN, USA). Subjects were required to wear tight fitting clothing such as a bathing suits or compression shorts as well as swim caps prior to entering the chamber. Subjects were evaluated twice, once in the baseline period and once after the sixth week of intervention, on both occasions they were tested after an overnight fast.

2.4. Clinical Parameters

Twelve-hour fasting blood samples were obtained by a licensed phlebotomist twice during the study. Whole blood was sent to the UC Davis Medical Center's clinical laboratory for analysis of glucose, lipids, cell counts, and iron status. The first collection occurred at baseline, the second occurred post intervention.

2.5. Gastrointestinal Symptoms Log Book

GI symptom log books were distributed and collected weekly with the market baskets. The goal of the logs was to monitor GI tolerability of the market basket products. Subjects were asked to record the day and time of each bowel movement and rate the consistency of each bowel movement using the Bristol stool scale [23]. There was also a short questionnaire in the log book that asked subjects to reflect over the past week when reporting their answers. The questions regarded frequency of experiencing gas, bloating, abdominal pain, nausea, or flatulence, and responses were recorded on a 5-point Likert scale [24]. There was a query about experiencing a change in stool and, if so, how they felt about the change.

2.6. Fecal Collection

A single bowel movement was collected by the subject at baseline and then again post intervention using a feces collection kit. The kit consisted of a plastic container lined with a ziplock bag, gloves, pens for labeling, and a hard-sided cooler with dry ice to keep their samples frozen until they could be delivered to the research center (WHNRC) for immediate storage at −20 °C.

2.7. Gut Microbial Community Analysis

The composition of the fecal microbiota was determined by sequencing of bacterial 16S rRNA genes. Comparisons of the fecal microbiota at baseline and post intervention were used to determine the change in relative abundance of specific taxa. Bacterial DNA was extracted as previously described [25]. Briefly, approximately 200 mg of fecal material was placed in a 2 mL screw cap tube containing 300 mg of 0.1 mm diameter zirconia/silica beads (Biospec Products, Bartlesville, OK, USA), the mixture was treated with lysozyme from the QIAamp DNA Stool Mini Kit (QIAGEN) and held for 30 min at 37 °C. Next mechanical lysis was performed by bead beating for 1 min, twice, at 6.5 m/s (FastPrep-24, BP Biomedicals, Santa Ana, CA, USA) in 1.5 mL ASL buffer [25,26]. Finally, the suspension was heated to 95 °C for 5 min while shaking at 500 rpm. DNA was then purified using the QIAamp DNA Stool Mini Kit (QIAGEN) according to the manufacturer's instructions.

The V4 region of the 16S rRNA gene was selected for PCR amplification because it has been shown to faithfully represent the taxonomic profile of microbial communities relative to characterization of the full length 16S gene sequences [27]. Primers F515 and R806 [28] were used to amplify the 16S rRNA V4 region from each purified DNA sample. An eight base pair (bp) barcode was present on the 5′ end of primer F515 [29] to facilitate demultiplexing of pooled sequence samples during downstream analysis. The PCR products were pooled and gel purified using the Wizard SV Gel and PCR Clean-Up System (Promega, Madison, WI, USA). Amplicons were then sent to the UC Davis Genome Center (http://www.genomecenter.ucdavis.edu/) for library preparation and paired-end 250 bp sequencing using the Illumina MiSeq platform (San Diego, CA, USA).

QIIME (Quantitative Insights into Microbial Ecology) [30] was used to join paired ends [31], quality filter, and demultiplex the sequencing data. Chimeras were identified using USEARCH [32,33] and removed. Operational Taxonomic Units (OTUs) were picked from the assembled sequences using the open reference OTU picking method and a threshold of 97% pairwise identity [30]. Very low abundance (0.005% or less) OTUs were removed prior to statistical analysis [34].

2.8. Statistical Methods

Microsoft Excel (Microsoft, Redmond, WA, USA)) was used to format data. JMP (JMP ®, Version 12.1.0. SAS Institute Inc., Cary, NC, USA) and R (R, Version 3.3.2, R Foundation for Statistical Computing, Vienna, Austria) were used for analysis. Data were tested for normal distribution using the Shapiro–Wilks test of normality and if non-normally distributed transformation using Box Cox was performed, if transformation was unsuccessful (w above 0.96) nonparametric testing was used. Body composition data and fasting blood data were analyzed using linear regression and analysis of variance using baseline measures as a cofactor in the regression model. Gastrointestinal symptoms, bowel movement frequency, Bristol scores of feces, and microbial abundance could not be normalized using Box Cox transformations so non-parametric Wilcoxon Signed Ranks tests were used to determine significance following logistical regression [35]. For the microbial data, OTU counts were rarefied to a depth of 15,000 sequences per sample prior to analysis. This number was chosen because at this sequencing depth the number of unique OTUs observed was no longer exponentially increasing. Samples from two subjects on the whole grain market basket intervention had fewer than 15,000 sequences and so were discarded prior to analysis. Taxa that were present in at least 2% relative abundance in at least one sample were analyzed for differential abundance between experimental groups using LefSe [36]. For the purposes of determining fold change, sequence counts of 0, when they occurred, were replaced with a sequence count of 1. Due to the increased risk of type 1 errors with multiple comparisons, the Benjamini–Hochberg False Discovery Rate Procedure was implemented to reduce the risk of false discovery [37].

3. Results

3.1. Market Basket Consumption

There was a wide range of consumption of the market baskets products with refined grain consumption ranging from 1.1% to 95.1% and whole grain consumption ranging from 18.1% to 97.5% (Figure 1).

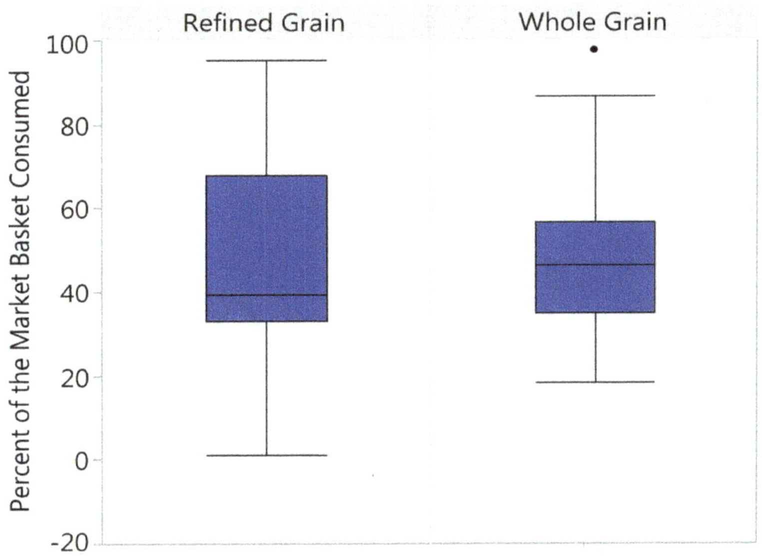

Figure 1. Range of Market Basket Consumption. Consumption of the refined grain market basket ranged from 1.1% to 95.1% with the average consumption being 44.7% and a standard error of the mean of 7.8. Consumption of the whole grain market basket ranged from 18.1% to 97.5% with the average consumption being 47.9% and a standard error of the mean of 3.0.

3.2. Changes in Body Composition from Baseline to Post-Intervention

Air displacement plethysmometry performed at baseline and post intervention was used to calculate the change in Body Mass Index (BMI), fat mass, and fat free mass between baseline and post intervention. Using baseline measures as a cofactor linear regression followed by analysis of variance were performed in the treatment groups and no significant differences were seen (Table 4). Similar analysis was performed on each treatment group relative to the percent of the market basket consumed and significant differences were still not observed (Figure 2).

Table 4. Change in body mass index and body composition over the six-week intervention for refined grain (RG) and whole grain (WG) and treatments [1,2].

Treatment	Change in BMI (kg/m^2)	Change in Fat Mass (kg)	Change in Fat Free Mass (kg)
RG	0.01 ± 0.11	1.13 ± 0.57	-0.45 ± 0.56
WG	0.05 ± 0.10	0.49 ± 0.31	-0.43 ± 0.37
p value	0.846	0.936	0.936

[1] Values are reported as the mean ± the standard error of the mean; [2] Change in BMI (RG: n = 11, WG: n = 34), change in Fat Mass and Fat Free Mass (RG: n = 10, WG: n = 33).

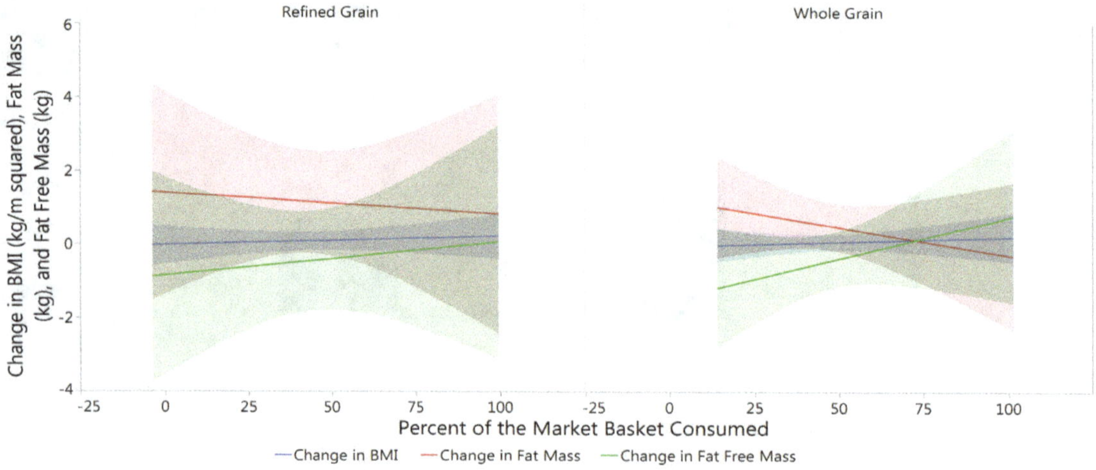

Figure 2. Changes in Body Composition with Percent Consumption of the Market Baskets. No significant differences were found using analysis of variance in the change of BMI (RG $p = 0.494$, WG $p = 0.658$), fat mass (RG $p = 0.962$, WG $p = 0.372$), or fat free mass (RG $p = 0.823$, WG $p = 0.561$) from baseline to post intervention.

3.3. Changes in Fasting Blood Glucose from Baseline to Post-Intervention

Similar to our findings with body composition, we found there was no significant impact of the type of market basket consumed on fasting blood glucose and the mean change for both treatment groups was negligible (RG = -3.00 ± 2.38 mg/dL; WG = -0.29 ± 1.62 mg/dL; $p = 0.250$). However, the percent of the WG market basket consumed trended with decreased fasting blood glucose when looking at the change in blood glucose from baseline to post intervention while controlling for baseline levels using linear regressions followed by analysis of variance ($p = 0.053$). This observation was not replicated with RG market basket consumption ($p = 0.590$), indicating that a certain quantity of whole grain consumption may be reducing fasting blood glucose (Figure 3).

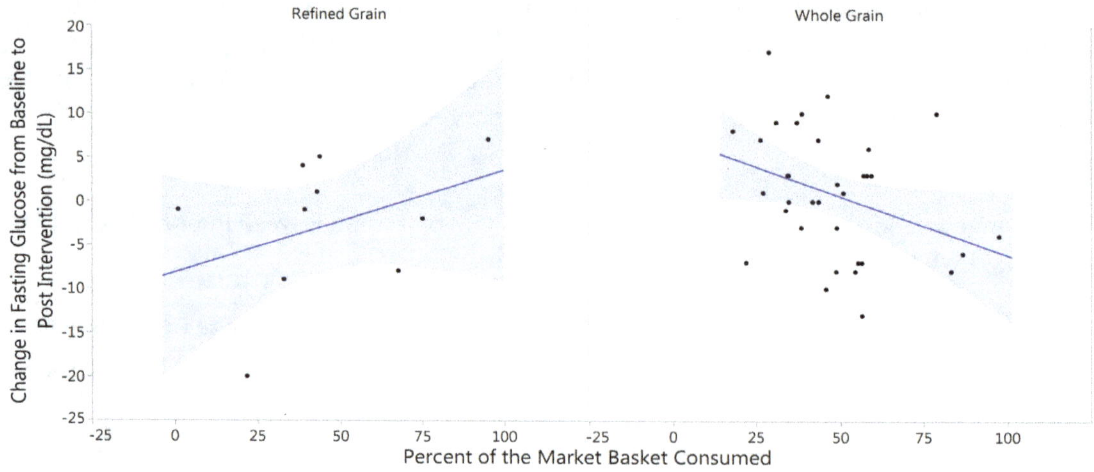

Figure 3. Percent of Market Basket Consumed Related to Change in Fasting Glucose. Increased consumption of the whole grain market basket was related to lower ($p = 0.053$) fasting blood glucose in the whole grain treatment, whereas there was a pattern of increased blood glucose with increased consumption of the refined grain market basket ($p = 0.590$).

3.4. Changes in Fasting Blood Lipids from Baseline to Post Intervention

When observing the changes in fasting blood lipids from baseline to post intervention between the RG and WG treatments, while controlling for baseline levels, significant differences were seen in total cholesterol ($p = 0.018$), LDL cholesterol ($p = 0.035$), and in non-high density lipoprotein (HDL) cholesterol ($p = 0.047$) (Figure 4). Negligible changes were seen in HDL cholesterol (RG = 1.55 ± 1.49 mg/dL; WG = −2.41 ± 1.31 mg/dL; $p = 0.178$) and triglycerides (RG = 2.73 ± 14.47 mg/dL; WG = 6.29 ± 8.97 mg/dL; $p = 0.799$).

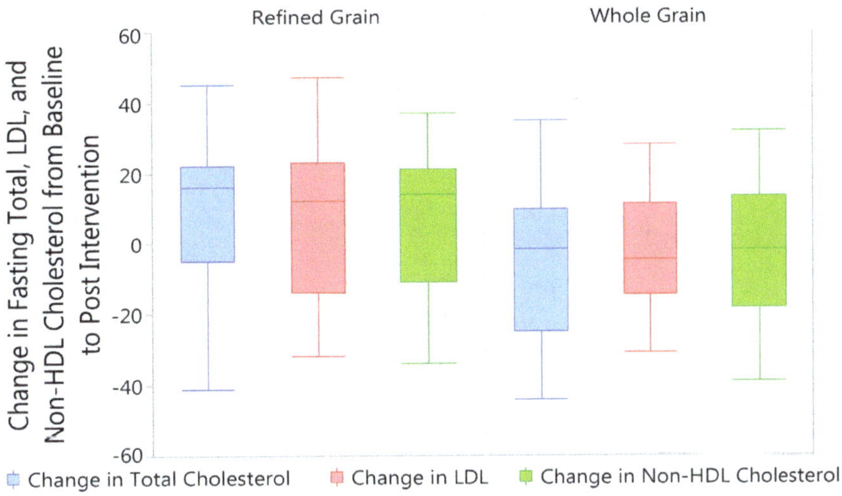

Figure 4. Consumption of the Whole or Refined Grain Market Basket Related to Change in Fasting Total, LDL, and Non-HDL Cholesterol. Consumption of the WG market basket was significantly associated with lower fasting levels of total cholesterol ($p = 0.018$), LDL cholesterol ($p = 0.035$), and non-HDL cholesterol ($p = 0.047$) when compared to subjects that consumed the RG market basket.

When comparing fasting lipid levels to percent consumption of the market baskets while controlling for baseline levels no significant differences were seen in the change in total (RG $p = 0.179$; WG $p = 0.122$), LDL (RG $p = 0.0682$; WG $p = 0.265$), HDL (RG $p = 0.972$; WG $p = 0.816$), or non-HDL (RG $p = 0.313$; WG $p = 0.313$) cholesterol, or triglycerides (RG $p = 0.790$; WG $p = 0.313$).

3.5. Gastrointestinal Tolerability

Gastrointestinal symptoms were reported by subjects in their weekly log books. Table 5 represents the self-reported gastrointestinal symptoms of bloating or gas, abdominal pain, nausea, flatulence, changes in stool, change in feelings about changes in stool, bowel movement frequency, and Bristol stool score for weeks one and six during the market basket intervention.

Table 5. GI symptoms reported at Weeks 1 and 6 of the refined grain (RG) ($n = 10$) and whole grain (WG) ($n = 27$) interventions [1,2].

Treatment	Bloating and Gas	Abdominal Pain	Nausea	Flatulence	Change in Stool	Feeling about Change in Stool	Bowel Movement Frequency	Average Bristol Score
Week 1 Responses								
RG	0.80 ± 0.29	0.70 ± 0.30	0.60 ± 0.31	0.90 ± 0.38	0.8 ± 0.25	2.14 ± 0.25	7.00 ± 0.61	3.18 ± 0.23
WG	0.78 ± 0.20	0.56 ± 0.12	0.38 ± 0.12	1.04 ± 0.24	1.17 ± 0.21	2.14 ± 0.23	8.28 ± 0.65	4.16 ± 0.54
p value	0.824	0.863	0.595	0.573	0.371	0.785	0.397	0.088
Week 6 Responses								
RG	0.40 ± 0.22	0.20 ± 0.13	0.10 ± 0.10	0.60 ± 0.31	0.90 ± 0.28	2.00± 0.19	7.00 ± 0.70	3.42 ± 0.25
WG	0.64 ± 0.14	0.44 ± 0.10	0.40 ± 0.14	0.68 ± 0.18	0.92 ± 0.20	2.18 ± 0.23	7.93 ± 0.59	3.41 ± 0.14
p value	0.307	0.198	0.187	0.774	0.952	0.518	0.535	0.959

[1] Values are means ± SEM. [2] Higher values represent increases in symptoms, frequency, changes, positive feelings, or firmness of feces while lower numbers represent decreases in symptoms, frequency, changes, positive feelings, or firmness of feces.

The average bowel movement frequency for subjects during the sixth week of the intervention was compared to the average grain product consumption (percent consumed) by rank (50% or higher consumption verses less than 50% consumption) by subject in each treatment group, respectively.

Using logistical regression and Wilcoxon Rank Sum testing, it was determined that there was a significant increase in bowel movement frequency with increased consumption of the whole grain market basket ($p = 0.046$). There was no association between increased frequency and the refined grain treatment ($p = 0.407$) (Figure 5).

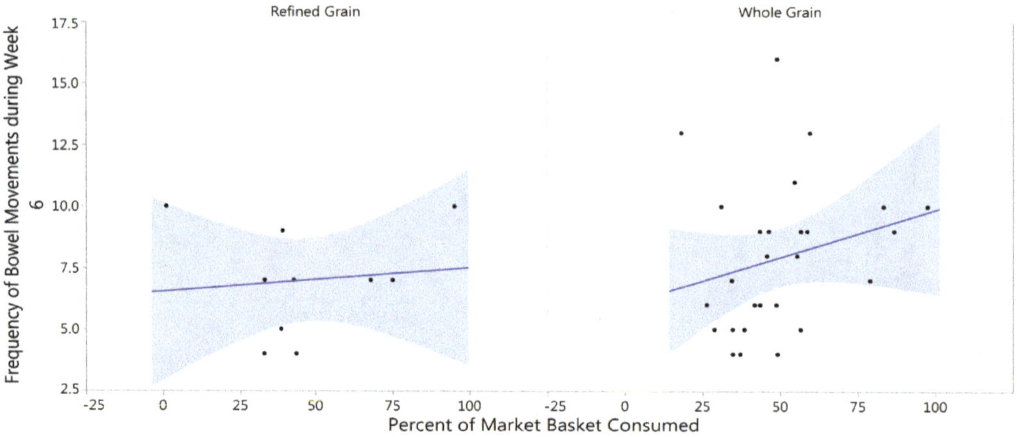

Figure 5. Percent of market basket consumed related to bowel movement frequency. The association between bowel movement frequency and percent of market basket consumed for refined grain consumers (**left** panel) and whole grain consumers (**right** panel) as determined by logistical regression and Wilcoxon Rank Sum testing. The refined grain treatment represents data from ten subjects; the whole grain treatment represents data from 27 subjects. There is a significant positive association with whole grain consumption ($p = 0.046$), but not with refined grain consumption ($p = 0.407$).

3.6. Fecal Microbiota Analysis

To determine if there were significant changes in the gut microbial community mediated by diet, which could then potentially influence changes in the health parameters observed, we sequenced the 16S rRNA V4 region of the bacterial DNA in subject stool collected at baseline and after six weeks of either WG or RG market basket consumption. A total of 2,983,060 sequences were obtained after quality filtering with an average of 48,100 sequences per sample. Two subjects in the WG market basket treatment were excluded from the microbiota analysis because one each of their samples was not sequenced sufficiently to effectively represent the overall community structure.

Overall, *Firmicutes* was the most relatively abundant phylum detected in our subjects, as has previously been observed in studies examining urban adult human gut microbiota using stool samples [38,39]. The second most abundant phylum was *Actinobacteria* with *Bacteroidetes* coming in third. The high proportion of *Actinobacteria* in our samples was driven primarily by a high representation of the genus *Bifidobacterium*, which composed as much as 40% of one sample prior to whole grain market basket consumption and was present at a median 10% and 16% relative abundance at baseline prior to WG and RG market basket consumption, respectively. Change in abundance during market basket consumption was not significant and this might be explained by the high levels present prior to consumption (Figure 6).

Although there was no significant difference in the relative abundance of any particular taxa between experimental groups, six of eight individuals consuming a high proportion (50% or greater) of the WG market basket showed increased relative abundance of *Akkermansia* and *Lactobacillus*, while two of three individuals consuming a high proportion of the RG market basket showed decreased relative abundance of this organism. There was also a trend for increased abundance of order *Erysipelotrichales* ($p = 0.023$) with high (50% or greater) RG market basket consumption. In our dataset, order *Erysipelotrichales* included unidentified members of family *Erysipelotrichaceae* and the genera *Eubacterium* and *Catenibacterium* (Figure 7).

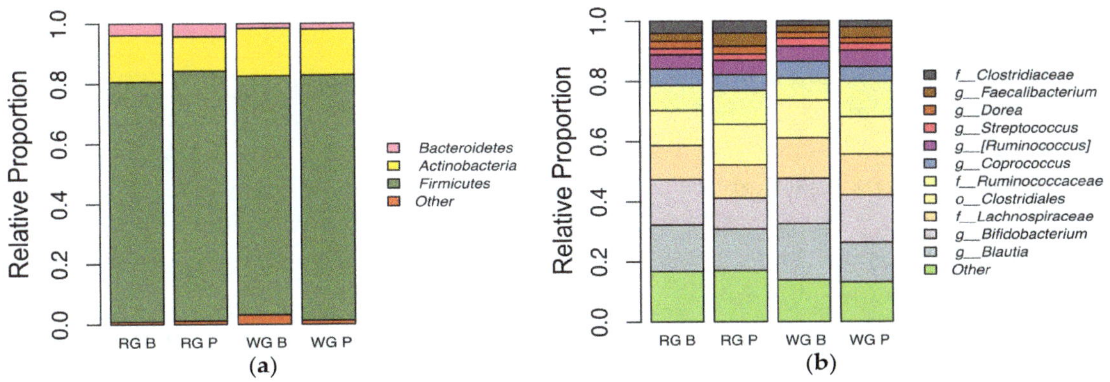

Figure 6. Relative proportion of taxa in each experimental group. The relative proportion of taxa at baseline (B) and post intervention (P) for the refined grain (RG) and whole (WG) treatments: (**a**) the relative proportion of bacteria at the phylum level; and (**b**) the relative abundance of bacteria at the most specific level of classification available. In both panels, taxa present at a median of 1% relative abundance in the data set are shown. Taxa present at lower than 1% median relative abundance are grouped into the "Other" category.

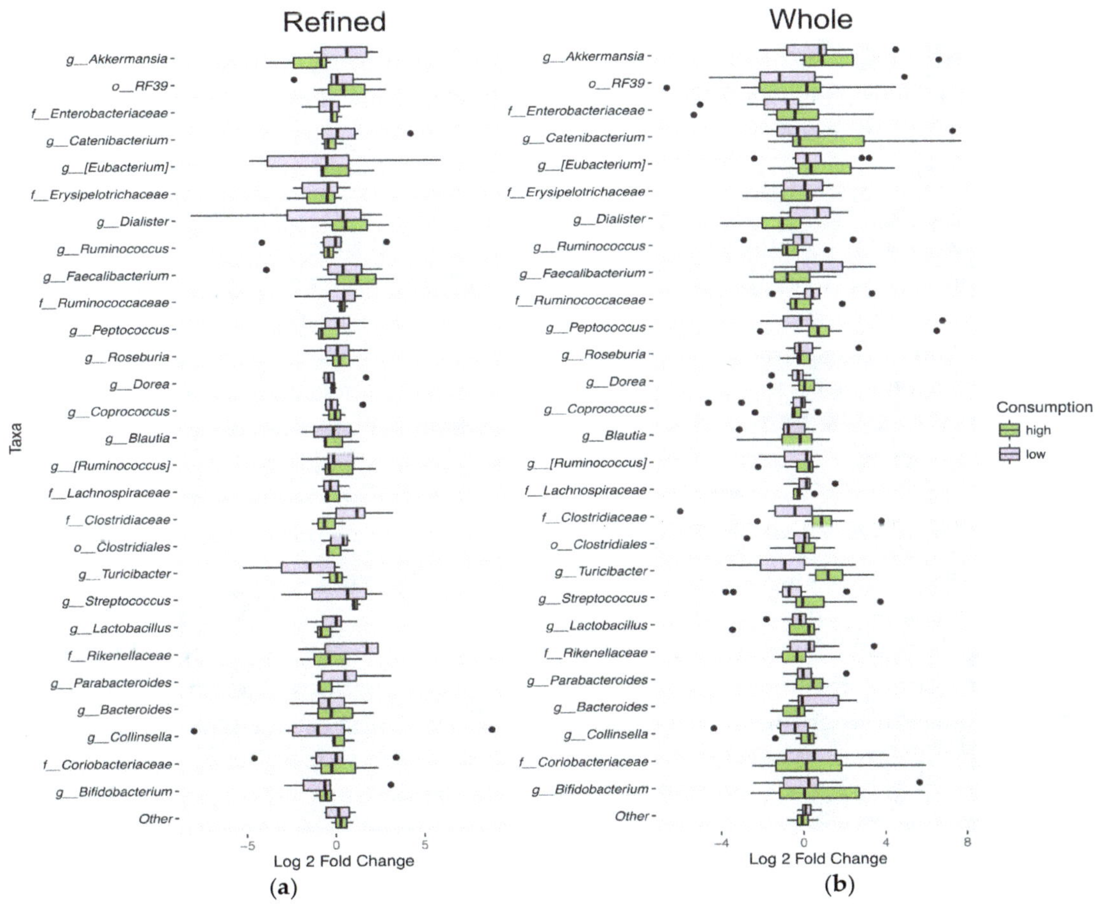

Figure 7. Variation in specific taxa during market basket consumption. Log2 fold change in abundance of bacteria at either high (50% or more) or low (49.99% or less) levels of consumption of the market baskets from baseline to post intervention for: refined grain (**a**); and whole grain (**b**). Taxa shown were present in at least 2% relative abundance in at least one sample. Dots seen in the graphs represent outliers. The findings of interest were an increase in the relative abundance of *Akkermansia* and *Lactobacillus* with high whole grain market basket consumption and a decrease with high refined grain consumption, as well as the increased abundance of the order *Erysipelotrichales* ($p = 0.023$) with high refined grain consumption.

4. Discussion

Consumption of the whole grain market basket products for six weeks was associated with a significant decrease in total, LDL, and non-HDL cholesterol compared to subjects consuming the refined grain market basket. Health parameters including fasting glucose, and bowel movement frequency were associated with a higher percentage of consumption of the whole grain market basket. No significant differences were seen when comparing the change from baseline to post intervention between treatment groups for the following parameters: BMI, fat mass, fat free mass, glucose, HDL, triglycerides, gas or bloating, abdominal pain, nausea, self-reported change in stool, feelings about changes in stool, bowel movement frequency, Bristol stool score, or abundance of microbiota.

4.1. Fiber Intake

Market baskets were designed to mimic the types of grain products typically consumed by Americans as closely as possible, which is why the baskets featured a majority of wheat products (~75%), some maize products (~15%), and rice (~10%), since those proportions are similar to the national availability of those grains as reported by USDA Economic Research Service [1]. The whole and the refined grain market baskets were matched as closely as possible in terms of types of foods provided, but the difference in the amount fiber between market baskets was substantial. At the 2000 kcal level, the whole grain market basket supplied 96 g of fiber, an average of 13.7 g per day, whereas the refined grain market basket supplied only 29.7 g of fiber, an average of 4.2 g per day, if all of the products were consumed. The average consumption of the market basket in this study, when rounded, was 47 percent. Thus, subjects in the refined grain group were consuming only about 2 g per day of fiber from the provided grain products whereas the whole grain subjects were consuming about 7 g per day of fiber from the grain products. Even though this is an average of a five-gram difference in fiber consumption between the grain treatments, whole grains at this percent consumption are not contributing a significant amount of fiber to the daily diet. Fibers such as beta glucan have been shown to reduce cholesterol and LDL with as small a dose as three grams per day [40]. However, the major sources of fiber in wheat are arabinoxylans, hemicellulose, and only very small amounts of beta glucan [41]; corn fibers are hemicellulose, arabinose, xylan, lignin, and resistant starch [42]; and rice contains cellulose, pectic fibers (arabinans, arabinogalactans, and galacturonans) and hemicellulose [21,43–46]. Not much is known about the dietary impacts of these individual fibers. Since background diet was not evaluated during the intervention it is possible that subjects in the whole and refined grain treatment groups were consuming vegetable and or fruit fiber at different levels from each other. Assuming we were successful at disqualifying habitual medium or high whole grain consumers, we were confident that the enrolled subjects were not consuming a large amount of cereal fiber outside of the intervention. Not having a reliable estimate of the subject's fiber intake outside of the intervention limits any conclusions we can draw about fiber intake during the study, and how the difference in fiber provided by the market baskets may have influenced the outcome of individual subjects.

4.2. Fasting Glucose

When comparisons were made taking into account what percentage of the market basket was consumed, a nearly significant trend was observed: as whole grain consumption increased fasting glucose levels decreased. A potential mechanism behind this theory is that due to the increased fiber of whole grains they remain as larger particles post mastication and so potentially are more challenging to mechanically and enzymatically degrade resulting in lower, longer releases of glucose into the blood stream and subsequently a more gradual secretion of insulin. However, this effect may not explain why a decrease in glucose might exist after something as long as a 12-h overnight fast [47–50]. Another potential mechanism that may explain the persistence of decreased glucose levels with increased consumption of whole grains, even after an overnight fast, is that the increase in fiber from whole grains may alter metabolism in the microbiota increasing the production of short chain fatty acids (SCFA) like propionate and acetate due to continued exposure to fiber from the whole grains. Propionate is known to stimulate enteroendocrine L cells to increase the release of glucagon-like peptide-1 (GLP-1) which increases the responsiveness of insulin to glucose as well as inhibiting gastric emptying [51–53]. In a human study, supplementation with propionate was shown to decrease glucose peaks and two-hour glucose area under the curve [54]. Acetate may be able to alter appetite and satiety signaling in the brain without use of gut hormone intermediaries, and has been shown to reduce fasting glucose levels in humans [55,56]. Reduced blood glucose has been seen postprandially in the literature with boiled barley, whole rye, whole wheat, and brown rice in comparison to refined grain interventions [46,57,58]. Fasting glucose has been shown to decrease with acute interventions of wheat bran in mice [50] and with acute interventions of whole wheat, whole oats, and whole barley in rats [59]. There is some literature suggesting that whole grains do not have an effect on glycemic control. For example Ampatzoglou and colleagues showed no significant impact of increasing whole grain consumption from 24 or more grams per day to at least 80 g per day for six weeks, on blood glucose [13]. Another study by Kristensen and colleagues compared acute whole grain wheat and refined grain wheat consumption and failed to show significant differences in blood glucose up to 180 min after feeding [60]. Since only a trend towards decreased glucose levels was observed in our study no strong conclusions can be drawn, but it is clear that future research will be needed to definitively understand if beginning or increasing whole grain consumption may effect glycemic control, and if so why.

4.3. Blood Lipids

Fasting total, LDL, and non-HDL cholesterol decreased with consumption of the whole grain market basket, whereas no significant changes were seen with these lipids in the refined grain group. Whole grain consumption has been shown to improve lipid profiles [12]. In rats diets high in maize have been shown to reduce LDL [61]. In humans diets rich in whole wheat have been shown to reduce total cholesterol when given at a dosage of 48 g per day [15,19]. Most of the research on the lipid lowering effects of whole grains has been performed with oats, which are rich in beta glucan, a fiber that has been clinically shown to lower cholesterol [40]. Oats were not featured in this study and while whole wheat contains very small amounts of beta glucan, maize and rice do not [21,41]. The current understanding of this lipid lowering property of whole grains is that it is due to their increased fiber content as compared to their refined grain counterparts [8,41].

Assuming whole grain intake replaces refined grain intake this diet alteration would be expected to increase fiber intake, thereby initiating the following signaling cascade. Fiber increases the viscosity of the foodstuffs in the stomach which may delay gastric emptying and affect satiety signaling. In the duodenum the increased viscosity may also alter nutrient release from the chyme and thus affect nutrient sensing, which could have far reaching consequences including lipid metabolism and processing [62]. The better established and accepted mechanism for increased fiber intake decreasing blood cholesterol levels is through sequestration of bile salts resulting in their loss in feces instead of their reabsorption back into the intestine, which results in the body needing to use cholesterol to manufacture more bile salts, thus decreasing blood cholesterol concentrations [58,63]. The existing literature suggests that in some cases increasing whole grains consumption does not affect lipid levels. This was seen in the previously discussed mixed increased whole grain consumption study by Ampatzoglou and colleagues [13]. Odes and colleagues also performed a study on humans using a mixed grain fiber supplement providing 12.5 g of fiber daily for two or four weeks and found that it had no effect on HDL or LDL cholesterol [64]. However, the findings of the current study indicate that inclusion of a combination of whole grain wheat, corn and rice in the diet for six weeks led to decreased fasting total, LDL, and non-HDL cholesterol levels compared to consuming the refined grain counterparts.

4.4. Fecal Frequency

While there was no difference in average bowel movement frequency across the six-week intervention, there was there a significant difference in frequency with relation to percent of the whole grain market basket consumed when looking at only the sixth week of intervention. Bowel movement frequency increased significantly with increased whole grain consumption in Week 6 while there was only a slight, non-significant increase in the refined grain intervention. Whole grains have been shown to decrease intestinal transit time, thereby increasing bowel movement frequency [8,41,65,66]. In a recent review of 65 intervention studies, it was found that intake of wheat fiber, such as is found in wheat bran, a component of whole grain wheat, was shown to decrease transit time by about 45 min per gram of wheat fiber consumed, if the initial transit time was more than 48 h [67]. In a meta-analysis of 65 intervention studies utilizing cereal fibers from wheat, rye, corn, oats, barley, sorghum, and rice, investigators reported that, if the initial transit time was more than 48 h, cereal fiber reduced transit time by 30 min per gram consumed [68]. The mechanism for this is generally thought to be fecal bulking due to the increased fiber from increasing whole grain intake causing water retention in the feces which improves transit time [8,69]. Consuming whole grain barley has been shown to increase average fecal weight compared to the stool weight of refined grain consumers [65] and consumption of a high fiber cereal made of wheat, corn, oats, and soybeans was shown to increase bowel movement frequency compared to a similar low fiber cereal in humans [70]. It must be noted that bowel movement frequency was self-reported in our study and was not measured pre-intervention at baseline. There was also a trend towards increased bowel movement frequency observed in the refined grain intervention, thus the validity of the increase should be interpreted with caution.

4.5. Microbiota

Increasing intake of whole grain wheat, maize, and barley have all been shown to alter the human gut microbiota, potentially through increasing the availability of fiber, but possibly due to other functional components in the whole grains such as polyphenols [14].

However, in this study no significant changes in microbial community composition were detected with consumption of the whole or refined grain market baskets. This is not necessarily surprising, given that in this pilot study subjects were free-living and the market basket comprised only about 16% of their expected calorie intake at the average level of consumption.

Although no significant differences were detected between the whole and refined grain treatments this does not empirically mean that there were not changes in the microbial community that were simply unable to reach statistical significance with our small sample size. Additionally, it is possible that changes occurred in the metabolic pathways or activity of the microbiota over the course of this investigation that could be detected with metatranscriptomic, metabolomics, or proteomic analysis [71]. For example, changes in the production of metabolic byproducts such as short chain fatty acids can occur without necessitating changes in bacterial composition [72–74]. Alterations in bacterial metabolism can occur due to changes in pH, oxygen tension, or substrate availability, to name a few [75].

Based on studies seen in the literature it was expected that the increase in dietary fiber from the consumption of 50% of more of the whole grain market basket would initiate an increase in the abundance in *Bifidobacterium* [19,76–78]. At baseline, high levels of *Actinobacteria* were seen, largely due to an enrichment of *Bifidobacterium*. Enrichment of *Actinobacteria* has previously been observed in expectant mothers in the third trimester of pregnancy [79], however since subjects were excluded if pregnant it is unclear to us why *Actinobacteria* was so abundant at baseline. It is possible that subjects were consuming a significant amount of dietary fiber from a non-whole grain source prior to the study, which could have selectively enriched *Bifidobacterium* [80]. If this were the case, background diet variability may have acted as a confounding factor obscuring the expected increase in the abundance of *Bifidobacterium*. The average fiber intake for American adults is 17.0 g per day with grain products as well as mixed dishes (containing grains) make up nearly half (46%) of the intake, whereas vegetables account for 16%, snacks and sweets for 13% and fruits 12% [81].

The trend towards increased relative abundance of *Akkermansia* and *Lactobacillus* with high whole grain consumption seen in this study has been previously observed with a whole grain barley feeding study in rats [82]. Increases in the abundance of *Lactobacillus* have also been seen in humans after a diet rich in whole grain barley [83] and whole grain wheat [19]. While this trend was not significant, we feel it is a noteworthy observation since increases in *Akkermansia* are associated with reduced endotoxemia, improved inflammatory tone, and potentially weight loss [84–87]. *Lactobacillus* are often taken as probiotics due to their ability to exclude pathogenic bacteria and prevent or shorten episodes of diarrhea [88].

An increase in the abundance of the order *Erysipelotrichales* was seen in this study in the three individuals that consumed 50% or more of the refined grain market basket. Increased abundance of *Erysipelotrichales* has also been reported in canines with a diet high in refined maize and low in fiber [89], in mice with high fat diets [90], in mouse models of acute inflammatory colitis [91], and in humans with Crohn's disease [92]. Within the order *Erysipelotrichales*, the genera *Eubacterium* and *Catenibacterium* as well as unidentified members of family *Erysipelotrichaceae* were observed, although no significant differences were detected at the family or genus levels. *Eubacterium* has been seen in lower abundance in individuals with metabolic syndrome [93] and advanced colorectal adenoma [94]. *Catenibacterium* has been observed to be enriched in individuals with end stage renal disease [95] and to be depleted in individuals with higher risk for cardiovascular disease [96]. *Erysipelotrichaceae* has been observed as being enriched with obesity, Western-type diets, and increased host cholesterol metabolites [97].

4.6. Limitations

A serious limitation of the study was the small sample size. The study enrolled 46 subjects but due to technical problems with instrumentation and only partial cooperation of some of our research volunteers, we have missing data for some variables reported here. Most notably fecal samples from only 28 subjects were available for microbiota analysis. Of those 28 subjects used for the microbiota analysis the ratio of sexes was not balanced. There was a 1:2 ratio of females to males in the refined grain treatment and about a 3:1 ratio of females to males in the whole grain treatment. When observing gut microbiota there is enormous variation between subjects, and within subjects, so it is difficult to detect the signal above the noise, as it were, especially with a small population of subjects. Only having one baseline and one post intervention blood draw and fecal collection was another limitation. Much of the data were collected through self-report which introduces its own complexities and errors, especially when it concerns dietary record keeping, however pre-weighing and re-weighing the market baskets was used to improve the accuracy of those data. Background diet was attempted to be assessed with phone interviews using the multi-pass 24 hour recall method, however subject cooperation was extremely poor so the data collected were not considered to be representative of the usual diet intake. Due to this limitation, we cannot say with certainty that subjects did maintain their habitual diet, creating another possible source of error. Estimated fiber intake from the market basket products was calculated, not determined directly by analysis, so it is possible that the quantity of grain fiber consumed was erroneous. However, since those values were then averaged across the week and by all subjects in the treatment group, this might improve the reliability of the estimations. Analysis was done for body composition, blood work, and GI symptoms using linear regression which can only be used to discover medium to large effects with a sample size as small as those utilized in this study; small changes many have occurred but would not have been detectable. This limits the ability to conclude with certainty that changes did not occur if no difference was detected in our analysis.

5. Conclusions

The results of this paper indicate that increasing the consumption of whole grains in habitual low-whole grain consumers may significantly lower fasting measures of total, LDL, and non-HDL cholesterol.

The trend towards decreased fasting glucose with increased whole grain consumption came tantalizingly close to significance, and was not seen when the same analysis was done with those receiving the refined grain intervention. Due to the tight regulation of blood glucose in healthy individuals, it is not surprising that changes to fasting levels would be subtle and challenging to detect without large groups of homogenous subjects. The fact that a strong trend was seen indicates that a true effect may be present and detectable with better study design.

The increase in bowel movement frequency seen with increased consumption of whole grains during the sixth week of the intervention is supported by existing literature and meta-analyses, however given that no baseline measurements were taken, the sample size was small (n = 37), the data rely solely on self-report, and that the same pattern was seen in the refined grain intervention this finding must be interpreted with some reservations.

Microbial analysis was conducted on 28 subjects, and we did not have the power needed to detect anything but very large changes in the microbial community. The only significant change seen was an increase in abundance of the order *Erysipelotrichales* in the three individuals that consumed 50% or more of the refined grain market basket. This finding cannot reasonably be interpreted to say that other changes to the microbiota were not occurring, since there was not enough power in the analysis to validate that inference. The microbial analysis performed in this study was exploratory and should not be interpreted without the many caveats discussed above.

6. Future Research

Given the small sample size and limited sample collection, future research would be necessary to definitively describe changes in health parameters seen with increased whole grain consumption. This study does indicate that whole grains may be an important food type for improving fasting cholesterol and glucose levels, as well as increasing bowel movement frequency. Due to the fact that some changes in health parameters only became apparent in subjects who consumed at least 50% of the whole grain market basket, another direction for future research would be to determine what level of whole grain consumption affords the most beneficial health effects. Due to differences in the composition and level of fibers, vitamins, minerals, and digestibility of different grains, it would also be important to consider exactly which whole grains are being studied and whether they are similar to the grains, and preparations of grains, seen in the population relevant to the study. Another possible direction for future research would be to compare the whole grains typically consumed in the US (wheat, corn, and rice) to other sources of whole grains such as oats, barley, and rye for which more definitive health effects have been documented. Then, recommendations could be further refined to include not only the total quantity of whole grains, but also more specifically for the types of grains consumed based on the potential health benefit.

It is likely that the improvements seen from increasing whole grain consumption come from the increases in fiber consumption, but future research is necessary to confirm this assertion and determine if other functional components of the whole grains contribute to health benefits. Regardless of how whole grains exert their effects, increasing whole grain consumption can reduce the gap between the recommended consumption of fiber and current fiber intake in the US.

Acknowledgments: Funding was contributed by USDA-ARS intramural funds from projects 5306-51530-019 and 2032-51530-022, as well as the University of California at Davis Henry A. Jastro Research Award (2012–2013).

Author Contributions: N.L.K., A.D.L., J.E.B. and B.R. conceived and designed the study; D.B. designed the sensory evaluation and market basket foods/recipes; A.D.L., B.R. and J.E.B. conducted the study visits; D.N.C., M.E.K. and W.H. performed sample analyses; A.D.L., M.E.K. and D.N.C. analyzed the data; N.L.K. and M.L.M. contributed reagents/materials/analysis tools; and D.N.C., M.E.K. and N.L.K. wrote the paper.

Appendix A

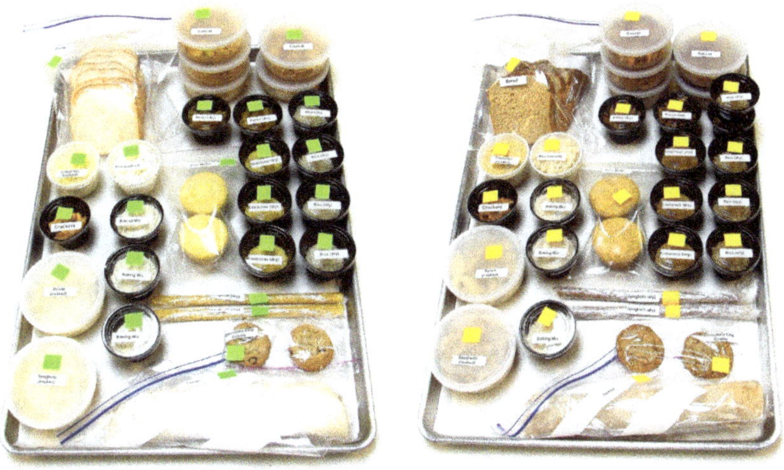

(a) (b)

Figure A1. Images of the 2000 kcal market baskets: (**a**) the refined grain basket; and (**b**) the whole grain basket.

References

1. Food Availability (Per Capita) Data System. Available online: http://ers.usda.gov/data-products/food-availability-per-capita-data-system.aspx (accessed on 20 April 2016).
2. Albertson, A.M.; Good, C.K.; Eldridge, A.L.; Holschuh, N.M. Whole grain consumption and food sources in the united states: Data from nhanes 1999–2000 and the usda's pyramid servings database for the usda survey food codes. *FASEB J.* **2005**, *19*, A87–A87.
3. McGill, C.; Fulgoni, V.L., III; Devareddy, L. Ten-year trends in fiber and whole grain intakes and food sources for the united states population: National health and nutrition examination survey 2001–2010. *Nutrients* **2015**, *7*, 1119–1130. [CrossRef] [PubMed]
4. Okarter, N.; Liu, R.H. Health benefits of whole grain phytochemicals. *Crit. Rev. Food Sci. Nutr.* **2010**, *50*, 193–208. [CrossRef] [PubMed]
5. Van der Kamp, J.W.; Poutanen, K.; Seal, C.J.; Richardson, D.P. The healthgrain definition of 'whole grain'. *Food Nutr. Res.* **2014**, *58*, 22100. [CrossRef] [PubMed]
6. International, AACC. Whole grain definition. *Cereal Foods World* **1999**, *45*, 79.
7. Bett-Garber, K.L.; Lea, J.M.; Champagne, E.T.; McClung, A.M. Whole-grain rice flavor associated with assorted bran colors. *J. Sens. Stud.* **2012**, *27*, 78–86. [CrossRef]
8. Slavin, J. Whole grains and digestive health. *Cereal Chem.* **2010**, *87*, 292–296. [CrossRef]
9. Slavin, J.L. Whole grains, refined grains and fortified refined grains: What's the difference? *Asia Pac. J. Clin. Nutr.* **2000**, *9*, S23–S27. [CrossRef] [PubMed]
10. Marquart, L.; Chan, H.W.; Orsted, M.; Schmitz, K.A.; Arndt, E.A.; Jacobs, D.R. Gradual incorporation of whole-grain flour into grain-based products. *Cereal Foods World* **2006**, *51*, 114–117. [CrossRef]
11. Montonen, J.; Knekt, P.; Jarvinen, R.; Aromaa, A.; Reunanen, A. Whole-grain and fiber intake and the incidence of type 2 diabetes. *Am. J. Clin. Nutr.* **2003**, *77*, 622–629. [PubMed]
12. Borneo, R.; Leon, A.E. Whole grain cereals: Functional components and health benefits. *Food Funct.* **2012**, *3*, 110–119. [CrossRef] [PubMed]
13. Ampatzoglou, A.; Atwal, K.K.; Maidens, C.M.; Williams, C.L.; Ross, A.B.; Thielecke, F.; Jonnalagadda, S.S.; Kennedy, O.B.; Yaqoob, P. Increased whole grain consumption does not affect blood biochemistry, body composition, or gut microbiology in healthy, low-habitual whole grain consumers. *J. Nutr.* **2015**, *145*, 215–221. [CrossRef] [PubMed]
14. Cooper, D.N.; Martin, R.J.; Keim, N.L. Does whole grain consumption alter gut microbiota and satiety? *Healthcare* **2015**, *3*, 364–392. [CrossRef] [PubMed]

15. Jackson, K.H.; West, S.G.; Vanden Heuvel, J.P.; Jonnalagadda, S.S.; Ross, A.B.; Hill, A.M.; Grieger, J.A.; Lemieux, S.K.; Kris-Etherton, P.M. Effects of whole and refined grains in a weight-loss diet on markers of metabolic syndrome in individuals with increased waist circumference: A randomized controlled-feeding trial. *Am. J. Clin. Nutr.* **2014**, *100*, 577–586. [CrossRef] [PubMed]
16. Modi, P. Benefits of low glycemic and high satiety index foods for obesity and diabetes control and management. In *Nutrients, Dietary Supplements, and Nutriceuticals;* Cost Analysis Versus Clinical Benefits; Springer: New York, NY, USA, 2011; pp. 403–424.
17. Zhou, A.L.; Hergert, N.; Rompato, G.; Lefevre, M. Whole grain oats improve insulin sensitivity and plasma cholesterol profile and modify gut microbiota composition in C57BL/6J mice. *J. Nutr.* **2015**, *145*, 222–230. [CrossRef] [PubMed]
18. Rebello, C.J.; Greenway, F.L.; Finley, J.W. Whole grains and pulses: A comparison of the nutritional and health benefits. *J. Agric. Food Chem.* **2014**, *62*, 7029–7049. [CrossRef] [PubMed]
19. Costabile, A.; Klinder, A.; Fava, F.; Napolitano, A.; Foglian, V.; Leonard, C.; Gibson, G.R.; Tuohy, K.M. Whole-grain wheat breakfast cereal has a prebiotic effect on the human gut microbiota: A double-blind, placebo-controlled, crossover study. *Br. J. Nutr.* **2008**, *99*, 110–120. [CrossRef] [PubMed]
20. Raninen, K.; Lappi, J.; Mykkanen, H.; Poutanen, K. Dietary fiber type reflects physiological functionality: Comparison of grain fiber, inulin, and polydextrose. *Nutr. Rev.* **2011**, *69*, 9–21. [CrossRef] [PubMed]
21. Nyman, M.; Siljestrom, M.; Pedersen, B.; Knudsen, K.E.B.; Asp, N.G.; Johansson, C.G.; Eggum, B.O. Dietary fiber content and composition in 6 cereals at different extraction rates. *Cereal Chem.* **1984**, *61*, 14–19.
22. Frankenfield, D.C.; Muth, E.R.; Rowe, W.A. The harris-benedict studies of human basal metabolism: History and limitations. *J. Am. Diet. Assoc.* **1998**, *98*, 439–445. [CrossRef]
23. Lewis, S.J.; Heaton, K.W. Stool form scale as a useful guide to intestinal transit time. *Scand. J. Gastroenterol.* **1997**, *32*, 920–924. [CrossRef] [PubMed]
24. Ferguson, L.W. A study of the likert technique of attitude scale construction. *J. Soc. Psychol.* **1941**, *13*, 51–57. [CrossRef]
25. Hsieh, Y.-H.; Peterson, C.M.; Raggio, A.; Keenan, M.J.; Martin, R.J.; Ravussin, E.; Marco, M.L. Impact of different fecal processing methods on assessments of bacterial diversity in the human intestine. *Front. Microbiol.* **2016**, *7*, 1–11. [CrossRef] [PubMed]
26. Salonen, A.; Nikkila, J.; Jalanka-Tuovinen, J.; Immonen, O.; Rajilic-Stojanovic, M.; Kekkonen, R.A.; Palva, A.; de Vos, W.M. Comparative analysis of fecal DNA extraction methods with phylogenetic microarray: Effective recovery of bacterial and archaeal DNA using mechanical cell lysis. *J. Microbiol. Methods* **2010**, *81*, 127–134. [CrossRef] [PubMed]
27. Wang, Q.; Garrity, G.M.; Tiedje, J.M.; Cole, J.R. Naive bayesian classifier for rapid assignment of rrna sequences into the new bacterial taxonomy. *Appl. Environ. Microbiol.* **2007**, *73*, 5261–5267. [CrossRef] [PubMed]
28. Caporaso, J.G.; Lauber, C.L.; Walters, W.A.; Berg-Lyons, D.; Lozupone, C.A.; Turnbaugh, P.J.; Fierer, N.; Knight, R. Global patterns of 16S rRNA diversity at a depth of millions of sequences per sample. *Proc. Natl. Acad. Sci. USA* **2011**, *108*, 4516–4522. [CrossRef] [PubMed]
29. Hamady, M.; Walker, J.J.; Harris, J.K.; Gold, N.J.; Knight, R. Error-correcting barcoded primers for pyrosequencing hundreds of samples in multiplex. *Nat. Methods* **2008**, *5*, 235–237. [CrossRef] [PubMed]
30. Caporaso, J.G.; Kuczynski, J.; Stombaugh, J.; Bittinger, K.; Bushman, F.D.; Costello, E.K.; Fierer, N.; Pena, A.G.; Goodrich, J.K.; Gordon, J.I.; et al. Qiime allows analysis of high-throughput community sequencing data. *Nat. Methods* **2010**, *7*, 335–336. [CrossRef] [PubMed]
31. Aronesty, E. Ea-utils: Command-Line Tools for Processing Biological Sequencing Data. Available online: https://github.com/ExpressionAnalysis/ea-utils (accessed on 17 April 2011).
32. Edgar, R.C.; Haas, B.J.; Clemente, J.C.; Quince, C.; Knight, R. Uchime improves sensitivity and speed of chimera detection. *Bioinformatics* **2011**, *27*, 2194–2200. [CrossRef] [PubMed]
33. Edgar, R.C. Search and clustering orders of magnitude faster than blast. *Bioinformatics* **2010**, *26*, 2460–2461. [CrossRef] [PubMed]
34. Bokulich, N.A.; Subramanian, S.; Faith, J.J.; Gevers, D.; Gordon, J.I.; Knight, R.; Mills, D.A.; Caporaso, J.G. Quality-filtering vastly improves diversity estimates from illumina amplicon sequencing. *Nat. Methods* **2013**, *10*, 57–59. [CrossRef] [PubMed]

35. Wu, G.D.; Lewis, J.D.; Hoffmann, C.; Chen, Y.Y.; Knight, R.; Bittinger, K.; Hwang, J.; Chen, J.; Berkowsky, R.; Nessel, L.; et al. Sampling and pyrosequencing methods for characterizing bacterial communities in the human gut using 16s sequence tags. *BMC Microbiol.* **2010**, *10*, 206. [CrossRef] [PubMed]
36. Segata, N.; Izard, J.; Waldron, L.; Gevers, D.; Miropolsky, L.; Garrett, W.S.; Huttenhower, C. Metagenomic biomarker discovery and explanation. *Genome Biol.* **2011**, *12*, R60. [CrossRef] [PubMed]
37. Kwong, K.S.; Holland, B.; Cheung, S.H. A modified benjamini-hochberg multiple comparisons procedure for controlling the false discovery rate. *J. Stat. Plan. Inference* **2002**, *104*, 351–362. [CrossRef]
38. De Filippo, C.; Cavalieri, D.; Di Paola, M.; Ramazzotti, M.; Poullet, J.B.; Massart, S.; Collini, S.; Pieraccini, G.; Lionetti, P. Impact of diet in shaping gut microbiota revealed by a comparative study in children from europe and rural africa. *Proc. Natl. Acad. Sci. USA* **2010**, *107*, 14691–14696. [CrossRef] [PubMed]
39. Mariat, D.; Firmesse, O.; Levenez, F.; Guimaraes, V.D.; Sokol, H.; Dore, J.; Corthier, G.; Furet, J.P. The firmicutes/bacteroidetes ratio of the human microbiota changes with age. *BMC Microbiol.* **2009**, *9*, 123. [CrossRef] [PubMed]
40. Lange, E. Oats products as functional food. *Zywnosc-Nauka Technol. Jakosc* **2010**, *17*, 7–24. [CrossRef]
41. Fardet, A. New hypotheses for the health-protective mechanisms of whole-grain cereals: What is beyond fibre? *Nutr. Res. Rev.* **2010**, *23*, 65–134. [CrossRef] [PubMed]
42. Bressani, R.; Breuner, M.; Ortiz, M.A. Acid-detergent and neutro-detergent fiber and mineral elements content of maize and tortilla. *Arch. Latinoam. Nutr.* **1989**, *39*, 382–391. [PubMed]
43. Sumczynski, D.; Bubelova, Z.; Fisera, M. Determination of chemical, insoluble dietary fibre, neutral-detergent fibre and in vitro digestibility in rice types commercialized in Czech markets. *J. Food Compos. Anal.* **2015**, *40*, 8–13. [CrossRef]
44. Lai, V.M.F.; Lu, S.; He, W.H.; Chen, H.H. Non-starch polysaccharide compositions of rice grains with respect to rice variety and degree of milling. *Food Chem.* **2007**, *101*, 1205–1210. [CrossRef]
45. Rose, D.J.; Patterson, J.A.; Hamaker, B.R. Structural differences among alkali-soluble arabinoxylans from maize (*Zea mays*), rice (*oryza sativa*), and wheat (*triticum aestivum*) brans influence human fecal fermentation profiles. *J. Agric. Food Chem.* **2010**, *58*, 493–499. [CrossRef] [PubMed]
46. Mohan, V.; Spiegelman, D.; Sudha, V.; Gayathri, R.; Hong, B.; Praseena, K.; Anjana, R.M.; Wedick, N.M.; Arumugam, K.; Malik, V.; et al. Effect of brown rice, white rice, and brown rice with legumes on blood glucose and insulin responses in overweight Asian Indians: A randomized controlled trial. *Diabetes Technol. Ther.* **2014**, *16*, 317–325. [CrossRef] [PubMed]
47. Tosh, S.M. Review of human studies investigating the post-prandial blood-glucose lowering ability of oat and barley food products. *Eur. J. Clin. Nutr.* **2013**, *67*, 310–317. [CrossRef] [PubMed]
48. Ranawana, V.; Clegg, M.E.; Shafat, A.; Henry, C.J. Postmastication digestion factors influence glycemic variability in humans. *Nutr. Res.* **2011**, *31*, 452–459. [CrossRef] [PubMed]
49. Bornhorst, G.M.; Stroebinger, N.; Rutherfurd, S.M.; Singh, R.P.; Moughan, P.J. Properties of gastric chyme from pigs fed cooked brown or white rice. *Food Biophys.* **2013**, *8*, 12–23. [CrossRef]
50. Oishi, K.; Yamamoto, S.; Itoh, N.; Nakao, R.; Yasumoto, Y.; Tanaka, K.; Kikuchi, Y.; Fukudome, S.; Okita, K.; Takano-Ishikawa, Y. Wheat alkylresorcinols suppress high-fat, high-sucrose diet-induced obesity and glucose intolerance by increasing insulin sensitivity and cholesterol excretion in male mice. *J. Nutr.* **2015**, *145*, 199–206. [CrossRef] [PubMed]
51. Arora, T.; Sharma, R.; Frost, G. Propionate. Anti-obesity and satiety enhancing factor? *Appetite* **2011**, *56*, 511–515. [CrossRef] [PubMed]
52. Everard, A.; Cani, P.D. Gut microbiota and GLP-1. *Rev. Endocr. Metab. Disord.* **2014**, *15*, 189–196. [CrossRef] [PubMed]
53. Chambers, E.S.; Viardot, A.; Psichas, A.; Morrison, D.J.; Murphy, K.G.; Sagen, E.K.; Varghese, Z.; MacDougall, K.; Preston, T. Effects of targeted delivery of propionate to the human colon on appetite regulation, body weight maintenance and adiposity in overweight adult. *BMJ* **2014**, 1–11. [CrossRef] [PubMed]
54. Todesco, T.; Rao, A.V.; Bosello, O.; Jenkins, D.J.A. Propionate lowers blood-glucose and alters lipid-metabolism in healthy-subjects. *Am. J. Clin. Nutr.* **1991**, *54*, 860–865. [PubMed]
55. Frost, G.; Sleeth, M.L.; Sahuri-Arisoylu, M.; Lizarbe, B.; Cerdan, S.; Brody, L.; Anastasovska, J.; Ghourab, S.; Hankir, M.; Zhang, S.; et al. The short-chain fatty acid acetate reduces appetite via a central homeostatic mechanism. *Nat. Commun.* **2014**, *5*, 3611. [CrossRef] [PubMed]

56. Venter, C.S.; Vorster, H.H.; Cummings, J.H. Effects of dietary propionate on carbohydrate and lipid-metabolism in healthy-volunteers. *Am. J. Gastroenterol.* **1990**, *85*, 549–553. [PubMed]
57. Johansson, E.V.; Nilsson, A.C.; Ostman, E.M.; Bjorck, I.M.E. Effects of indigestible carbohydrates in barley on glucose metabolism, appetite and voluntary food intake over 16 h in healthy adults. *Nutr. J.* **2013**, *12*, 46. [CrossRef] [PubMed]
58. McIntosh, G.H.; Noakes, M.; Royle, P.J.; Foster, P.R. Whole-grain rye and wheat foods and markers of bowel health in overweight middle-aged men. *Am. J. Clin. Nutr.* **2003**, *77*, 967–974. [PubMed]
59. Youn, M.; Csallany, A.S.; Gallaher, D.D. Whole grain consumption has a modest effect on the development of diabetes in the goto-kakisaki rat. *Br. J. Nutr.* **2012**, *107*, 192–201. [CrossRef] [PubMed]
60. Kristensen, M.; Jensen, M.G.; Riboldi, G.; Petronio, M.; Bugel, S.; Toubro, S.; Tetens, I.; Astrup, A. Wholegrain vs. Refined wheat bread and pasta. Effect on postprandial glycemia, appetite, and subsequent ad libitum energy intake in young healthy adults. *Appetite* **2010**, *54*, 163–169. [CrossRef] [PubMed]
61. Cano, J.M.M.; Aguilar, A.C.; Hernandez, J.C. Lipid-lowering effect of maize-based traditional mexican food on a metabolic syndrome model in rats. *Lipids Health Dis.* **2013**, *12*, 35. [CrossRef] [PubMed]
62. Mackie, A.; Bajka, B.; Rigby, N. Roles for dietary fibre in the upper gi tract: The importance of viscosity. *Food Res. Int.* **2016**, *88*, 234–238. [CrossRef]
63. Knudsen, K.E.B.; Laerke, H.N. Whole grain cereals and gut health. *Agro Food Ind. Hi-Tech* **2008**, *19*, 6–8.
64. Odes, H.S.; Lazovski, H.; Stern, I.; Madar, Z. Double-blind trial of a high dietary fiber, mixed grain cereal in patients with chronic constipation and hyperlipidemia. *Nutr. Res.* **1993**, *13*, 979–985. [CrossRef]
65. Bird, A.R.; Vuaran, M.S.; King, R.A.; Noakes, M.; Keogh, J.; Morell, M.K.; Topping, D.L. Wholegrain foods made from a novel high-amylose barley variety (himalaya 292) improve indices of bowel health in human subjects. *Br. J. Nutr.* **2008**, *99*, 1032–1040. [CrossRef] [PubMed]
66. Kim, J.Y.; Son, B.K.; Lee, S.S. Effects of adlay, buckwheat, and barley on transit time and the antioxidative system in obesity induced rats. *Nutr. Res. Pract.* **2012**, *6*, 208–212. [CrossRef] [PubMed]
67. De Vries, J.; Miller, P.E.; Verbeke, K. Effects of cereal fiber on bowel function: A systematic review of intervention trials. *World J. Gastroenterol.* **2015**, *21*, 8952–8963. [CrossRef] [PubMed]
68. De Vries, J.; Birkett, A.; Hulshof, T.; Verbeke, K.; Gibes, K. Effects of cereal, fruit and vegetable fibers on human fecal weight and transit time: A comprehensive review of intervention trials. *Nutrients* **2016**, *8*, 130. [CrossRef] [PubMed]
69. Slavin, J. Health aspects of dietary fibre. *Fibre-Rich Wholegrain Foods Improv. Qual.* **2013**, *237*, 61–75.
70. Belobrajdic, D.P.; Bird, A.R. The potential role of phytochemicals in wholegrain cereals for the prevention of type-2 diabetes. *Nutr. J.* **2013**, *12*, 62. [CrossRef] [PubMed]
71. Coughlin, S.S. Toward a road map for global -omics: A primer on -omic technologies. *Am. J. Epidemiol.* **2014**, *180*, 1188–1195. [CrossRef] [PubMed]
72. Scott, K.P.; Martin, J.C.; Duncan, S.H.; Flint, H.J. Prebiotic stimulation of human colonic butyrate-producing bacteria and bifidobacteria, in vitro. *Fems Microbiol. Ecol.* **2014**, *87*, 30–40. [CrossRef] [PubMed]
73. Mirande, C.; Kadlecikova, E.; Matulova, M.; Capek, P.; Bernalier-Donadille, A.; Forano, E.; Bera-Maillet, C. Dietary fibre degradation and fermentation by two xylanolytic bacteria bacteroides xylanisolvens xb1at and roseburia intestinalis xb6b4 from the human intestine. *J. Appl. Microbiol.* **2010**, *109*, 451–460. [PubMed]
74. Hamer, H.M.; De Preter, V.; Windey, K.; Verbeke, K. Functional analysis of colonic bacterial metabolism: Relevant to health? *Am. J. Physiol.-Gastrointest. Liver Physiol.* **2012**, *302*, G1–G9. [CrossRef] [PubMed]
75. Lozupone, C.A.; Stombaugh, J.I.; Gordon, J.I.; Jansson, J.K.; Knight, R. Diversity, stability and resilience of the human gut microbiota. *Nature* **2012**, *489*, 220–230. [CrossRef] [PubMed]
76. Bosscher, D.; Breynaert, A.; Pieters, L.; Hermans, N. Food-based strategies to modulate the composition of the intestinal microbiota and their associated health effects. *J. Physiol. Pharmacol.* **2009**, *60*, 5–11. [PubMed]
77. Cani, P.D.; Neyrinck, A.M.; Fava, F.; Knauf, C.; Burcelin, R.G.; Tuohy, K.M.; Gibson, G.R.; Delzenne, N.M. Selective increases of bifidobacteria in gut microflora improve high-fat-diet-induced diabetes in mice through a mechanism associated with endotoxaemia. *Diabetologia* **2007**, *50*, 2374–2383. [CrossRef] [PubMed]
78. Christensen, E.G.; Licht, T.R.; Kristensen, M.; Bahl, M.I. Bifidogenic effect of whole-grain wheat during a 12-week energy-restricted dietary intervention in postmenopausal women. *Eur. J. Clin. Nutr.* **2013**, *67*, 1316–1321. [CrossRef] [PubMed]

79. Koren, O.; Goodrich, J.K.; Cullender, T.C.; Spor, A.; Laitinen, K.; Backhed, H.K.; Gonzalez, A.; Werner, J.J.; Angenent, L.T.; Knight, R.; et al. Host remodeling of the gut microbiome and metabolic changes during pregnancy. *Cell* **2012**, *150*, 470–480. [CrossRef] [PubMed]
80. Gibson, G.R.; Probert, H.M.; Van Loo, J.; Rastall, R.A.; Roberfroid, M.B. Dietary modulation of the human colonic microbiota: Updating the concept of prebiotics. *Nutr. Res. Rev.* **2004**, *17*, 259–275. [CrossRef] [PubMed]
81. Mobley, A.R.; Jones, J.M.; Rodriguez, J.; Slavin, J.; Zelman, K.M. Identifying practical solutions to meet america's fiber needs: Proceedings from the food & fiber summit. *Nutrients* **2014**, *6*, 2540–2551. [PubMed]
82. Zhong, Y.; Nyman, M.; Fak, F. Modulation of gut microbiota in rats fed high-fat diets by processing whole-grain barley to barley malt. *Mol. Nutr. Food Res.* **2015**, *59*, 2066–2076. [CrossRef] [PubMed]
83. De Angelis, M.; Montemurno, E.; Vannini, L.; Cosola, C.; Cavallo, N.; Gozzi, G.; Maranzano, V.; Di Cagno, R.; Gobbetti, M.; Gesualdo, L. Effect of whole-grain barley on the human fecal microbiota and metabolome. *Appl. Environ. Microbiol.* **2015**, *81*, 7945–7956. [CrossRef] [PubMed]
84. Everard, A.; Belzer, C.; Geurts, L.; Ouwerkerk, J.P.; Druart, C.; Bindels, L.B.; Guiot, Y.; Derrien, M.; Muccioli, G.G.; Delzenne, N.M.; et al. Cross-talk between akkermansia muciniphila and intestinal epithelium controls diet-induced obesity. *Proc. Natl. Acad. Sci. USA* **2013**, *110*, 9066–9071. [CrossRef] [PubMed]
85. Joyce, S.A.; Gahan, C.G.M. The gut microbiota and the metabolic health of the host. *Curr. Opin. Gastroenterol.* **2014**, *30*, 120–127. [CrossRef] [PubMed]
86. Greer, R.L.; Dong, X.X.; Moraes, A.C.F.; Zielke, R.A.; Fernandes, G.R.; Peremyslova, E.; Vasquez-Perez, S.; Schoenborn, A.A.; Gomes, E.P.; Pereira, A.C.; et al. Akkermansia muciniphila mediates negative effects of ifn gamma on glucose metabolism. *Nat. Commun.* **2016**, *7*, 13329. [CrossRef] [PubMed]
87. Remely, M.; Tesar, I.; Hippe, B.; Gnauer, S.; Rust, P.; Haslberger, A.G. Gut microbiota composition correlates with changes in body fat content due to weight loss. *Benef. Microbes* **2015**, *6*, 431–439. [CrossRef] [PubMed]
88. Sarao, L.K.; Arora, M. Probiotics, prebiotics, and microencapsulation: A review. *Crit. Rev. Food Sci. Nutr.* **2017**, *57*, 344–371. [CrossRef] [PubMed]
89. Hang, I.; Rinttila, T.; Zentek, J.; Kettunen, A.; Alaja, S.; Apajalahti, J.; Harmoinen, J.; de Vos, W.M.; Spillmann, T. Effect of high contents of dietary animal-derived protein or carbohydrates on canine faecal microbiota. *BMC Vet. Res.* **2012**, *8*, 90. [CrossRef] [PubMed]
90. Magnusson, K.R.; Hauck, L.; Jeffrey, B.M.; Elias, V.; Humphrey, A.; Nath, R.; Perrone, A.; Bermudez, L.E. Relationships between diet-related changes in the gut microbiome and cognitive flexibility. *Neuroscience* **2015**, *300*, 128–140. [CrossRef] [PubMed]
91. Schwab, C.; Berry, D.; Rauch, I.; Rennisch, I.; Ramesmayer, J.; Hainzl, E.; Heider, S.; Decker, T.; Kenner, L.; Muller, M.; et al. Longitudinal study of murine microbiota activity and interactions with the host during acute inflammation and recovery. *ISME J.* **2014**, *8*, 1101–1114. [CrossRef] [PubMed]
92. Gevers, D.; Kugathasan, S.; Denson, L.A.; Vazquez-Baeza, Y.; Van Treuren, W.; Ren, B.Y.; Schwager, E.; Knights, D.; Song, S.J.; Yassour, M.; et al. The treatment-naive microbiome in new-onset crohn's disease. *Cell Host Microbe* **2014**, *15*, 382–392. [CrossRef] [PubMed]
93. Haro, C.; Garcia-Carpintero, S.; Alcala-Diaz, J.F.; Gomez-Delgado, F.; Delgado-Lista, J.; Perez-Martinez, P.; Zuniga, O.A.R.; Quintana-Navarro, G.M.; Landa, B.B.; Clemente, J.C.; et al. The gut microbial community in metabolic syndrome patients is modified by diet. *J. Nutr. Biochem.* **2016**, *27*, 27–31. [CrossRef] [PubMed]
94. Chen, W.G.; Liu, F.L.; Ling, Z.X.; Tong, X.J.; Xiang, C. Human intestinal lumen and mucosa-associated microbiota in patients with colorectal cancer. *PLoS ONE* **2012**, *7*, e39743. [CrossRef] [PubMed]
95. Vaziri, N.D.; Wong, J.; Pahl, M.; Piceno, Y.M.; Yuan, J.; DeSantis, T.Z.; Ni, Z.M.; Nguyen, T.H.; Andersen, G.L. Chronic kidney disease alters intestinal microbial flora. *Kidney Int.* **2013**, *83*, 308–315. [CrossRef] [PubMed]
96. Kelly, T.N.; Bazzano, L.A.; Ajami, N.J.; He, H.; Zhao, J.Y.; Petrosino, J.F.; Correa, A.; He, J. Gut microbiome associates with lifetime cardiovascular disease risk profile among bogalusa heart study participants. *Circ. Res.* **2016**, *119*, 956–964. [CrossRef] [PubMed]
97. Kaakoush, N.O. Insights into the role of erysipelotrichaceae in the human host. *Front. Cell. Infect. Microbiol.* **2015**, *5*, 84. [CrossRef] [PubMed]

7

Analysis of the Anti-Cancer Effects of Cincau Extract (*Premna oblongifolia* Merr) and Other Types of Non-Digestible Fibre Using Faecal Fermentation Supernatants and Caco-2 Cells as a Model of the Human Colon

Samsu U. Nurdin [1,2,3], Richard K. Le Leu [3,4], Graeme P. Young [3], James C. R. Stangoulis [1], Claus T. Christophersen [4,5] and Catherine A. Abbott [1,3,*]

1 School of Biological Sciences, Flinders University, Adelaide, SA 5042, Australia; samsu.udayana@fp.unila.ac.id (S.U.N.); james.stangoulis@flinders.edu.au (J.C.R.S.)

2 Department of Agricultural Product Technology, Lampung University, Bandar Lampung 35145, Indonesia

3 Flinders Centre for Innovation in Cancer, Adelaide, SA 5042, Australia; Richard.LeLeu@sa.gov.au (R.K.L.L.); graeme.young@flinders.edu.au (G.P.Y.)

4 CSIRO Food and Nutrition, Adelaide, SA 5000, Australia; c.christophersen@ecu.edu.au

5 School of Medical and Health Sciences, Edith Cowan University, Joondalup, WA 6027, Australia

* Correspondence: cathy.abbott@flinders.edu.au;

Abstract: Green cincau (*Premna oblongifolia* Merr) is an Indonesian food plant with a high dietary fibre content. Research has shown that dietary fibre mixtures may be more beneficial for colorectal cancer prevention than a single dietary fibre type. The aim of this study was to investigate the effects of green cincau extract on short chain fatty acid (SCFA) production in anaerobic batch cultures inoculated with human faecal slurries and to compare these to results obtained using different dietary fibre types (pectin, inulin, and cellulose), singly and in combination. Furthermore, fermentation supernatants (FSs) were evaluated in Caco-2 cells for their effect on cell viability, differentiation, and apoptosis. Cincau increased total SCFA concentration by increasing acetate and propionate, but not butyrate concentration. FSs from all dietary fibre sources, including cincau, reduced Caco-2 cell viability. However, the effects of all FSs on cell viability, cell differentiation, and apoptosis were not simply explainable by their butyrate content. In conclusion, products of fermentation of cincau extracts induced cell death, but further work is required to understand the mechanism of action. This study demonstrates for the first time that this Indonesian traditional source of dietary fibre may be protective against colorectal cancer.

Keywords: dietary fibre; colorectal cancer; fermentation; cincau; short chain fatty acids

1. Introduction

Colorectal cancer (CRC) incidence is rising significantly in most countries due to increasing prosperity [1]. Compounds such as short chain fatty acids (SCFAs), which are produced by bacterial fermentation of undigested dietary fibre, are capable of inhibiting cancer in vitro and in vivo [2–6]. The type of dietary fibre consumed influences the proportion and distribution of SCFAs in the gastrointestinal tract [7–10]. Rapidly fermentable dietary fibre is fermented in the proximal colon and results in increased SCFA levels in this region of the gut; conversely, slow fermentable dietary fibre will reach the distal colon and modulate SCFA production at this site [7,11].

Many researchers have shown mixtures of multiple dietary fibre types are more beneficial than a single dietary fibre [7,12–14]. Rats administered diets containing guar gum or pectin produced low proportions of butyrate in comparison to rats fed mixtures of both [12,13]. Compared with control or wheat bran diets alone, diets containing a combination of wheat bran and resistant starch produced higher wet and dry output, a lower pH and ammonia, as well as lower levels of phenol [13]. An in vitro fermentation study showed that a combination of Raftilose (oligofructose) and guar gum results in higher total SCFAs than individual guar gum [14]. Following 24 h culture, the SCFA production rate from individual Raftilose or guar gum fermentation decreased, but when these fibres were combined, the production rate kept increasing, indicating that a combination of fibre sources may be more beneficial.

The inulin-type compound fructan has also been well studied for its ability to protect against colorectal cancer when included in the diet [15–18]. In combination with lycopene and probiotics, inulin induced apoptosis, and inhibited cell proliferation and aberrant crypt formation (ACF) in rat colon when the chemical 1,2-dimethylhydrazine (DMH) was used to induce cancer [19]. Inulin intake reduced CRC levels in rats fed a high lipid diet or chemical-induced CRC through decreasing enzyme activity and bile acid concentration [20,21]. The dietary fibre pectin is fermentable by human faecal bacteria and produces high proportions of acetic acid in vitro and in vivo [22]. Fermentation supernatant from incubation of human faecal slurry with apple pectin was found to be rich in butyrate and inhibited histone deacetylase in nucleus extracted from tumour cell lines [23].

Green cincau (*Premna oblongifolia* Merr) is a tropical plant belonging to the Verbenaceae family which is a traditional food source in Indonesia. Extracts from green leaf of the cincau plant contain about 20% pectin and have free radical scavenging activity [24]. Research on cincau extracts indicates they have the ability to induce cell-mediated immune responses in vitro [25]. As a dietary fibre, cincau extracts have laxative properties and can effectively induce the growth of lactic acid producing bacteria in the colon [26]. This study aimed to compare the efficacy of cincau extracts as a traditional source of dietary fibre with other dietary fibre combinations known to be protective against CRC. Our study found that, when fermented, cincau extracts were able to reduce Caco-2 cell viability, but the mechanism was unclear. In addition, this study found that when two different dietary fibres were combined, the benefits were not always additive.

2. Materials and Methods

2.1. Green Cincau Extracts

Green cincau leaves (*Premna oblongifolia* Merr.) were collected from traditional farmers in Indonesia. The fresh leaves were dried in an oven at 50 °C (water content around 12%), ground into fine powder, and imported into Australia using an AQIS permit (IP07024278). To prepare extracts for this study, 5 g of dried cincau leaf powder was placed in a glass beaker, then boiled water was added until the final volume was 100 mL, and the mixture was stirred for 5 min at maximum speed. The mixture was then filtered and allowed to set at room temperature [24]. The resulting jelly like extract was then freeze dried (Dynavac) and ground with mortar and pestle before use. Table 1 shows the freeze dried cincau extract composition as determined by CSIRO analytical tests (Adelaide, South Australia), as described in Belobrajdic [27]. A modification of the AOACI Method 994.13 [28] was used to determine dietary fibre composition as soluble and insoluble non-starch polysaccharides (NSPs) [27].

Table 1. Composition of dried green cincau extract (g/100 g dry weight).

Dietary Component	Concentration
Moisture	4.4
Fat	4.4
Protein	13.3
Ash	12.2
Starch	1.8
Resistant starch	0.5
Soluble NSP	5.8
Insoluble NSP	46.3
Total non-starch polysaccharides (NSPs)	52.1

2.2. *In Vitro Fermentation of Dietary Fibre*

Seven substrates as a single or a mixture of two dietary fibres (50:50) were tested following a CSIRO protocol (Adelaide, Australia): pectin, inulin, cellulose, pectin-cellulose mixture, inulin-cellulose, pectin-inulin, and green cincau extract (Table 2). The anaerobic batch fermentation was carried out as described in Charoendsiddhi et al. [29] and was adapted from Zhou et al. [30]. Briefly, 150 mg of each dietary fibre source or a 50:50 mixture was placed in a 15 mL capped tube, then 9 mL of sterile fermentation media was added. The media contained 0.25% (*w*/*v*) Tryptone, 125 ppm (*v*/*v*) micro-mineral solution (containing $CaCl_2 \cdot H_2O$ 13.2%, $MnCl_2 \cdot 4H_2O$ 10%, $CoCl_2 \cdot 6H_2O$ 1%, and $FeCl_3 \cdot 6H_2O$ 8%), 25% (*v*/*v*) carbonate buffer solution (0.4% NH_4HCO_3 and 3.5% $NaHCO_3$), 25% (*v*/*v*) macro-mineral solution (containing Na_2HPO_4 0.57%, KH_2PO_4 0.62%, and $MgSO_4 \cdot 7H_2O$ 0.06%), and 3.35% (*v*/*v*) reducing solution (containing cysteine hydrochloride 0.625%, $Na_2S \cdot 9H_2O$ 0.625%, and NaOH 0.04 M). After addition of the dietary fibre/s to the fermentation media, the pH was adjusted to pH 7.0. For inoculums, fresh faecal slurry from three healthy volunteers was pooled and diluted in phosphate buffer to produce 10% (*w*/*v*) inoculums. Signed consent was obtained from staff volunteers for the collection of fresh faecal samples. The faecal collection process was approved by the CSIRO Human Ethics Committee. Final concentration of inoculums was 1% (*w*/*v*) after mixing of 1 mL of 10% inoculums with 9 mL of media containing dietary fibre/s. A negative control containing only fermentation media and inoculum was prepared as a faecal blank (FB). All processes were carried out in anaerobic chamber with rocking (SL Bactron IV, Cornelius, OR, USA) to maintain anaerobic conditions set at 37 °C for 24 h. To help monitor that the chamber was maintained under anaerobic conditions, 1.25 ppm (*w*/*v*) of resazurine solution (Sigma-Aldrich, St Louis, MO, USA) was added to the initial fermentation media. Supernatants were sterilized by filtration (pore size 0.22 μm) (Minisart®, Sartorius AG, Dandenong South, Victoria, Australia) and stored at −80 °C until use.

Table 2. Type of dietary fibre and combinations used for batch in vitro fermentation.

Dietary Fibre	Ratio (%)
Pectin	100
Inulin	100
Cellulose	100
Pectin + cellulose	50:50
Pectin + inulin	50:50
Inulin + cellulose	50:50
Cincau extract	100
Faecal blank (FB)	-

2.3. *Cell Culture*

Human colorectal carcinoma cells Caco-2 were obtained from the American Type Culture Collection (ATCC Number CCL-247). Experiments were conducted on Caco-2 cells passage number 76 to 85 and were performed three to four passages post thawing. Cultures were maintained in Dulbecco's modified Eagle's medium (DMEM) (Sigma-Aldrich) supplemented with 10% fetal bovine serum (Bovogen, Victoria, Australia), 100 U/mL penicillin-streptomycin (Sigma-Aldrich), 1% nonessential amino acids (Sigma-Aldrich), and 20 mM 4-(2-hydroxyethyl)-1-piperazineethanesulfonic acid (HEPES, Sigma-Aldrich) in a CO_2 incubator (37 °C and 5% CO_2). For each assay, cells were seeded so that following the 24 h attachment and 48 h experimental time, cells reached 80%–90% confluence.

2.4. SCFA Analysis

Fermentation supernatant (FS) samples were homogenized in three volumes of internal standard solution (heptanoic acid, 1.68 mmol/L) (Sigma-Aldrich) and centrifuged at 3000× *g* for 10 min. The supernatant was then distilled and 0.3 μL was injected into a gas chromatograph (Hewlett-Packard 5890 Series II A, Wilmington, DE, USA) equipped with a flame ionization detector and a capillary column (Zebron ZB-FFAP, 30 m × 0.53 mm i.d., 1-μm film, SGE, Phenomenex, Torrance, CA, USA). Helium was used as the carrier gas; the initial oven temperature was 120 °C and was increased at 30 °C/min to 190 °C; the injector temperature was 210 °C and the detector temperature was 210 °C. A standard SCFA mixture containing acetate, propionate, and butyrate (Sigma-Aldrich) was used for calculations, and the results are expressed as μmol/g of sample [31].

2.5. MTT Proliferation Assay

Caco-2 cells were seeded into a 96-well plate (Costar®, Corning incorporated, Corning, NY, USA) at a density of 1.5 × 10^4 cells per well 24 h before treatment with FS (day 0) to allow adherence, then incubated for 48 h in media containing 20% FS. For standard curves, 1:2 serial dilutions were prepared to generate a standard curve of 5000–80,000 cells per well, in final volume of 100 μL [32].

After 48 h treatment, media was removed and 100 μL of medium containing 0.5 mg/mL 3-4,5-dimethylthiazol-2-yl)2,5-diphenyl-tetrazolium bromide (MTT) (Sigma-Aldrich) solution was added to each well and incubated (37 °C, 5% CO_2) for 1 h (to allow MTT to be metabolized). The formazan (MTT metabolic product) was resuspended in 80 μL of 20% sodium dodecyl sulfate (SDS, Amresco, Solon, OH, USA) in 0.02 M HCl (Sigma-Aldrich), and the plate was incubated in the dark for 1 h at room temperature. The optical density was read at 570 nm with background absorbance at 630 nm (FLUOstar omega, BMG Labtech GmbH, Ortenberg, Germany). Optical densities were converted to a total number of live cells using a linear regression plot. Results were expressed as the number of live cells in wells containing treatment compared with the number of cells in control wells (medium alone).

2.6. Alkaline Phosphatase (AP) Activity Assay

For the AP assay, 3.0 × 10^5 cells were seeded into each well of a six-well plate with supplemented media (as described above) and allowed to adhere for 24 h. The medium was removed and replaced with media containing 20% FS. After 48 h incubation, the medium was removed and cells were detached by incubation with 1× Trypsin-EDTA solution (Sigma-Aldrich) for 5 min at 37 °C. Detached cells were resuspended in 50 mM Tris-HCl buffer, pH 10.0, and homogenized by sonification. The homogenized cells were centrifuged at 100,000 rpm for 30 min to remove cell debris.

AP activity was measured by hydrolysis of *p*-nitro phenol phosphate (5 mM) (Sigma-Aldrich) and expressed in units (the number of μmol *p*-nitrophenol liberated in 1 min measured at 400 nm per mg protein). *p*-nitrophenol (0–200 μM) was used to generate a standard curve [33].

2.7. Caspase 3–7 and Lactate Dehydrogenase (LDH) Assay

Caco-2 cells were seeded into 96-well white plates (Costar®) at a density of 1.5 × 10^4 cells per well in supplemented media. The cells were incubated 24 h to allow the cells to adhere prior to treatment with 20% FS or control. After FS treatment, the cells were incubated for 48 h. Staurosporine 5 μM (Sigma) was used as a positive control to induce apoptosis (data not shown). The CytoTox-ONE™ Homogeneous Membrane Integrity assay kit (Promega, Madison, WI, USA) was employed to quantify the LDH enzyme activity, where 70 μL of cell culture supernatant was mixed with 70 μL CytoTox-ONE™ Reagent and shaken for 30 s, then incubated for 10 min. The stop solution (35 μL) was added to each well, and fluorescence was measured at excitation wavelength of 560 nm and an emission wavelength of 590 nm. In parallel, quantification of caspase-3/7 activities was carried out using the Caspase-GloR 3/7 assay kit (Promega). The FS treatments were also applied to separate Caco-2 cells cultured in 96-well plates for determination of cell proliferation using the MTT assay.

To confirm the role of caspase 3/7 in the cell death mechanism, FS from the inulin, cincau extract, and faecal blank fermentation were applied to the Caco-2 cells in combination with 10 μM caspase inhibitor (Ac-DEVD-CHO, Promega). Cells were seeded in 96-well plates as outlined above and the inhibitor was added 1 h preceding FS treatment.

2.8. Statistical Analysis

All cell culture experiments were performed on three different occasions, and the results are expressed as the mean ± standard error of mean (SEM). Statistical analysis was carried out with the statistical program SPSS version 19. One way-ANOVA with Least Significant Difference test was used. Results were considered significant if $p < 0.05$.

3. Results

3.1. SCFA Content of Dietary Fibre Fermentation Supernatant

Fermentation with cellulose alone had no significant effect on SCFA production. In contrast, fermentation of all other dietary fibres, individually or in combination, increased the yields of total SCFA, acetate, and propionate levels in the FS in comparison to the FB ($p < 0.05$) (Figure 1A–C). Cincau as the dietary fibre source significantly increased total SCFA, acetate, and propionate, but not butyrate levels. Butyrate levels were only significantly increased in the FS after fermentation with inulin, inulin-cellulose, and inulin-pectin (Figure 1D).

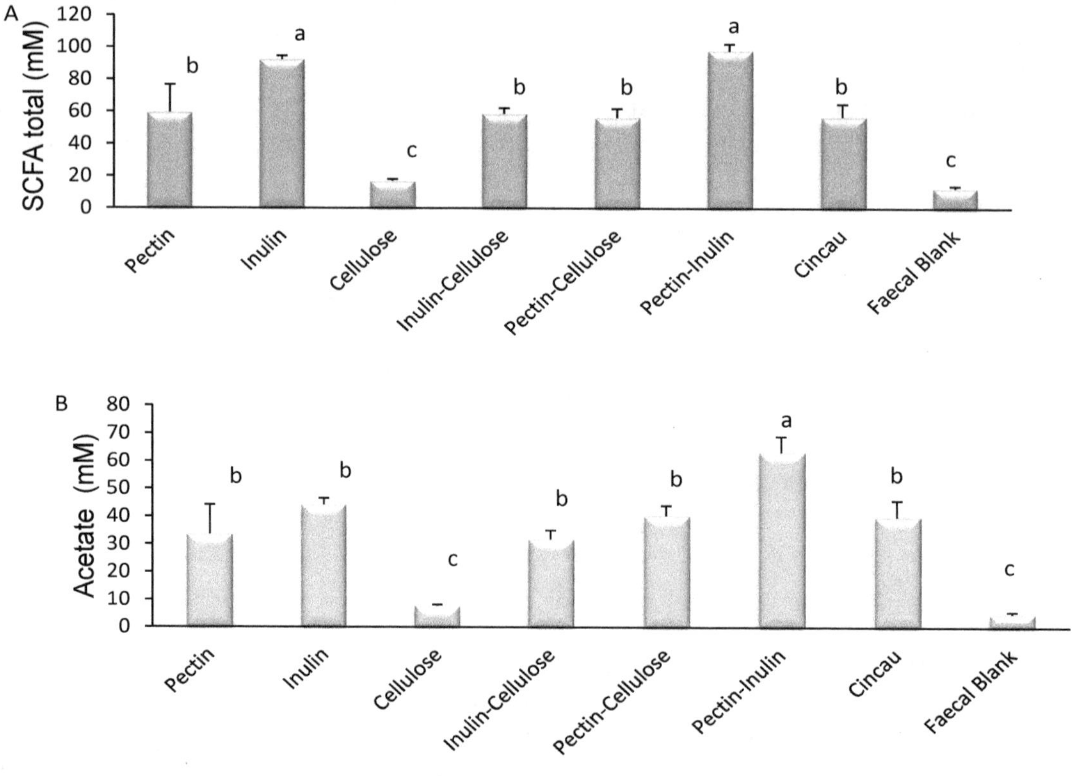

Figure 1. *Cont.*

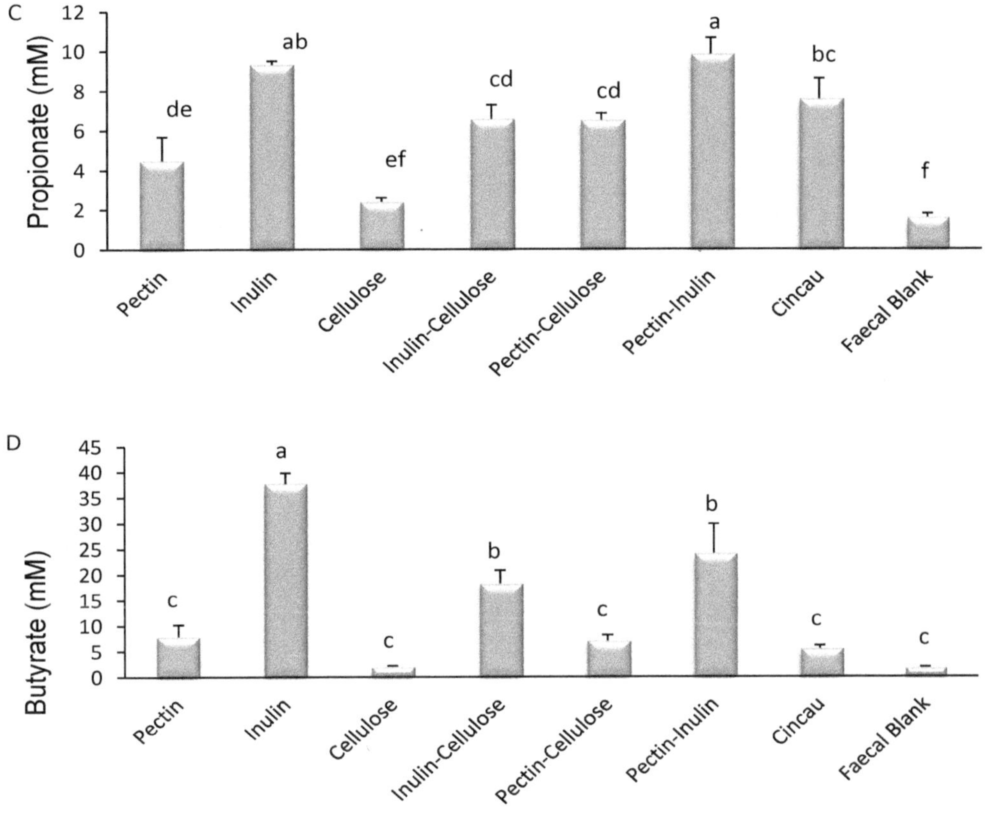

Figure 1. Effect of dietary fibre on the concentration of short chain fatty acid (SCFA) total (**A**), acetate (**B**), propionate (**C**), and butyrate (**D**) in fermentation supernatants. Dietary fibre/s were fermented with human faecal bacteria at 37 °C for 24 h in anaerobic conditions. The bars represent the mean, and the lines are SEM of four replicates. Data points denoted by different superscripts (letters above the bar) differ significantly when $p < 0.05$.

3.2. Effect of Dietary Fibre FS on Caco-2 Cell Viability

Due to the increased production of SCFA in the FS from the different fibre fermentations, we examined the effects of the FS on Caco-2 cell viability. As cellulose alone had no effect on SCFA production and inhibited SCFA production when mixed with inulin, no further studies were performed on FS from these two dietary fibre groups. In addition, as SCFA production was no different between the faecal blank (FB) and the cellulose group, for the remaining studies the blank served as the negative control. Treatment of Caco-2 cells with the remaining five FSs affected cell viability. Caco-2 cell number was significantly reduced after incubation of cells with 20% FS after incubation with cincau and with other dietary fibre/s compared to control FB (Figure 2, $p < 0.05$). Incubation with inulin FS inhibited cell growth the most when compared to FB. Combining pectin with inulin in the FS had no significant effect on the ability of inulin or pectin to inhibit cell growth.

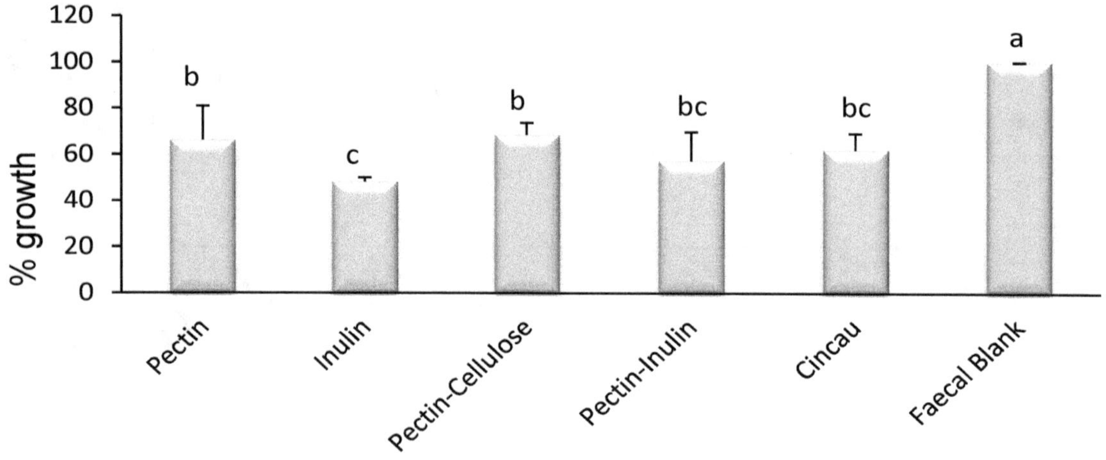

Figure 2. All dietary fibre sources reduced Caco-2 cell viability. Cells were seeded 1 day before the treatment with (fermentation supernatant) FS (day 0), then incubated for 48 h in media containing 20% FS. The bars represent the mean, and the lines are SEM of three independent experiments each performed in triplicate. Data points denoted by different superscripts (letters above the bar) differ significantly with $p < 0.05$.

3.3. *Effect of Dietary Fibre FS on Cell Differentiation*

Cell differentiation was assessed by measuring cellular levels of the enzyme alkaline phosphatase (AP) [34]. FSs from all dietary fibre sources, including cincau, failed to increase alkaline phosphatase enzyme levels but unexpectedly some caused significant decreases in alkaline phosphatase levels (Figure 3, $p < 0.05$). Cells that were incubated in FS after fermentation with inulin and mixtures of pectin and inulin had significantly lower alkaline phosphatase activity compared to FB, whereas cells incubated with FS from pectin, mixture of pectin-cellulose, and cincau displayed similar alkaline phosphatase activities to FB ($p < 0.05$).

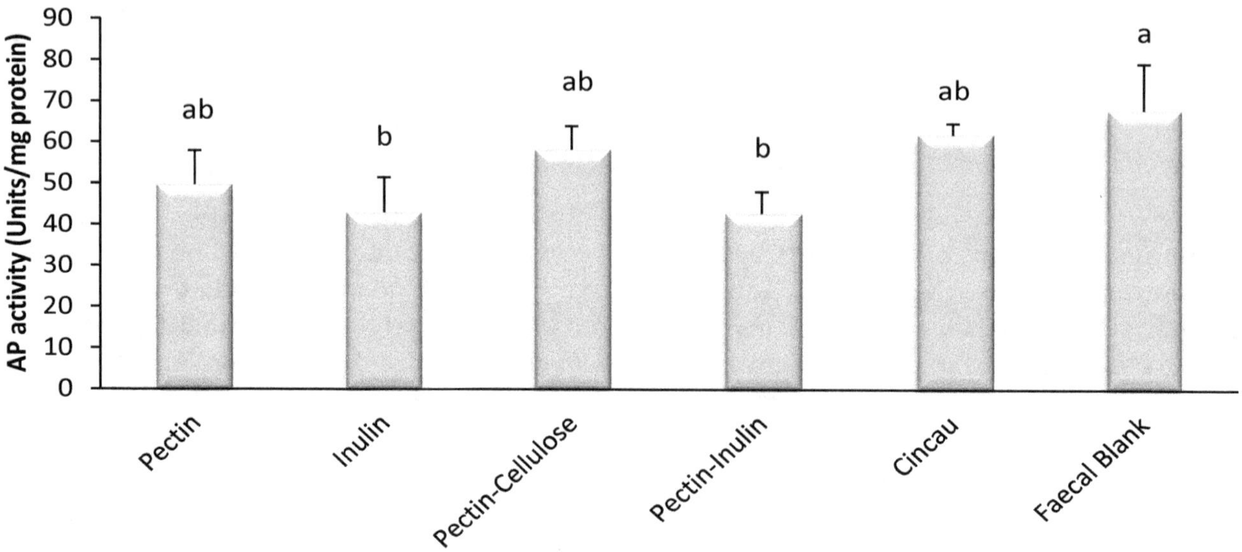

Figure 3. Effect of dietary fibre FS on alkaline phosphatase (AP) enzyme levels. AP enzyme activity was measured by hydrolysis of *p*-nitro phenol phosphate (5 mM) and expressed in units (the number of μmol *p*-nitrophenol liberated in 1 min measured at 400 nm per mg protein). The bars represent the mean, and the lines are SEM of three independent experiments each performed in triplicates. Data points denoted by different superscripts (letters above the bar) differ significantly with $p < 0.05$.

3.4. *Effect of Dietary Fibre FS on Caspase 3/7 Activity*

SCFAs have been shown to reduce proliferation and induce apoptosis in colorectal cell lines [2]. Caspase 3 and 7 are key effectors of apoptosis, therefore their activity was measured in Caco-2 cells after incubation with FS. Caspase 3/7 activity was affected by the type of dietary fibre fermented by colon microbiota (Figure 4, $p < 0.05$). Pectin, individually or in combination with inulin, induced higher caspase 3/7 activity compared to no treatment (control). In contrast, cincau extracts and the faecal blank suppressed caspase 3/7 activity ($p < 0.05$).

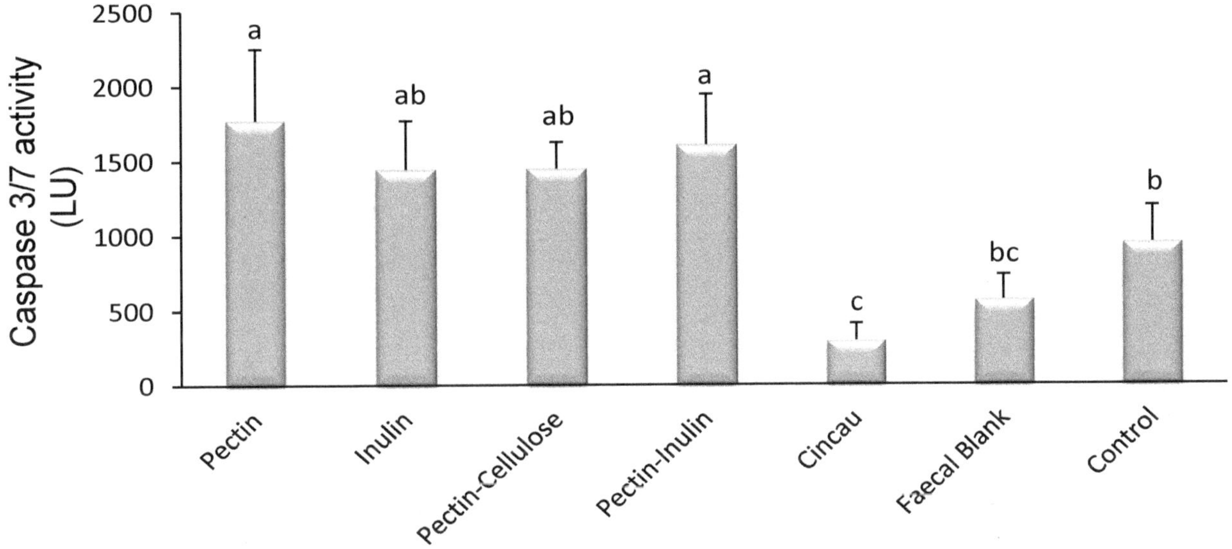

Figure 4. Effects of dietary fibre/s FS on caspase 3/7 activity. Cells were seeded 1 day before the treatment with FS (day 0), then incubated for 48 h in media containing 20% FS. Caspase-3 and 7 activities were measured using the Caspase-GloR 3/7 assay kit (Promega, USA). Control is cells incubated in media without FS. The bars represent the mean, and the lines are SEM of three independent experiments each performed in triplicate. Data points denoted by different superscripts (letters above the bar) differ significantly with $p < 0.05$. LU, Luminescence units.

3.5. *Mechanism of Cell Death Induced by FSs Containing SCFAs*

To further examine the increase in caspase 3/7 activity triggered by FSs from different dietary fibres above, a caspase inhibitor was utilised. Extracellular release of lactate dehydrogenase (LDH) was utilised as an additional measure of Caco-2 cell death. The caspase inhibitor significantly inhibited the ability of FSs from both inulin and the faecal blank to induce caspase 3/7 activity. In contrast, when cells were incubated with FS from cincau fermentation, very little caspase activity was detected and the inhibitor had no significant effect on this activity (Figure 5A; $p < 0.05$). LDH release in cells treated with FS when cincau was the fibre source was lower compared to that from inulin FS and FB (Figure 5B; $p < 0.05$). LDH release was not affected by the addition of the caspase inhibitor. Both inulin and cincau FS inhibited cell growth compared to the FB, and the caspase inhibitor was able to partially prevent this inhibition when inulin was the dietary fibre (Figure 5C; $p < 0.05$).

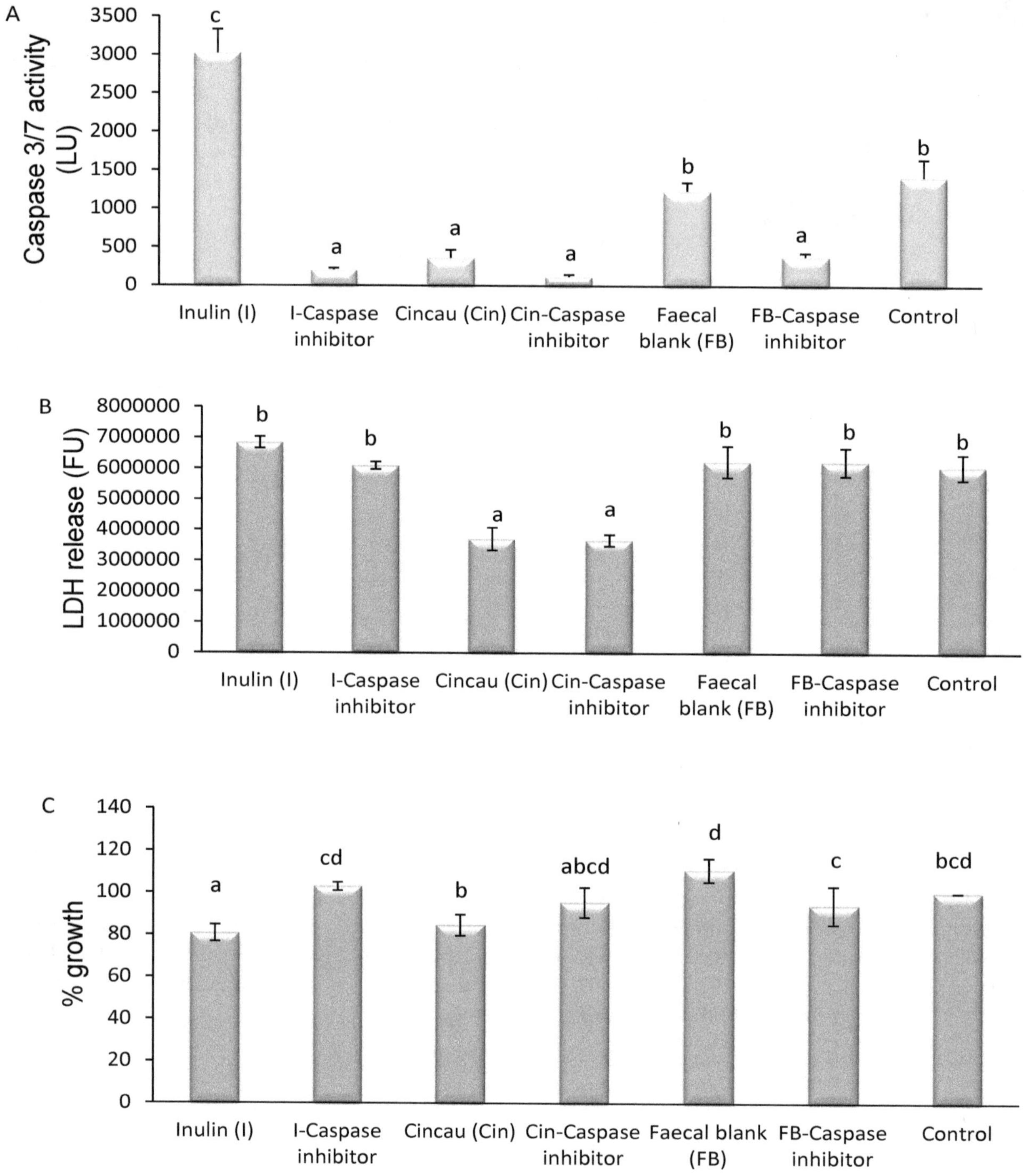

Figure 5. Effect of inulin and cincau on caspase 3/7 activity (**A**), LDH release (**B**), and Caco-2 cell viability (**C**) with or without caspase inhibitor. Cells were seeded 1 day before the treatment with FS (day 0), then incubated for 48 h in media containing 20% FS. Caspase inhibitor (10 μM) was added 1 h preceding FS treatment. Caspase 3–7 activity was measured using the Caspase-GloR 3/7 assay kit (Promega), the LDH activity was quantified using the CytoTox-ONE™ Homogeneous Membrane Integrity assay kit (Promega), and cell viability was measured using the MTT (dimethylthiazol-2-yl)2,5-diphenyl-tetrazolium bromide) assay and expressed as % growth against control. Control is cells incubated in media without FS. The bars represent the mean, and the lines are SEM of three independent experiments performed in triplicates. Data points denoted by different superscripts (letters above the bar) differ significantly with $p < 0.05$. LU, Luminescence units; FU, fluorescence units.

4. Discussion

This work demonstrates for the first time that green cincau, a traditional food that is indigenous to Indonesia, can be fermented to produce SCFAs which, when tested on colon cancer cells, can inhibit cell growth in vitro. In particular, cincau fermentation resulted in increased acetate and propionate production as assessed by their concentrations, but not butyrate. Furthermore, this study demonstrates that pectin and inulin alone, or in combination, had the greatest influence on individual and total SCFA production after fermentation by gut microbiota. Inulin produced the highest concentration of butyrate among the dietary fibres tested. Butyrate levels in FS from cellulose and pectin increased significantly if these dietary fibres were mixed with inulin. Inulin is known to stimulate butyrate-producing bacteria (*Roseburia intestinalis, Eubacterium rectale, Anaerostipes caccae*), which in turn leads to higher concentrations and proportions of butyrate [35].

The concentration of total SCFA, acetate, and butyrate produced in culture from the cincau extract was very similar to that produced when pectin or pectin-cellulose was added as the dietary fibre. Cellulose is a non-fermentable fibre and as a result has little effect on SCFA concentrations. Given that cincau extracts are known to contain 20% pectin [24], the increases in SCFA concentrations observed may be produced by the fermentation of the pectin component of this extract. However, when analysed these hot water extracts contained 5.8% soluble NSPs and 46.3% insoluble NSPs, thus it appears that the heating, cooling, and freeze drying process may have modified chemical and physical properties of the non-starch polysaccharides including pectin to form insoluble NSPs [36]. These now insoluble NSPs may also contribute to SCFA production during the in vitro fermentation.

SCFAs, and particularly butyrate, are well known for their ability to inhibit proliferation and induce apoptosis of colorectal cancer cells [2,3], but in this study high levels of butyrate in FS did not always affect cell viability. The butyrate content in pectin-inulin FS was nearly two-fold higher than pectin alone FS, while the propionate and acetate content from pectin-inulin FS was nearly double of pectin FS, however, the effect on Caco-2 cell growth when cultured in media containing these fermentation supernatants was no different. This indicates that butyrate or combinations of butyrate with propionate or acetate are not the main factors in fermentation supernatant that affect cell growth, and that non-SCFA compounds also contained in the FS may be involved [33]. Interestingly, cincau extract and pectin-cellulose FSs which had lower concentrations of total or individual SCFAs than pectin-inulin FS, inhibited Caco- 2 cell growth to the same extent as pectin-inulin FS.

Cell differentiation is one of the mechanisms by which SCFAs act in order to slow cancer cell growth [37]. This process requires cells to enter G1/G0 phase arrest, and cell proliferation is then inhibited [38]. Our results indicate that FS from pectin, inulin, pectin-cellulose mixture, pectin-inulin mixture, or cincau extract do not induce alkaline phosphatase, a marker of cell differentiation. Surprisingly, FS from blank (FB) induced higher alkaline phosphatase levels than pectin, inulin, or pectin-inulin, even though all of these dietary fibre FSs had high SCFA concentrations. There are some possibilities to explain these observations. First, the effect of butyrate on cell differentiation is dose dependent. It was previously observed that butyrate induced cell differentiation of Caco-2 cells at a concentration of 0.1 mM, but when the butyrate level was increased to 5 mM, activity of this enzyme decreased [39]. In the present study, the inulin and pectin-inulin FSs contained 37.7 and 24.2 mM of butyrate, respectively. When 20% of these FSs were added to the media, the final concentration of butyrate in the media would be 7.5 and 4.8 mM, respectively, whereas the final concentration of butyrate in media containing pectin, pectin-cellulose, and cincau was only 1.6, 1.4, and 1.1 mM, respectively. It is suggested that high levels of butyrate in inulin and pectin-inulin FSs may have led to the downregulation of AP activity. However, this explanation is not likely, as the blank (FB) which contains very little SCFA, elicited higher AP levels. Therefore, a second possibility needs to be considered to rationally explain the effects of FB. Previous researchers have also found that FB had an effect that was unexplainable by SCFA content in FS [16,33,40]. For example, Sauer et al. found that metabolic activity of HT-29 cells was increased by 15% by FB supplementation, with levels increasing similarly to those from inulin FS [16]. Moreover, these authors also found that FB enhanced gene expression of GSTA4, but inulin FS or SCFA mixture had no effects on this gene. GSTA4 is a gene encoding a glutathione S-transferase belonging to the alpha class 4 that has high catalytic efficiency with 4-hydroxyalkenals and other cytotoxic and mutagenic products of radical reactions and lipid peroxidation [41]. Taking this into account, data from this study indicate that the effect of FSs from dietary fibre on cell differentiation may depend on several factors including SCFA pattern and unidentified products formed during the fermentation process or that originally exist in the fresh faecal sample as a source of inoculums.

The ability of pectin, inulin, pectin-inulin, and pectin-cellulose FSs to induce apoptosis was confirmed by their ability to increase caspase 3/7 activity compared to control (Figure 4; $p < 0.05$). In contrast, cincau and FB, when compared to control, decreased levels of caspase 3/7. Previous research has shown that inulin induced apoptosis in HT-29 cells [42] or in a colon cancer rat model [43]. Our results support that inulin or pectin-inulin FSs are able to induce apoptosis through caspases, as caspase 3/7 activity increased in Caco-2 cells incubated with these FSs (Figure 4, $p < 0.05$).

Pectin or pectin-cellulose mixtures also increased caspase 3/7 activity (Figure 4, $p < 0.05$), and this may support a role for pectin via its increase in SCFAs as a dietary fibre that can affect the apoptosis process. Butyrate or other SCFAs produced by the fermentation of pectin may be able to inhibit histone deacetylase activity in order to induce gene transcription of caspase 3 and induce apoptosis [6,44–46].

Butyrate is the most potent SCFA for modulating colorectal cancer growth, including the induction of apoptosis [6,47]. However, our data indicate that modulation of apoptosis is not always dependant on butyrate content. The effect of FSs on caspase 3/7 activity was also unexplainable by total SCFA content of FS. Therefore, some factors other than SCFAs might be involved in modulating caspase 3/7 activity [23,42].

FSs from inulin, cincau, and FB were chosen to further elucidate the role of caspase 3/7 on cell death using the caspase inhibitor (Ac-DEVD-CHO) before the application of FS. LDH is an accurate method to assay cell death with membrane damage such as necrosis, while the MTT assay can measure differences in cell viability, but it cannot tell whether cells are being killed via apoptosis or necrosis [45]. The FS from inulin induced cell death through a caspase 3/7-dependent pathway, as the release of caspase 3/7 could be inhibited by the addition of the caspase inhibitor, and this led to an observed increase in Caco-2 cell viability. Cincau extract FS suppressed Caco-2 cell growth compared to FB (Figure 5C, $p < 0.05$), but the mechanism appeared to be different to that observed with inulin. Compared to FB, cincau did not induce caspase 3/7 activity (Figure 5A, $p < 0.05$), and indeed less LDH was released from cells treated with either cincau or cincau and caspase inhibitor (Figure 5B, $p < 0.05$), suggesting that cincau could protect cells from necrotic cell death. However, these cells were less viable than the control cells. Previously, Huang et al. [48] found that *Solanum nigrum* Linn leaf extract, rich in polyphenols and anthocyanidin, caused cell death due to the induction of autophagy and apoptosis. Acetone and ethyl acetate extracts from *Eupatorium odoratum* induced autophagic cell death in MCF-7 and Vero cell lines [49]. Cincau was extracted from green cincau leaves (*Premna oblongifolia* Merr.). The extract contains alkaloids, saponins, phenol hydroquinones, molisch, benedict, and tannins [50]. Supernatants collected after the non-digestible fraction of cooked common bean (*Phaseolus vulgaris* L.), when fermented with gut microbes, were able to induce apoptosis of HT-29 colon cells, and this was thought to be due to the participation of other phenolic fatty acid derivatives and biopeptides and not the SCFA contained in the supernates [51] Therefore, it may be possible that the phytochemical compounds from cincau or cincau fermentation induce autophagic cell death which cannot be measured by either the caspase or LDH assay, but would be worth investigating in future studies.

Our research implies that the beneficial effects of mixed dietary fibre as experienced in most human diets will depend on how each dietary fibre consumed interacts with the colon microbiota, and suggests the important role of unidentified compounds produced during fermentation by gut microbes in modulation of the effect of dietary fibre on CRC carcinogenesis. Furthermore, for the first time we show that Green cincau, a traditional Indonesian food, is not only able to inhibit colon cancer cell growth, but by an apoptosis-independent pathway. Further work should be conducted to assess the ability of this novel traditional dietary fibre as a chemopreventative.

Acknowledgments: This work was partially funded by an anonymous Philanthropic grant to Graeme P. Young (G.P.Y.) and by a Ph.D. scholarship from the Indonesian government to support Samsu U. Nurdin (S.U.N.). We would also like to thank Samsul Rizal from the University of Lampung, Indonesia for supplying the green cincau.

Author Contributions: S.U.N., R.K.L.L., G.P.Y., J.C.R.S. and C.A.A. all contributed to the design of this study. S.U.N. conducted all of the research and analysed all data. C.T.C. and R.K.L.L. helped S.U.N with setting up the in vitro fermentation and the SCFA measurements. S.U.N., R.K.L.L., G.P.Y. and C.A.A. contributed to the writing of the paper.

References

1. Center, M.M.; Jemal, A.; Ward, E. International trends in colorectal cancer incidence rates. *Cancer Epidemiol. Biomarkers Prev.* **2009**, *18*, 1688–1694. [CrossRef] [PubMed]
2. Fung, K.Y.; Cosgrove, L.; Lockett, T.; Head, R.; Topping, D.L. A review of the potential mechanisms for the lowering of colorectal oncogenesis by butyrate. *Br. J. Nutr.* **2012**, *108*, 820–831. [CrossRef] [PubMed]
3. Encarnacao, J.C.; Abrantes, A.M.; Pires, A.S.; Botelho, M.F. Revisit dietary fiber on colorectal cancer: Butyrate and its role on prevention and treatment. *Cancer Metastasis Rev.* **2015**, *34*, 465–478. [CrossRef] [PubMed]
4. Scharlau, D.; Borowicki, A.; Habermann, N.; Hofmann, T.; Klenow, S.; Miene, C.; Munjal, U.; Stein, K.; Glei, M. Mechanisms of primary cancer prevention by butyrate and other products formed during gut flora-mediated fermentation of dietary fibre. *Mutat. Res.* **2009**, *682*, 39–53. [CrossRef] [PubMed]
5. Whitehead, R.H.; Young, G.P.; Bhathal, P.S. Effects of short chain fatty acids on a new human colon carcinoma cell line (lim1215). *Gut* **1986**, *27*, 1457–1463. [CrossRef] [PubMed]
6. Medina, V.; Edmonds, B.; Young, G.P.; James, R.; Appleton, S.; Zalewski, P.D. Induction of caspase-3 protease activity and apoptosis by butyrate and trichostatin a (inhibitors of histone deacetylase): Dependence on protein synthesis and synergy with a mitochondrial/cytochrome c-dependent pathway. *Cancer Res.* **1997**, *57*, 3697–3707. [PubMed]
7. Juskiewicz, J.; Zdunczyk, Z. Effects of cellulose, carboxymethylcellulose and inulin fed to rats as single supplements or in combinations on their caecal parameters. *Comp. Biochem. Phys. A* **2004**, *139*, 513–519. [CrossRef] [PubMed]
8. Pompei, A.; Cordisco, L.; Raimondi, S.; Amaretti, A.; Pagnoni, U.M.; Matteuzzi, D.; Rossi, M. In vitro comparison of the prebiotic effects of two inulin-type fructans. *Anaerobe* **2008**, *14*, 280–286. [CrossRef] [PubMed]
9. Nilsson, U.; Nyman, M.; Ahrne, S.; Sullivan, E.O.; Fitzgerald, G. Bifidobacterium lactis bb-12 and lactobacillus salivarius ucc500 modify carboxylic acid formation in the hindgut of rats given pectin, inulin, and lactitol. *J. Nutr.* **2006**, *136*, 2175–2180. [PubMed]
10. McIntyre, A.; Young, G.P.; Taranto, T.; Gibson, P.R.; Ward, P.B. Different fibers have different regional effects on luminal contents of rat colon. *Gastroenterology* **1991**, *101*, 1274–1281. [CrossRef]
11. Pluske, J.R.; Durmic, Z.; Pethick, D.W.; Mullan, B.P.; Hampson, D.J. Confirmation of the role of rapidly fermentable carbohydrates in the expression of swine dysentery in pigs after experimental infection. *J. Nutr.* **1998**, *128*, 1737–1744. [PubMed]
12. Henningsson, A.M.; Bjorck, I.M.; Nyman, E.M. Combinations of indigestible carbohydrates affect short-chain fatty acid formation in the hindgut of rats. *J. Nutr.* **2002**, *132*, 3098–3104. [PubMed]
13. Muir, J.G.; Yeow, E.G.; Keogh, J.; Pizzey, C.; Bird, A.R.; Sharpe, K.; O'Dea, K.; Macrae, F.A. Combining wheat bran with resistant starch has more beneficial effects on fecal indexes than does wheat bran alone. *Am. J. Clin. Nutr.* **2004**, *79*, 1020–1028. [PubMed]
14. Khan, K.M.; Edwards, C.A. In vitro fermentation characteristics of a mixture of raftilose and guar gum by human faecal bacteria. *Eur. J. Nutr.* **2005**, *44*, 371–376. [CrossRef] [PubMed]

15. Pool-Zobel, B.L. Inulin-type fructans and reduction in colon cancer risk: Review of experimental and human data. *Br. J. Nutr.* **2005**, *93*, S73–S90. [CrossRef] [PubMed]
16. Pool-Zobel, B.L.; Sauer, J. Overview of experimental data on reduction of colorectal cancer risk by inulin-type fructans. *J. Nutr.* **2007**, *137*, 2580s–2584s. [PubMed]
17. Qamar, T.R.; Syed, F.; Nasir, M.; Rehman, H.; Zahid, M.N.; Liu, R.H.; Iqbal, S. Novel combination of prebiotics galacto-oligosaccharides and inulin-inhibited aberrant crypt foci formation and biomarkers of colon cancer in wistar rats. *Nutrients* **2016**, *8*. [CrossRef] [PubMed]
18. Wu, W.T.; Yang, L.C.; Chen, H.L. Effects of konjac glucomannan, inulin and cellulose on acute colonic responses to genotoxic azoxymethane. *Food Chem.* **2014**, *155*, 304–310. [CrossRef] [PubMed]
19. Dias, M.C.; Vieiralves, N.F.; Gomes, M.I.; Salvadori, D.M.; Rodrigues, M.A.; Barbisan, L.F. Effects of lycopene, synbiotic and their association on early biomarkers of rat colon carcinogenesis. *Food Chem. Toxicol.* **2010**, *48*, 772–780. [CrossRef] [PubMed]
20. Wu, W.T.; Chen, H.L. Effects of konjac glucomannan on putative risk factors for colon carcinogenesis in rats fed a high-fat diet. *J. Agric. Food Chem.* **2011**, *59*, 989–994. [CrossRef] [PubMed]
21. Bertkova, I.; Hijova, E.; Chmelarova, A.; Mojzisova, G.; Petrasova, D.; Strojny, L.; Bomba, A.; Zitnan, R. The effect of probiotic microorganisms and bioactive compounds on chemically induced carcinogenesis in rats. *Neoplasma* **2010**, *57*, 422–428. [CrossRef] [PubMed]
22. Rao, C.V.; Chou, D.; Simi, B.; Ku, H.; Reddy, B.S. Prevention of colonic aberrant crypt foci and modulation of large bowel microbial activity by dietary coffee fiber, inulin and pectin. *Carcinogenesis* **1998**, *19*, 1815–1819. [CrossRef] [PubMed]
23. Waldecker, M.; Kautenburger, T.; Daumann, H.; Veeriah, S.; Will, F.; Dietrich, H.; Pool-Zobel, B.L.; Schrenk, D. Histone-deacetylase inhibition and butyrate formation: Fecal slurry incubations with apple pectin and apple juice extracts. *Nutrition* **2008**, *24*, 366–374. [CrossRef] [PubMed]
24. Nurdin, S.U.; Zuidar, S.A.; Suharyono. Dried extract from green cincau leaves as potential fibre sources for food enrichment. *Afr. Crop. Sci. J.* **2005**, *7*, 655–658.
25. Nurdin, S.U.; Hwang, J.K.; Hung, P. Effect of green cincau leaf (*Premna oblongifolia* merr.) water extracts on cytokines production in whole cell culture of mouse splenocytes. *Indo Food Nutr. Prog.* **2003**, *10*, 70–74.
26. Nurdin, S.U. Evaluation of laxative effect and fermentability of gel forming component of green cincau leaves (*Premna oblongifolia* merr.). *Teknologi dan Industri Pangan* **2007**, *18*, 10–16.
27. Belobrajdic, D.P.; Hino, S.; Kondo, T.; Jobling, S.A.; Morell, M.K.; Topping, D.L.; Morita, T.; Bird, A.R. High wholegrain barley beta-glucan lowers food intake but does not alter small intestinal macronutrient digestibility in ileorectostomised rats. *Int. J. Food Sci. Nutr.* **2016**, *67*, 678–685. [CrossRef] [PubMed]
28. Association of Official Analytical Chemists (AOAC). *Official Methods of Analysis, Method 994.13, Supplement Total Dietary Fibre (Determined as Neutral Sugar Residues, Uronic Acid Residues and Klason Lignin)*; AOAC: Arlington, VA, USA, 1995.
29. Charoensiddhi, S.; Conlon, M.A.; Vuaran, M.S.; Franco, C.M.M.; Zhang, W. Impact of extraction processes on prebiotic potential of the brown seaweed ecklonia radiata by in vitro human gut bacteria fermentation. *J. Funct. Foods* **2016**, *24*, 221–230. [CrossRef]
30. Zhou, Z.; Cao, X.; Zhou, J.Y.H. Effect of resistant starch structure on short-chain fatty acids production by human gut microbiota fermentation in vitro. *Starch Stärke* **2013**, *65*, 509–516. [CrossRef]
31. Le Leu, R.K.; Brown, I.L.; Hu, Y.; Bird, A.R.; Jackson, M.; Esterman, A.; Young, G.P. A synbiotic combination of resistant starch and bifidobacterium lactis facilitates apoptotic deletion of carcinogen-damaged cells in rat colon. *J. Nutr.* **2005**, *135*, 996–1001. [PubMed]
32. Young, F.M.; Phungtamdet, W.; Sanderson, B.J. Modification of mtt assay conditions to examine the cytotoxic effects of amitraz on the human lymphoblastoid cell line, wil2ns. *Toxicol. In Vitro* **2005**, *19*, 1051–1059. [CrossRef] [PubMed]
33. Beyer-Sehlmeyer, G.; Glei, M.; Hartmann, E.; Hughes, R.; Persin, C.; Bohm, V.; Rowland, I.; Schubert, R.; Jahreis, G.; Pool-Zobel, B.L. Butyrate is only one of several growth inhibitors produced during gut flora-mediated fermentation of dietary fibre sources. *Br. J. Nutr.* **2003**, *90*, 1057–1070. [CrossRef] [PubMed]
34. Matsumoto, H.; Erickson, R.H.; Gum, J.R.; Yoshioka, M.; Gum, E.; Kim, Y.S. Biosynthesis of alkaline-phosphatase during differentiation of the human colon cancer cell-line caco-2. *Gastroenterology* **1990**, *98*, 1199–1207. [CrossRef]

35. Van den Abbeele, P.; Gerard, P.; Rabot, S.; Bruneau, A.; El Aidy, S.; Derrien, M.; Kleerebezem, M.; Zoetendal, E.G.; Smidt, H.; Verstraete, W.; et al. Arabinoxylans and inulin differentially modulate the mucosal and luminal gut microbiota and mucin-degradation in humanized rats. *Environ. Microbiol.* **2011**, *13*, 2667–2680. [CrossRef] [PubMed]
36. Lovegrove, A.; Edwards, C.H.; De Noni, I.; Patel, H.; El, S.N.; Grassby, T.; Zielke, C.; Ulmius, M.; Nilsson, L.; Butterworth, P.J.; et al. Role of polysaccharides in food, digestion, and health. *Crit. Rev. Food Sci. Nutr.* **2017**, *57*, 237–253. [CrossRef] [PubMed]
37. Lanneau, D.; de Thonel, A.; Maurel, S.; Didelot, C.; Garrido, C. Apoptosis versus cell differentiation: Role of heat shock proteins hsp90, hsp70 and hsp27. *Prion* **2007**, *1*, 53–60. [CrossRef] [PubMed]
38. Ding, Q.M.; Ko, T.C.; Evers, B.M. Caco-2 intestinal cell differentiation is associated with g(1) arrest and suppression of cdk2 and cdk4. *Am. J. Physiol.* **1998**, *275*, C1193–C1200. [PubMed]
39. Orchel, A.; Dzierzewicz, Z.; Parfiniewicz, B.; Weglarz, L.; Wilczok, T. Butyrate-induced differentiation of colon cancer cells is pkc and jnk dependent. *Dig. Dis. Sci.* **2005**, *50*, 490–498. [CrossRef] [PubMed]
40. Kiefer, J.; Beyer-Sehlmeyer, G.; Pool-Zobel, B.L. Mixtures of scfa, composed according to physiologically available concentrations in the gut lumen, modulate histone acetylation in human ht29 colon cancer cells. *Br. J. Nutr.* **2006**, *96*, 803–810. [CrossRef] [PubMed]
41. Hubatsch, I.; Ridderstrom, M.; Mannervik, B. Human glutathione transferase a4-4: An alpha class enzyme with high catalytic efficiency in the conjugation of 4-hydroxynonenal and other genotoxic products of lipid peroxidation. *Biochem. J.* **1998**, *330 Pt 1*, 175–179. [CrossRef] [PubMed]
42. Munjal, U.; Glei, M.; Pool-Zobel, B.L.; Scharlau, D. Fermentation products of inulin-type fructans reduce proliferation and induce apoptosis in human colon tumour cells of different stages of carcinogenesis. *Br. J. Nutr.* **2009**, *102*, 663–671. [CrossRef] [PubMed]
43. Hughes, R.; Rowland, I.R. Stimulation of apoptosis by two prebiotic chicory fructans in the rat colon. *Carcinogenesis* **2001**, *22*, 43–47. [CrossRef] [PubMed]
44. Anh, T.D.; Ahn, M.Y.; Kim, S.A.; Yoon, J.H.; Ahn, S.G. The histone deacetylase inhibitor, trichostatin a, induces g2/m phase arrest and apoptosis in yd-10b oral squamous carcinoma cells. *Oncol. Rep.* **2012**, *27*, 455–460. [PubMed]
45. Hwang, J.J.; Kim, Y.S.; Kim, M.J.; Jang, S.J.; Lee, J.H.; Choi, J.; Ro, S.; Hyun, Y.L.; Lee, J.S.; Kim, C.S. A novel histone deacetylase inhibitor, cg0006, induces cell death through both extrinsic and intrinsic apoptotic pathways. *Anti-Cancer Drug* **2009**, *20*, 815–821. [CrossRef] [PubMed]
46. Wallace, D.M.; Donovan, M.; Cotter, T.G. Histone deacetylase activity regulates apaf-1 and caspase 3 expression in the developing mouse retina. *Investig. Ophth. Vis. Sci.* **2006**, *47*, 2765–2772. [CrossRef] [PubMed]
47. Matthews, G.M.; Howarth, G.S.; Butler, R.N. Short-chain fatty acids induce apoptosis in colon cancer cells associated with changes to intracellular redox state and glucose metabolism. *Chemotherapy* **2012**, *58*, 102–109. [CrossRef] [PubMed]
48. Huang, H.C.; Syu, K.Y.; Lin, J.K. Chemical composition of solanum nigrum linn extract and induction of autophagy by leaf water extract and its major flavonoids in au565 breast cancer cells. *J. Agric. Food Chem.* **2010**, *58*, 8699–8708. [CrossRef] [PubMed]
49. Harun, F.B.; Jamalullail, S.M.S.S.; Yin, K.B.; Othman, Z.; Tilwari, A.; Balaram, P. Autophagic cell death is induced by acetone and ethyl acetate extracts from eupatorium odoratum in vitro: Effects on mcf-7 and vero cell lines. *Sci. World J.* **2012**, *2012*, 1–9. [CrossRef] [PubMed]
50. Aryudhani, N. Mechanism of Antitumor Activity of Powdered Leaf Green Grass Jelly (*Premna blongifolia* merr.) in Mice Transplanted c3h Breast Tumor Cells. Master's Thesis, Bogor Agricultural University, Bogor, Indonesia, 2011.
51. Cruz-Bravo, R.K.; Guevara-Gonzalez, R.G.; Ramos-Gomez, M.; Oomah, B.D.; Wiersma, P.; Campos-Vega, R.; Loarca-Pina, G. The fermented non-digestible fraction of common bean (*Phaseolus vulgaris* L.) triggers cell cycle arrest and apoptosis in human colon adenocarcinoma cells. *Genes Nutr.* **2014**, *9*, 359. [CrossRef] [PubMed]

8

Effect of Consuming Oat Bran Mixed in Water before a Meal on Glycemic Responses in Healthy Humans

Robert E. Steinert [1,*], Daniel Raederstorff [1] and Thomas M. S. Wolever [2]

[1] DSM Nutritional Products Ltd., R & D Human Nutrition and Health, Basel 4057, Switzerland; daniel.raederstorff@dsm.com

[2] Glycemic Index Laboratories, Inc., Toronto, ON M5C 2N8, Canada; thomas.wolever@utoronto.ca

* Correspondence: robert.steinert@dsm.com

Abstract: Background: Viscous dietary fibers including oat β-glucan are one of the most effective classes of functional food ingredients for reducing postprandial blood glucose. The mechanism of action is thought to be via an increase in viscosity of the stomach contents that delays gastric emptying and reduces mixing of food with digestive enzymes, which, in turn, retards glucose absorption. Previous studies suggest that taking viscous fibers separate from a meal may not be effective in reducing postprandial glycemia. Methods: We aimed to re-assess the effect of consuming a preload of a commercially available oat-bran (4.5, 13.6 or 27.3 g) containing 22% of high molecular weight oat β-glucan (O22 (OatWell®22)) mixed in water before a test-meal of white bread on glycemic responses in 10 healthy humans. Results: We found a significant effect of dose on blood glucose area under the curve (AUC) ($p = 0.006$) with AUC after 27.3 g of O22 being significantly lower than white bread only. Linear regression analysis showed that each gram of oat β-glucan reduced glucose AUC by 4.35% ± 1.20% ($r = 0.507$, $p = 0.0008$, $n = 40$) and peak rise by 6.57% ± 1.49% ($r = 0.582$, $p < 0.0001$). Conclusion: These data suggest the use of oat bran as nutritional preload strategy in the management of postprandial glycemia.

Keywords: postprandial glycemia; dietary fibre; blood glucose; type 2 diabetes mellitus; preload

1. Introduction

In current obesogenic societies with many people having mild or moderate hyperglycemia, postprandial blood glucose patterns account for the majority of variability of overall glycemic control [1,2]. This is not surprising considering that most individuals spend perhaps only about three to four hours before breakfast in a truly fasted state [1,3]. Dietary means to lower postprandial glycemic responses are, thus, urgently needed for the prevention of Type 2 Diabetes mellitus (T2DM). Viscous dietary fibers including high molecular weight (HMW) oat β-glucan are one of the most effective classes of functional food ingredients for reducing postprandial glucose [4]. The mechanism of action is thought to be their ability to increase the viscosity of the contents of the upper gastrointestinal (GI) tract and, hence, slow gastric emptying (GE) [5]. The rate of GE has a substantial impact on postprandial glycemia by determining glucose absorption and incretin hormone secretion [6,7]. In addition, an increase in viscosity of GI contents reduces the rate of digestion of starch by pancreatic amylase and the rate of absorption of glucose in the small intestine by increasing the thickness of the unstirred water layer [5].

Previous studies suggest that taking viscous fibers separate from a main meal may not be effective in reducing postprandial glycemia [8,9]. One potential solution to this problem may be to consume, before eating, a fiber "preload", which develops viscosity slowly, so that it can be consumed in a palatable form, and remains liquid in the stomach long enough to be able to mix effectively with the main meal, but becomes viscous by the time the stomach starts to empty the meal. OatWell®22 (O22) is a commercially available oat-bran including 44% dietary fiber and 22% HMW oat β-glucan, which forms a palatable drink when mixed with water and which becomes viscous after several minutes. Therefore, we evaluated the dose-response effect of O22 mixed in water and consumed before a white bread meal on glycemic responses in healthy humans.

2. Subjects and Methods

2.1. Subjects

Ten healthy normal-weight, overweight and obese subjects (5 male/5 female, mean age (years): 48.0 ± 15.3 (range 22–65), BMI (kg/m^2): 29.5 ± 4.4 (range 23.2–36.9)) were studied using an open-label, randomized block design. The study was performed according to accepted standards and the Declaration of Helsinki. Ethical approval was obtained from the Western Institutional Review Board, and the study was registered as a clinical trial with clinical trials.gov (registration number NCT02801916). Written informed consent was obtained from all participants.

2.2. Study Outline

Each subject underwent 4 treatments on separate days, with each subject performing up to 3 tests per week separated by at least one day. On each test day, subjects came to the laboratory in the morning after a 10–14 h overnight fast. Two fasting blood samples (t = −5 min and t = 0 min) were obtained by finger-prick. After the first fasting blood sample, subjects consumed a preload consisting of 200 mL water either alone or mixed with 4.5, 13.6 or 27.3 g of O22 containing 0.9, 2.6, and 5.3 g of oat β-glucan, respectively (DSM Nutritional Products, Table 1). After the second fasting blood sample (t = 0 min), subjects were asked to consume a test meal consisting of a portion (119 g) of white bread containing 50 g available carbohydrate (Table 1). The time taken to consume the bread was between 7 and 12 min. Further blood samples were obtained at 15, 30, 45, 60, 90 and 120 min after meal onset. Subjects remained seated quietly during the 2 h of the test. After the last blood sample was obtained, subjects were offered a snack and then permitted to leave.

Table 1. Nutrient content of test meal ingredients.

Test Meal	Energy (kcal)	Weight (g)	Protein (g)	Fat (g)	tCHO [1] (g)	Fibre (g)		avCHO [1] (g)
						Total	β-Glucan	
White Bread [1]	245	119	9.0	1.0	52.6	2.6	0	50.0
OatWell®22 [2]	13.1	4.5	1.0	0.2	3.0	2.2	0.9	0.8
	39.7	13.6	3.1	0.6	8.8	6.5	2.6	2.3
	79.7	27.3	6.2	1.1	17.7	13.1	5.3	4.6

[1] Baked at Glycemic Index Laboratories using an automatic bread maker; values represent the mean of 5 proximate analyses performed by Gelda Scientific, Mississauga, ON, Canada; [2] Nutritional analysis, including β-glucan content, was performed by SGS Institute Fresenius GmbH, Im Maisel, Taunusstein, Germany.

2.3. Measurements

After consuming the test meal, subjects rated the palatability of the test meal using a visual analogue scale consisting of a 100-mm line anchored at the left end by "very unpalatable" and at the right end by "very palatable". Subjects made a vertical mark along the line to indicate their perceived palatability. The distance from the left end of the line to the mark made by the subject is the palatability rating; the higher the value, the higher the perceived palatability.

Blood samples (2–3 drops each) were collected into 5 mL tubes containing ~500 µg sodium fluoride and 400 µg potassium oxalate. The samples were mixed and refrigerated immediately during the testing session. After completion of the test session, samples were stored at −20 °C prior to glucose analysis. Blood glucose analysis, using a YSI (Yellow Spring Instruments, Yellow Springs, OH, USA) analyzer, took place within five days of collection.

2.4. Data and Statistical Analysis

The primary endpoint was incremental area under the blood glucose curve (AUC) which was calculated using the trapezoid rule, ignoring area beneath the baseline. Baseline blood glucose was calculated as mean of values obtained at $t = -5$ min and $t = 0$ min. AUC and peak rise were analyzed using repeated-measures analysis of variance (RMANOVA) examining for the main effects of treatment dose. In case of significant heterogeneity, differences among different doses were tested using Tukey's test to adjust for multiple comparisons. AUC and peak rises for each dose of O22 were expressed relative to the AUC or peak rise after the test of white bread alone taken by the same subject. The glycemic response of 1 subject with a relative response after the 13.6 g dose of 2.55 × SD above the mean was considered to be an outlier and the data removed; the values were replaced using a procedure described by Snedecor and Cochran [10], and the error degrees of freedom in RMANOVA reduced by one. Blood glucose concentrations at each time were subjected to RMANOVA examining for the main effects of time and treatment and the time × treatment interaction; after demonstrating a highly significant time × treatment interaction ($p = 1.2 \times 10^{-17}$), blood glucose concentrations at each time were subjected to RMANOVA followed by Tukey's test, as described above for AUC. Differences were considered to be statistically significant if 2-tailed $p < 0.05$.

3. Results

There were significant differences in blood glucose concentration among doses at 15 ($p = 0.0015$), 30 ($p < 0.0001$), 45 ($p = 0.0003$) and 120 min ($p = 0.0004$). At 15 min, blood glucose concentration after 27.3 g was significantly lower than those after 0 g and 4.5 g. At 30 min, blood glucose after the 27.3 g dose was significantly lower than after 13.6 g, which, in turn, was significantly lower than the 0 and 4.5 g doses. At 45 min blood glucose concentration after 27.3 g of O22 was significantly lower than those after the 0, 4.5 and 13.6 g doses. At 120 min, blood glucose after 27.3 g of O22 was significantly higher than that after the 0 and 4.5 g doses (Figure 1A). There was a significant effect of dose on blood glucose AUC ($p = 0.006$) with AUC after 27.3 g of O22 (141 ± 21 mmol × min/L) being significantly lower than both the 4.5 g and 0 g doses (174 ± 1 7 and 185 ± 18 mmol × min/L, respectively) and the AUC after 13.6 g being intermediate (167 ± 19 mmol × min/L). When AUC was expressed relative to that of bread alone, the relative responses for the 4.5, 13.6 and 27.3 g doses of O22, respectively, were 95.0% ± 4.1%, 90.3% ± 4.7% and 76.3% ± 7.7% with the only significant reduction being seen with the highest dose. However, linear regression analysis showed that each gram of oat β-glucan reduced glucose AUC by 4.35% ± 1.20% ($r = 0.507$, $p = 0.0008$, $n = 40$; Figure 1B). There was also a significant effect of dose for blood glucose peak rise ($p < 0.0001$) with the peak rise after 27.3 g of O22, 1.96 ± 0.29 mmol/L, being significantly lower than that after all the other doses (3.07 ± 0.25, 2.83 ± 0.30 and 2.72 ± 0.30 g for the 0, 4.5 and 13.6 g doses of O22, respectively). When peak rise was expressed relative to that for bread alone, the relative responses for the 4.5, 13.6 and 27.3 g doses of O22, respectively, were 92.5% ± 6.8%, 88.5% ± 7.2% and 63.8% ± 7.1% with the only significant reduction being seen with the highest dose. However, linear regression analysis showed that each gram of oat β-glucan reduced glucose peak rise by 6.57% ± 1.49% ($r = 0.582$, $p < 0.0001$, $n = 40$; Figure 1C).

There was a significant main effect of dose on palatability, with all 3 doses of O22 rated as being less palatable than white bread alone (palatability in mm: 71 ± 7 for white bread alone; 38 ± 9 for 4.5 g O22; 33 ± 10 for 13.6 g O22; 31 ± 9 for 27.3 g O22; $p = 0.0003$). Although palatability tended to decrease as the dose increased, this difference was not significant. There was no significant relationship between palatability and glucose AUC (expressed as % of that after white bread) for 4.5 g ($r = 0.439$, $p = 0.20$, $n = 10$), 13.6 g ($r = 0.502$, $p = 0.14$, $n = 10$) or 27.3 g ($r = 0.398$, $p = 0.25$, $n = 10$) doses of O22.

No adverse effects were observed.

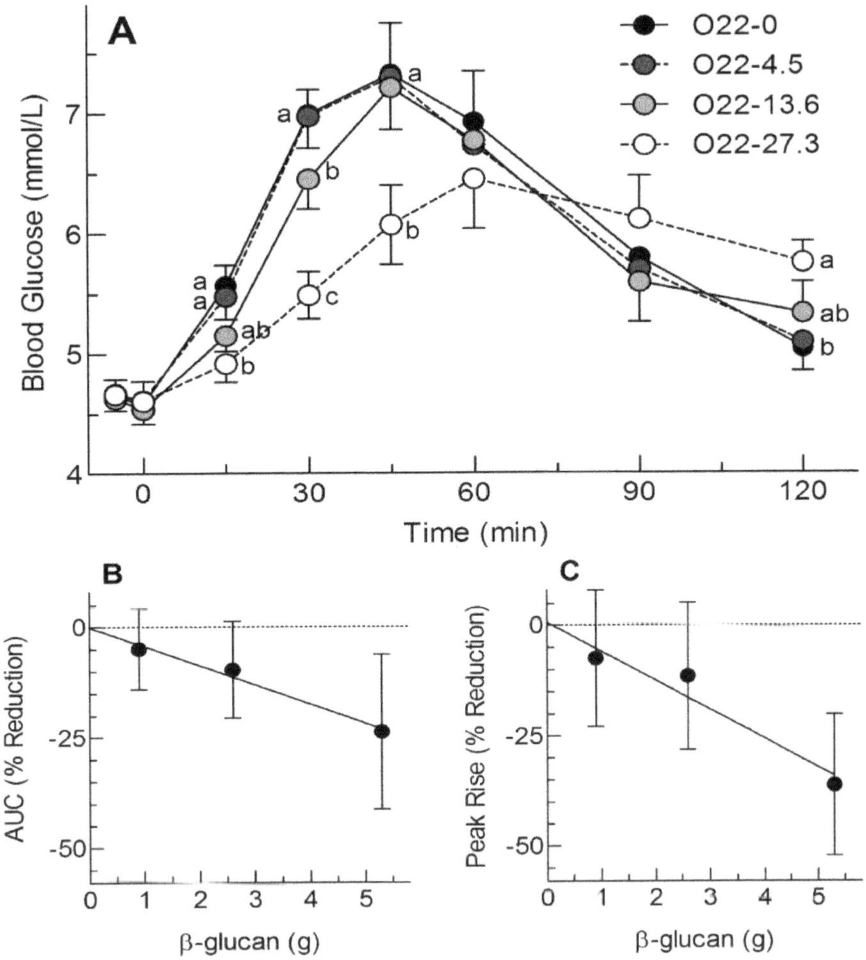

Figure 1. Panel (**A**): Blood glucose concentrations after taking 0, 4.5, 13.6 and 27.3 g, respectively, of OatWell®22 (O22-0, O22-4.5, O22-13.6 and O22-27.3) at −5 min followed by 50 g available carbohydrate from white bread at 0 min. Values are means ± SEM for $n = 10$ subjects. [a–c] Means at the same time containing different letters within the superscripts differ significantly by Tukey's test $p < 0.05$; (**B**,**C**): Percentage reduction from control in incremental areas under the curve (AUC); (**B**) and peak rise in blood glucose; (**C**) after taking 0, 4.5, 13.6 and 27.3 g of OatWell®22 (containing 0, 0.9, 2.6 and 5.3 g oat β-glucan, respectively) at −5 min followed by 50 g available carbohydrate from white bread at 0 min. Values are means ± 95% confidence interval for $n = 9$ or 10 subjects (after excluding outlying values).

4. Discussion

We demonstrated that consuming a commercially available oat-bran containing 22% of HMW oat β-glucan mixed in water before a white bread meal significantly lowers postprandial glycemia in a dose dependent manner with 27.3 g of O22 being significantly lower than white bread only. Linear regression analysis, in addition, showed that each gram of oat β-glucan reduced glucose AUC by ~4% and peak rise by ~7%. Given that the magnitude of this reduction would be similar in patients with T2DM, these data may have considerable implications for nutritional strategies in the management of diabetes, however, this concept warrants further investigation. The mechanism of action of oat beta-glucan to reduce postprandial glycemia is well established. In their native form, oat beta-glucan consists of very high molecular weight polysaccharides that exhibit high viscosities at low concentrations [11]. An increase in viscosity of a meal bolus in the stomach delays gastric emptying and reduces mixing of food with digestive enzymes. This retards absorption of glucose making oat β-glucan one of the most effective classes of functional food ingredients to reduce postprandial blood glucose and insulin responses [4,5].

Previous studies have suggested that taking viscous fibers, such as psyllium or guar gum, separate from a main meal may not be effective in reducing postprandial glycemia [12,13]. In contrast, the concept of a "preload" that refers to administration of a small load of nutrient at a fixed interval before a main meal to lower postprandial blood glucose via the slowing of GE has been confirmed several times [14–16]. While in the classical sense of the preload concept, the slowing of GE is related primarily to a nutrient-induced neuroendocrine feedback [14–16], the present findings suggest that the preload concept also applies to fibers such as oat beta-glucan that delay GE via increases in meal bolus viscosity. It requires consideration, however, that the oat bran also contained about 20% protein that may have contributed to the slowing of GE via neuroendocrine feedbacks. In addition, the protein may have lowered postprandial blood glucose independently of the preload effect because a reduction in postprandial blood glucose was observed also in studies with protein ingested simultaneously with carbohydrate-rich meals [17]. The discrepancy between the current results and those of previous investigations mentioned above suggests that proper control of method of administration of the preload such as timing (i.e., interval between preload administration and meal onset) and the physicochemical properties of the fiber at meal onset, as well as other macronutritional components, are important. Ideally the fiber preload remains liquid in the stomach long enough to be able to mix effectively with the meal, but becomes viscous by the time the stomach starts to empty the meal.

The present results are in line with the health claim that has previously been evaluated by the European Food Safety Authority (EFSA) and authorized by the European commission for β-glucans from oats and barley and reduction of postprandial glycemia [18]. The conditions of use state that in order to obtain the claimed effect, 4 g of beta-glucans for each 30 g of available carbohydrates should be consumed per meal. Our results further indicate that lower doses of HMW oat β-glucan may be sufficient to impact postprandial glycemia when consumed in a suitable manner (e.g., several smaller doses/day, correct timing/preload paradigm). This approach is in line with a recent systematic review by Tosh et al. [4], including 119 treatments from 34 publications that finds that the efficacy of oat and barley β-glucan in lowering postprandial blood glucose is more strongly related to β-glucan content alone than to the ratio of β-glucan/available carbohydrate. In addition, when authors actually calculated a ratio, 4 g of β-glucan per meal were found to be sufficient to reduce post-prandial blood glucose in a clinical relevant amount for meals with up to 80 g of available carbohydrate.

A limitation of this pilot trial that requires consideration is that it was not powered to detect small differences seen with the lower doses used here (i.e., 4.5 and 13.6 g). We only found a significant effect with 27.3 g of O22, however, the results show that the expected reduction in AUC and peak rise for the 13.6 g dose were 11.3% and 17.1%, respectively. Therefore, based on the results of this study, 27 subjects would be required to have 80% power to detect an 11.3% reduction in AUC and 14 subjects to detect a 17.1% reduction in peak rise. The additional energy intake associated with an oat bran preload should also be considered if using such a strategy over the long term, althoughsubjects usually tend to compensateat least in part, for extra energy by eating less at a subsequent ad libitum meal. There is good evidence for particularly viscous fibers to reduce appetite and eating. For example, a recent systematic review including 58 original studies by Wanders et al. [19] reports a reduction in appetite perception by 7.4% over a 4 h time interval when dietary fiber is added as part of a preload. Similarly, a recent meta-analysis including 6 human studies shows that polydextrose fiber as part of a mid-morning preload reduces energy intake at a subsequent ad libitum meal at lunch time by 12.5% [20]. Finally, there is evidence from epidemiological studies that show associations between high fiber intakes and weight loss [21,22].

In conclusion, consuming O22 mixed in water before a meal reduces glycemic response in a dose-dependent manner with each gram of oat β-glucan reducing glucose AUC by about 4%. This suggests the use of O22 as a nutritional preload strategy in the management of postprandial glycemia.

Author Contributions: Robert E. Steinert, Thomas M. S. Wolever and Daniel Raederstorff conceptualized the study. Thomas M. S. Wolever conducted the experiments and statistical analysis. Robert E. Steinert, Thomas M. S. Wolever and Daniel Raederstorff interpreted the data. Robert E. Steinert and Thomas M. S. Wolever drafted the manuscript. All authors reviewed and approved the manuscript.

References

1. Monnier, L.; Lapinski, H.; Colette, C. Contributions of fasting and postprandial plasma glucose increments to the overall diurnal hyperglycemia of type 2 diabetic patients: Variations with increasing levels of HbA(1c). *Diabetes Care* **2003**, *26*, 881–885. [CrossRef] [PubMed]
2. Peter, R.; Dunseath, G.; Luzio, S.D.; Owens, D.R. Estimates of the relative and absolute diurnal contributions of fasting and post-prandial plasma glucose over a range of hyperglycaemia in type 2 diabetes. *Diabetes Metab.* **2013**, *39*, 337–342. [CrossRef] [PubMed]
3. Monnier, L.; Colette, C.; Owens, D. Postprandial and basal glucose in type 2 diabetes: Assessment and respective impacts. *Diabetes Technol. Ther.* **2011**, *13*, S25–S32. [CrossRef] [PubMed]
4. Tosh, S.M. Review of human studies investigating the post-prandial blood-glucose lowering ability of oat and barley food products. *Eur. J. Clin. Nutr.* **2013**, *67*, 310–317. [CrossRef] [PubMed]
5. Würsch, P.; Pi-Sunyer, F.X. The role of viscous soluble fiber in the metabolic control of diabetes: A review with special emphasis on cereals rich in beta-glucan. *Diabetes Care* **1997**, *20*, 1774–1780. [CrossRef] [PubMed]
6. Horowitz, M.; Edelbroek, M.A.; Wishart, J.M.; Straathof, J.W. Relationship between oral glucose tolerance and gastric emptying in normal healthy subjects. *Diabetologia* **1993**, *36*, 857–862. [CrossRef] [PubMed]
7. Marathe, C.S.; Rayner, C.K.; Jones, K.L.; Horowitz, M. Relationships between gastric emptying, postprandial glycemia, and incretin hormones. *Diabetes Care* **2013**, *36*, 1396–1405. [CrossRef] [PubMed]
8. Fuessl, S.; Adrian, T.E.; Bacarese-Hamilton, A.J.; Bloom, S.R. Guar in NIDD: Effect of different modes of administration on plasma glucose and insulin responses to a starch meal. *Pract. Diabetes Int.* **1986**, *3*, 258–260. [CrossRef]
9. Jenkins, D.J.; Nineham, R.; Craddock, C.; Craig-McFeely, P.; Donaldson, K.; Leigh, T.; Snook, J. Fibre in diabetes. *Lancet* **1979**, *1*, 434–435. [CrossRef]
10. Snedecor, G.W.; Cochran, W.G. *Statistical Methods*, 7th ed.; Iowa State University Press: Ames, IA, USA, 1980.
11. Ren, Y.; Ellis, P.R.; Sutherland, I.W.; Ross-Murphy, S.B. Dilute and semi-dilute solution properties of an exopolysaccharide from *Escherichia coli* strain S61. *Carbohydr. Polym.* **2003**, *52*, 189–195. [CrossRef]
12. Wolever, T.M.; Vuksan, V.; Eshuis, H.; Spadafora, P.; Peterson, R.D.; Chao, E.S.; Storey, M.L.; Jenkins, D.J. Effect of method of administration of psyllium on glycemic response and carbohydrate digestibility. *J. Am. Coll. Nutr.* **1991**, *10*, 364–371. [CrossRef] [PubMed]
13. Cohen, M.; Leong, V.W.; Salmon, E.; Martin, F.I. Role of guar and dietary fibre in the management of diabetes mellitus. *Med. J. Aust.* **1980**, *1*, 59–61. [PubMed]
14. Gentilcore, D.; Chaikomin, R.; Jones, K.L.; Russo, A.; Feinle-Bisset, C.; Wishart, J.M.; Rayner, C.K.; Horowitz, M. Effects of fat on gastric emptying of and the glycemic, insulin, and incretin responses to a carbohydrate meal in type 2 diabetes. *J. Clin. Endocrinol. Metab.* **2006**, *91*, 2062–2067. [CrossRef] [PubMed]
15. Ma, J.; Stevens, J.E.; Cukier, K.; Maddox, A.F.; Wishart, J.M.; Jones, K.L.; Clifton, P.M.; Horowitz, M.; Rayner, C.K. Effects of a protein preload on gastric emptying, glycemia, and gut hormones after a carbohydrate meal in diet-controlled type 2 diabetes. *Diabetes Care* **2009**, *32*, 1600–1602. [CrossRef] [PubMed]
16. Ma, J.; Jesudason, D.R.; Stevens, J.E.; Keogh, J.B.; Jones, K.L.; Clifton, P.M.; Horowitz, M.; Rayner, C.K. Sustained effects of a protein "preload" on glycaemia and gastric emptying over 4 weeks in patients with type 2 diabetes: A randomized clinical trial. *Diabetes Res. Clin. Pract.* **2015**, *108*, e31–e34. [CrossRef] [PubMed]
17. Lan-Pidhainy, X.; Wolever, T.M.S. The hypoglycemic effect of fat and protein is not attenuated by insulin resistance. *Am. J. Clin. Nutr.* **2010**, *91*, 98–105. [CrossRef] [PubMed]
18. Panel on Dietetic Products, Nutrition and Allergies (NDA). Scientific Opinion on the substantiation of health claims related to beta-glucans from oats and barley and maintenance of normal blood LDL-cholesterol concentrations (ID 1236, 1299), increase in satiety leading to a reduction in energy intake (ID 851, 852),

reduction of post-prandial glycaemic responses (ID 821, 824), and "digestive function" (ID 850) pursuant to Article 13(1) of Regulation (EC) No 1924/2006. *EFSA J.* **2011**, *9*. [CrossRef]

19. Wanders, A.J.; van den Borne, J.J.G.C.; de Graaf, C.; Hulshof, T.; Jonathan, M.C.; Kristensen, M.; Mars, M.; Schols, H.A.; Feskens, E.J.M. Effects of dietary fibre on subjective appetite, energy intake and body weight: A systematic review of randomized controlled trials. *Obes. Rev. Off. J. Int. Assoc. Study Obes.* **2011**, *12*, 724–739. [CrossRef] [PubMed]
20. Ibarra, A.; Astbury, N.M.; Olli, K.; Alhoniemi, E.; Tiihonen, K. Effect of polydextrose on subjective feelings of appetite during the satiation and satiety periods: A systematic review and meta-analysis. *Nutrients* **2016**, *8*. [CrossRef] [PubMed]
21. Howarth, N.C.; Saltzman, E.; Roberts, S.B. Dietary fiber and weight regulation. *Nutr. Rev.* **2001**, *59*, 129–139. [CrossRef] [PubMed]
22. Alfieri, M.A.; Pomerleau, J.; Grace, D.M.; Anderson, L. Fiber intake of normal weight, moderately obese and severely obese subjects. *Obes. Res.* **1995**, *3*, 541–547. [CrossRef] [PubMed]

9

Associations between Dietary Fiber Intake in Infancy and Cardiometabolic Health at School Age

Rafaëlle M. A. van Gijssel [1,2,†], Kim V. E. Braun [1,†], Jessica C. Kiefte-de Jong [1,3], Vincent W. V. Jaddoe [1,2,4], Oscar H. Franco [1] and Trudy Voortman [1,*]

1 The Department of Epidemiology, Erasmus MC, University Medical Center, Office Na-2909, P.O. Box 2040, Rotterdam 3000 CA, The Netherlands; rmavgijssel@gmail.com (R.M.A.v.G.); k.braun@erasmusmc.nl (K.V.E.B.); j.c.kiefte-dejong@erasmusmc.nl (J.C.K.-d.J.); v.jaddoe@erasmusmc.nl (V.W.V.J.); o.franco@erasmusmc.nl (O.H.F.)
2 The Generation R Study Group, Erasmus MC, University Medical Center, Rotterdam 3000 CA, The Netherlands
3 Department of Global Public Health, Leiden University, The Hague 3595 DG, The Netherlands
4 The Department of Pediatrics, Erasmus MC, University Medical Center, Rotterdam 3000 CA, The Netherlands
* Correspondence: trudy.voortman@erasmusmc.nl;
† These authors contributed equally to this work.

Abstract: Dietary fiber (DF) intake may be beneficial for cardiometabolic health. However, whether this already occurs in early childhood is unclear. We investigated associations between DF intake in infancy and cardiometabolic health in childhood among 2032 children participating in a population-based cohort in The Netherlands. Information on DF intake at a median age of 12.9 months was collected using a food-frequency questionnaire. DF was adjusted for energy intake using the residual method. At age 6 years, body fat percentage, high-density lipoprotein (HDL)-cholesterol, insulin, triglycerides, and blood pressure were assessed and expressed in age- and sex-specific standard deviation scores (SDS). These five factors were combined into a cardiometabolic risk factor score. In models adjusted for several parental and child covariates, a higher DF intake was associated with a lower cardiometabolic risk factor score. When we examined individual cardiometabolic factors, we observed that a 1 g/day higher energy-adjusted DF intake was associated with 0.026 SDS higher HDL-cholesterol (95% CI 0.009, 0.042), and 0.020 SDS lower triglycerides (95% CI −0.037, −0.003), but not with body fat, insulin, or blood pressure. Results were similar for DF with and without adjustment for energy intake. Our findings suggest that higher DF intake in infancy may be associated with better cardiometabolic health in later childhood.

Keywords: body fat; blood pressure; cohort; dietary fiber; early childhood; HDL-C; insulin; triglyceride

---

1. Introduction

Several studies suggest that dietary fiber (DF) is beneficial for various aspects of cardiometabolic health in adults, such as lower insulin and cholesterol concentrations, and a lower blood pressure [1,2]. High DF intake has been proposed to lower cardiometabolic risk through lower absorption of cholesterol and fat, improved glucose and insulin metabolism after meals, or via increased satiety and a subsequent lower energy intake [3]. However, many of the cardiometabolic health consequences in adulthood are preceded by abnormalities that might begin in childhood [4]. For example, overweight often already occurs in early childhood and is associated with a higher risk of overweight, type 2 diabetes, hypertension, dyslipidemia, and atherosclerosis in later life [4,5]. Small changes in other cardiometabolic risk factors can also already start during childhood and predict later cardiometabolic disease risk [6,7]. Therefore, it is important to focus on cardiometabolic health and its determinants already in childhood. A few previous studies in children suggested that the beneficial effect of DF on cardiometabolic health may already be present in childhood: a higher DF intake was, for example, associated with a lower body fat percentage in children around the age of 9 years [8], and with lower serum total cholesterol in children at ages of 13 months to 9 years [9].

However, these previous studies on DF intake in children in relation to body composition and metabolic risk factors focused on school-age children and adolescents [8–16], whereas diet might be important for cardiometabolic health already earlier in childhood [17]. Whether DF intake in early childhood is associated with cardiometabolic risk remains unknown and there is a lack of well-founded guidelines for adequate DF intake in young children [18–20]. Potential effects of DF intake might also differ by type of DF, such as soluble versus insoluble DF [3,21–24]. An observational study in adolescents showed that a higher intake of specifically soluble DF was associated with a reduction of visceral body fat over a period of 2 years [13]. However, data about the effects of different sources of DF is scarce [3].

Therefore, we investigated the association between DF intake in infancy and cardiometabolic health at the age of 6 years in a large prospective cohort. Additionally, we examined whether associations were explained by differences in energy intake and we explored whether associations differ for DF from different food sources.

2. Subjects and Methods

2.1. Study Design and Subjects

In this study we examined data from The Generation R Study, a population-based prospective cohort study from fetal life onward in Rotterdam, The Netherlands [25]. Pregnant women were enrolled between April 2002 and January 2006, and 7893 live-born children were available for postnatal follow-up, of whom 4215 had a Dutch ethnic background [25].

Because the food-frequency questionnaire (FFQ) was designed for dietary assessment of a Dutch population and was validated in Dutch children, we restricted our analyses to Dutch children. Children without information on diet (n = 1778) or any of the cardiometabolic health measurements (n = 405) were excluded, resulting in a study population of 2032 children (Figure 1). Because not all of these children had information available on all outcomes, the population for analysis ranged from 1314 to 1995 per cardiometabolic outcome. The study was approved by the local Medical Ethics Committee of Erasmus Medical Center, Rotterdam (MEC 198.782/2001/31, 2001), and written consent was given by parents.

2.2. Dietary Intake Assessment

Dietary data were collected using a 211-item semiquantitative FFQ, as described in detail elsewhere [26,27]. This FFQ was validated against three 24 h-recalls and the intraclass correlation coefficient was 0.7 for DF intake [27]. The median age of the children was 12.9 (interquartile range (IQR) 12.6–13.9) months. Total DF intake was calculated using the Dutch Food Composition Table (NEVO), where DF is defined as plant cell wall components that are not digestible by human digestive enzymes, including for example, lignin, cellulose, hemicellulose, and pectin [28]. Thereafter, we divided DF intake in DF from four different food groups, based on the different types of DF that are mainly present in these food groups [3,22]: (1) DF from cereals, as proxy for insoluble DF, defined as fiber from bread, cereals, pasta, rice, cookies, cakes, pastries, crackers, and ready-to-eat meals; (2) DF from potatoes and potato products, containing resistant starch; (3) DF from fruits and vegetables; and (4) DF from legumes, containing different types of soluble DF, insoluble DF, and resistant starch [29].

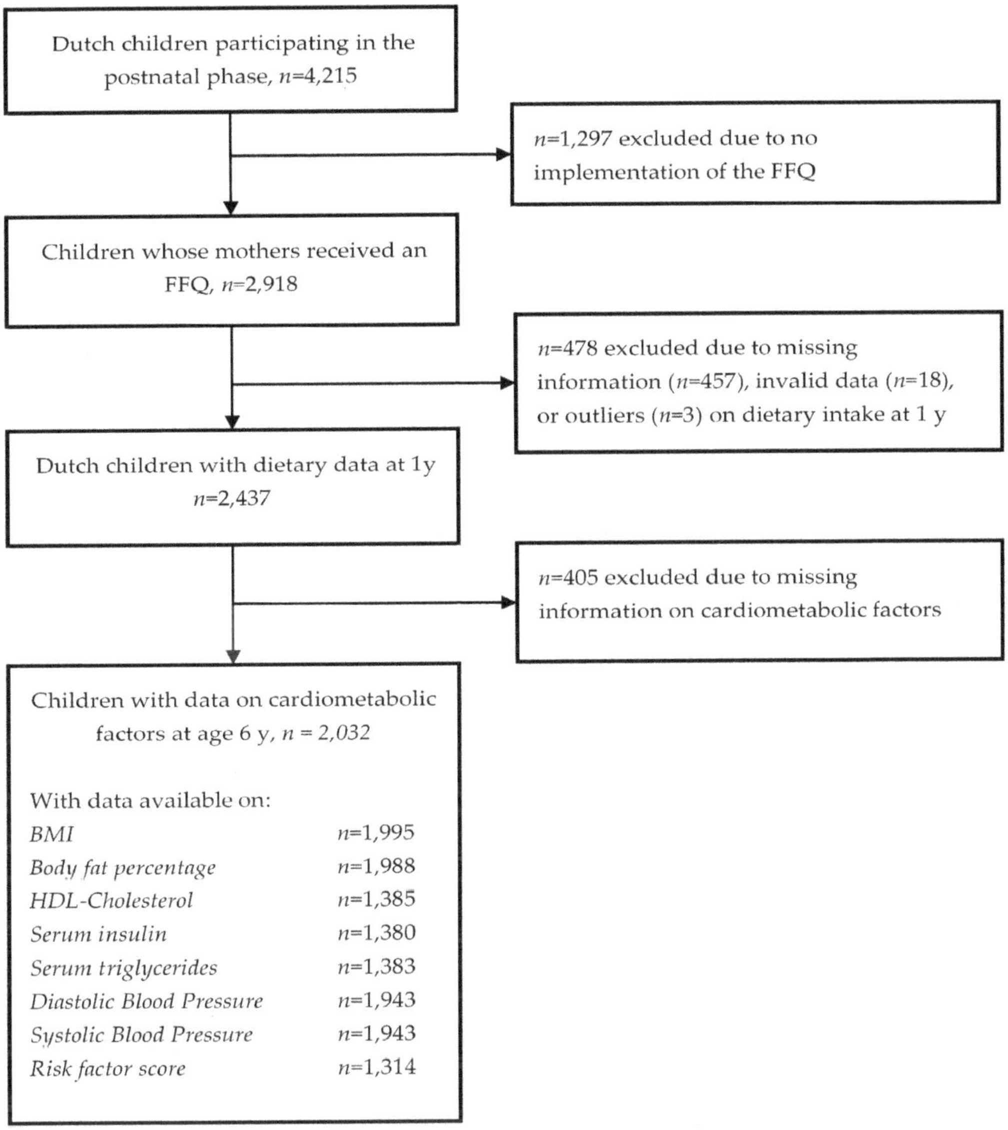

Figure 1. Flow chart of study participants included in the analysis.

2.3. *Cardiometabolic Health Assessment*

Children's height and weight up to the age of 4 years were repeatedly measured during routine visits to Child Health Centers [30]. At a median age of 5.9 (IQR 5.8–6.1) years, children visited our dedicated research center in the Sophia Children's Hospital in Rotterdam where they were examined in detail. As a primary outcome we used a cardiometabolic risk factor score including the components body fat percentage (BF%), high-density lipoprotein cholesterol (HDL-C), insulin, and triglyceride concentrations, and diastolic blood pressure (DBP) and systolic blood pressure (SBP). Body weight, measured with a mechanical personal scale (SECA), and body height, without shoes and heavy clothes, were measured to the nearest 0.1 kg or 0.1 cm, respectively, and BMI was calculated (kg/m^2). Body fat was determined using a dual-energy X-ray absorptiometry scanner (iDXA; General Electrics-Lunar, 2008, Madison, WI, USA) and enCORE software v.13.6 (GE Healthcare, Little Chalfont, UK) [31]. Total body fat was expressed as percentage of total body weight to define BF%. Additionally, we calculated fat mass index (FMI) as fat mass (kg)/m^2.

Non-fasting blood samples were drawn for measurements of HDL-C, insulin, and triglyceride concentrations, using enzymatic methods (using a Cobas 8000 analyzer, Roche, Almere, The Netherlands) [32]. Quality control samples demonstrated intra-assay and inter-assay coefficients of variation ranging from 0.77% to 1.69%. DBP and SBP were measured, while the children were lying down, at the right brachial artery, using the validated automatic sphygmomanometer Datascope

Accutorr Plus™ (Paramus, NJ, USA) [33]. Measurements were repeated four times with 1 min intervals and we used the mean of DBP and the mean of SBP of the last three measurements.

For all outcomes we calculated age- and sex-specific standard deviation scores (SDS) on the basis of our study population. Outliers, defined as the SDS $\geq |3.29|$ [34], were excluded (n = 0–7 per outcome). Individual cardiometabolic outcomes were combined into a continuous cardiometabolic risk factor score as described elsewhere [17,35]. This score included the sum of age- and sex-specific SD scores of BF%, the inverse of HDL-C, insulin, triglycerides, SBP, and DBP and was transformed into an SD score. A higher score is indicative of a less favorable cardiometabolic profile.

2.4. Covariates

Maternal age, household income, educational levels of both parents, and proxies for mother's pre-pregnancy cardiometabolic health (i.e., hypercholesterolemia, diabetes mellitus, or hypertension) were obtained with a questionnaire at enrolment in the study. Educational level of both parents was assessed with the same questionnaire and highest finished education was categorized into: no higher education; one parent with higher education; or both parents finished higher education, with higher education defined as higher vocational training, a Bachelor's degree, or university degree [36].

Maternal height and weight were measured at the research center at enrollment in the study, and BMI was calculated. Information about smoking, alcohol intake, and folic acid supplementation during pregnancy, as markers of health-conscious behavior of the mother, was obtained with questionnaires during pregnancy [27]. Information about pregnancy complications (i.e., gestational hypertension, preeclampsia, or gestational diabetes mellitus) was retrieved from medical records.

Medical records and hospital registries were used to collect information about child's sex, birth weight and gestational age. Sex- and gestational age-specific z-scores for birth weight were calculated using reference data [37]. Information about receiving breastfeeding at 4 months and timing of introduction of fruit and vegetables was collected with postnatal questionnaires [27].

A food-based diet score for preschool children was used to assess overall diet quality [27] and macronutrient intakes and glycemic load of the diet were calculated [38] from data obtained with the FFQ. Information about receiving dietary supplements (e.g., vitamins and mineral supplements) as a proxy of health-conscious behavior, was retrieved using the FFQ. Information about average screen time as proxy for sedentary behavior and about time spent walking or bicycling to school and playing outside as proxies for physical activity, and smoking in the household (categorized into never; less than once per week; or once per week or more) was obtained with a questionnaire at the child's age of 6 years.

2.5. Statistical Analysis

To explore whether potential associations of DF intake with cardiometabolic health were explained by energy intake, we examined both absolute DF (i.e., not adjusted for energy intake) and energy-adjusted DF intake. DF was adjusted for energy intake using the residual method [39]. Insulin was root-transformed, to obtain a normal distribution. Potential nonlinearity of the associations was assessed using natural cubic spline models with two to four degrees of freedom [40]. Because there were no indications for nonlinear associations for any of the outcomes (all $p > 0.05$), we assessed all associations using linear regression analyses only. In these models, we analyzed total DF intake and DF intake from different sources (per 1 g/day) and the cardiometabolic risk factor score and individual cardiometabolic health components at the age of 6 years.

In the crude model, we included child's age at FFQ and sex. To identify potential dietary confounders, we first examined correlations of DF intake with intake of total protein, vegetable protein, animal protein, fat, polyunsaturated fatty acids, monounsaturated fatty acids, saturated fatty acids, carbohydrates, glycemic load, and the diet quality score. We observed a strong correlation for energy intake, glycemic load, and the diet score with DF intakes, and therefore included these variables in the analyses. To avoid overadjustment, the diet quality score and glycemic load were adjusted for DF intake using the residual method. All other covariates described in the Covariates section were included as potential confounders using the manual forward stepwise method starting with the crude model. Variables were retained in the covariate-adjusted model when they resulted in a ≥5% change of the effect estimates of absolute or energy-adjusted DF intake on at least one of the outcomes. Following this procedure, all variables were retained, so covariate-adjusted models were adjusted for: maternal age, maternal BMI, household income, educational level of the parents, smoking, alcohol intake and folic acid supplementation during pregnancy, pregnancy complications, child's birth weight, sex, receiving breastfeeding at 4 months, timing of introduction of fruit and vegetables, age at FFQ, receiving dietary supplements, glycemic load, diet quality score, physical activity, screen time, and smoking in the household.

We tested for potential effect modification by child's sex, age at FFQ, and overweight status at the age of 6 years in the crude and covariate-adjusted models. We additionally explored whether DF intake was associated with repeatedly measured height, weight, and BMI using multivariable linear mixed models including the same covariates as in the main models. For the cardiometabolic risk factor score, we performed sensitivity analyses in which we excluded individual components from the score one at a time. Furthermore, we repeated the analyses in a selection of the children with complete data on all cardiometabolic outcomes ($n = 1314$).

Missing values of covariates were multiply imputed ($n = 10$ imputations) according to the Fully Conditional Specification method (predictive mean matching), with the assumption of no monotone missing pattern [41]. Effect estimates and population characteristics (Supplementary Materials Table S1) were similar before and after imputation and we report the pooled results after the multiple imputation procedure. Statistical analyses were performed using SPSS 21.0 (IBM Corp., version 21.0, Armonk, NY, USA) and R (The R Foundation for Statistical Computing, version 3.2.0, Aalborg, Denmark) and results were considered statistically significant at a p-value < 0.05.

3. Results

3.1. Population Characteristics

The population characteristics are shown in Table 1. At the age of 1 year, mean ± SD intake of total DF was 15.0 ± 4.3 g/day, with a range of 3.0–38.6 g/day, with 46.4% of the children having a DF intake above the Dutch recommended intake of 15 g/day for 1–3 year old children [42]. Most of the DF in the diet of our study population came from cereal products (median (IQR) 8.0 (6.2–10.0) g/day) and from fruits and vegetables (4.7 (3.2–6.2) g/day). Overall, parents of most of the children had a high educational level and a high income.

Table 1. Population characteristics ($n = 2032$).

	Mean ± SD, Median (IQR), or n (%)
Infancy Characteristics	
Gestational age at birth (weeks)	40.1 (39.3–41.1)
Birth weight (g)	3499 ± 563
Girls (n)	1031 (50.7%)
Receiving breastfeeding	
• Never	272 (13.3%)
• Partial in the first 4 months	1154 (56.8%)
• Exclusively in the first 4 months	606 (29.9%)
Timing of introduction of fruits and vegetables	
• <4 months	162 (7.9%)
• 4–6 months	1716 (84.4%)
• ≥6 months	154 (7.7%)
Characteristics at Dietary Assessment	
Age (months)	12.9 (12.6–13.9)

Table 1. Population characteristics (n = 2032).

	Mean ± SD, Median (IQR), or n (%)
Dietary fiber (DF) intake (g/day)	15.0 ± 4.3
• DF from cereals	8.0 (6.2–10.0)
• DF from potatoes	1.1 (0.4–1.9)
• DF from fruit and vegetables	4.7 (3.2–6.2)
• DF from legumes	0.2 (0.0–0.6)
Energy intake (kcal/day)	1267 (1070–1491)
Receiving any dietary supplements	973 (47.9%)
Characteristics at Cardiometabolic Health Assessment	
Age (year)	5.9 (5.8–6.1)
Height (cm)	118 (115–122)
Weight (kg)	21.8 (20.2–23.8)
BMI (kg/m^2) (n = 1995)	15.6 (15.0–16.5)
Body fat percentage (n = 1988)	23.1 (20.4–26.4)
Serum HDL-cholesterol (mmol/L) (n = 1385)	1.33 ± 0.30
Serum insulin (pmol/L) (n = 1380)	114 (63.8–183.6)
Serum triglycerides (mmol/L) (n = 1383)	0.98 (0.72–1.29)
Diastolic blood pressure (mmHg) (n = 1943)	60 ± 6
Systolic blood pressure (mmHg) (n = 1943)	102 ± 8
Physical activity (h/day)	1.60 (1.00–2.43)
Screen time (h/day)	1.14 (0.75–1.71)
Seldom or no smoking in household	1829 (90.0%)
Parental Characteristics	
Maternal age at enrolment (year)	32.3 (29.7–34.6)
Maternal BMI at enrolment (kg/m^2)	23.3 (21.7–25.8)
Household income ≥ €2,200 per month	1586 (78.0%)
Educational level parents	
• No higher education	421 (20.7%)
• One parent higher education	495 (24.4%)
• Both parents higher education	1116 (54.9%)
Maternal hypercholesterolemia, diabetes mellitus, or hypertension	93 (4.6%)
Smoking during pregnancy	
• Never	1606 (79.0%)
• Until pregnancy was known	213 (10.5%)
• Continued	213 (10.5%)
Alcohol consumption during pregnancy	
• Never	627 (30.9%)
• Until pregnancy was known	364 (17.9%)
• Continued	1041 (51.2%)
Use of folic acid supplements during pregnancy	
• Start periconceptional	1245 (61.3%)
• Start in first 10 weeks of pregnancy	599 (29.4%)
• No	188 (9.3%)
Gestational hypertension, preeclampsia, or gestational diabetes mellitus	183 (9.1%)

Abbreviations: DF, dietary fiber; HDL, high density lipoprotein; IQR, interquartile range.

3.2. *Associations between DF Intake and Cardiometabolic Health*

Table 2 presents the crude and covariate-adjusted associations between DF intake and energy-adjusted DF intake and age- and sex-adjusted outcomes of cardiometabolic health. In covariate-adjusted models, a 1 g/day higher energy-adjusted DF intake was associated with a 0.022 (95% CI −0.038, −0.006) SD lower cardiometabolic risk factor score. The effect estimate for DF without adjustment for energy was similar (−0.022 SDS; 95% CI −0.037, −0.006).

Table 2. Crude and covariate-adjusted associations between DF intake and energy-adjusted DF intake and cardiometabolic outcomes.

	DF Intake (per 1 g/day)		Energy-Adjusted DF Intake (per 1 g/day) [1]	
	Crude Model [2]	Covariate-Adjusted Model [3]	Crude Model [2]	Covariate-Adjusted Model [3]
Cardiometabolic risk factor score n = 1314	−0.014 * (−0.024, −0.003)	−0.022 * (−0.037, −0.006)	−0.023 * (−0.038, −0.007)	−0.022 * (−0.038, −0.006)
BF% (SDS) n = 1988	−0.005 (−0.014, 0.004)	−0.005 (−0.017, 0.007)	−0.004 (−0.016, 0.008)	−0.003 (−0.015, 0.010)
HDL-C (SDS) n = 1385	0.018 * (0.012, 0.024)	0.027 * (0.011, 0.044)	0.023 * (0.007, 0.039)	0.026 [*,4] (0.009, 0.043)
Insulin (SDS) n = 1380	0.001 (−0.005, 0.007)	0.002 (−0.014, 0.019)	−0.005 (−0.013, 0.003)	−0.003 (−0.020, 0.015)
Triglycerides (SDS) n = 1383	−0.008 (−0.020, 0.004)	−0.019 * (−0.035, −0.003)	−0.015 (−0.031, 0.001)	−0.018 [*,4] (−0.036, −0.002)
DBP (SDS) n = 1943	−0.006 (−0.015, 0.004)	−0.006 (−0.019, 0.008)	−0.004 (−0.017, 0.009)	−0.003 (−0.017, 0.011)
SBP (SDS) n = 1943	−0.001 (−0.006, 0.004)	−0.007 (−0.020, 0.007)	−0.009 (−0.022, 0.005)	−0.009 (−0.023, 0.005)

Values are based on multivariable linear regression models and reflect differences (95% confidence interval) in individual cardiometabolic outcomes and in cardiometabolic risk factor score (age- and sex-adjusted SDS) per 1 g/day increase in DF intake. [1] DF was analyzed as energy-adjusted DF using the residual method and models were additionally adjusted for energy intake; [2] Crude model is adjusted for child's sex and age at FFQ; [3] Covariate-adjusted model additionally includes maternal cardiometabolic health, age, BMI, smoking, alcohol intake and folic acid supplementation during pregnancy, pregnancy complications, household income, parental education, child's birth weight, breastfeeding, timing of introduction of fruit and vegetables, receiving dietary supplements, glycemic load, diet quality score, physical activity, screen time, and smoking in the household; [4] In our study population, a 0.026 SDS higher HDL-C corresponds to approximately 0.008 mmol/L or 0.31 mg/dL; and a 0.020 SDS lower triglyceride concentrations to approximately 0.010 mmol/L or 0.89 mg/dL; * p-value $<$ 0.05. Abbreviations: BF%, body fat percentage; DBP, diastolic blood pressure; DF, dietary fiber; HDL-C, high-density lipoprotein cholesterol; SBP, systolic blood pressure; SDS, standard deviation score.

Thereafter, we analyzed the components of the cardiometabolic risk factor score separately (Table 2). A 1 g/day higher energy-adjusted DF intake was associated with 0.026 SDS (95% CI 0.089, 0.042) higher HDL-C concentrations. In addition, a higher energy-adjusted DF intake were associated with 0.020 SDS lower triglyceride concentrations (95% CI −0.037, −0.003). DF intake was not associated with BF%, insulin, DBP, or SBP. Intake of DF was also not associated with repeatedly measured height (−0.004 (95% CI −0.012, 0.005)), weight (−0.007 (95% CI −0.017, 0.003)), or BMI (−0.001 (95% CI −0.010, 0.008)), or with FMI at 6 years (−0.003 (95% CI −0.009, 0.009)). Also for the individual cardiometabolic outcomes, effect estimates with and without energy adjustment were similar (Table 2).

3.3. Associations between DF Intake from Different Sources and Cardiometabolic Health

Table 3 presents the covariate-adjusted associations between intake of DF from different sources and cardiometabolic health. A 1 g/day higher energy-adjusted DF intake from potatoes was associated with a 0.051 SDS (95% CI −0.094, −0.009) lower cardiometabolic risk factor score, and a 0.076 SDS lower triglyceride concentration (95% CI −0.121, −0.031). Effect estimates without energy adjustment were similar and in addition, there was a positive association between DF intake from potatoes and HDL-C (0.028 SDS; 95% CI 0.016, 0.072).

We observed that a 1 g/day higher energy-adjusted DF intake from fruit and vegetables was associated with a 0.028 SDS (95% CI 0.001, 0.054) higher HDL-C (similar without energy adjustment). Effect estimates for DF from legumes were similar to those obtained for total DF, however, the confidence intervals were wide and none of the associations for DF from legumes was statistically significant. For DF intake from cereals, we observed no associations with any of the outcomes.

Table 3. Covariate-adjusted associations between DF intake and energy-adjusted DF intake from cereals, from potatoes, from fruits and vegetables, and from legumes (per 1 g/day) and cardiometabolic outcomes.

	Cereals (per 1 g/day)		Potatoes (per 1 g/day)		Fruit & Vegetables (per 1 g/day)		Legumes (per 1 g/day)	
	DF Intake	Energy-Adjusted DF Intake [1]	DF Intake	Energy-Adjusted DF Intake [1]	DF Intake [1]	Energy-Adjusted DF Intake [1]	DF Intake	Energy-Adjusted DF Intake [1]
Cardiometabolic risk factor score (SDS) $n = 1311$	−0.006 (−0.026, 0.014)	−0.004 (−0.026, 0.019)	−0.050 * (−0.093, −0.008)	−0.051 * (−0.096, −0.009)	−0.009 (−0.034, 0.017)	−0.009 (−0.034, 0.016)	−0.032 (−0.111, 0.048)	−0.03 (−0.110, 0.049)
BF% (SDS) $n = 1984$	−0.009 (−0.024, 0.005)	−0.005 (−0.022, 0.011)	0 (−0.032, 0.032)	−0.001 (−0.033, 0.032)	0.006 (−0.012, 0.025)	0.006 (−0.013, 0.025)	−0.001 (−0.061, 0.059)	0 (−0.059, 0.060)
HDL-C (SDS) $n = 1383$	0.008 (−0.013, 0.029)	0.002 (−0.021, 0.024)	0.028 * (0.016, 0.072)	0.033 (−0.012, 0.077)	0.027 * (0.000, 0.054)	0.028 * (0.002, 0.054)	0.035 (−0.047, 0.117)	0.033 (−0.048, 0.115)
Insulin (SDS) $n = 1378$	0.001 (−0.019, 0.022)	−0.008 (−0.030, 0.015)	−0.018 (−0.055, 0.033)	−0.01 (−0.053, 0.034)	0.012 (−0.015, 0.039)	0.013 (−0.014, 0.040)	−0.015 (−0.097, 0.067)	−0.016 (−0.098, 0.066)
Triglycerides (SDS) $n = 1381$	0.011 (−0.010, 0.032)	−0.007 (−0.015, 0.000)	−0.075 * (−0.120, −0.030)	−0.076 * (−0.121, −0.032)	−0.02 (−0.048, 0.007)	−0.021 (−0.050, 0.006)	−0.015 (−0.098, 0.068)	−0.014 (−0.098, 0.069)
DBP (SDS) $n = 1939$	−0.007 (−0.024, 0.009)	−0.003 (−0.021, 0.016)	−0.001 (−0.038, 0.035)	−0.0034 (−0.040, 0.033)	−0.004 (−0.025, 0.017)	−0.005 (−0.026, 0.016)	−0.016 (−0.052, 0.084)	0.017 (−0.051, 0.085)
SBP (SDS) $n = 1939$	−0.009 (−0.026, 0.009)	−0.012 (−0.032, 0.008)	0.004 (−0.034, 0.041)	0.004 (−0.033, 0.042)	0.001 (−0.021, 0.023)	0.002 (−0.021, 0.024)	−0.008 (−0.028, 0.012)	−0.008 (−0.028, 0.012)

Values are based on multivariable linear regression models and reflect differences (95% confidence intervals) in individual cardiometabolic outcomes and in cardiometabolic risk factor score (age- and sex-adjusted SD scores) per 1 g/day increase in DF intake from different sources. All models are adjusted for maternal cardiometabolic health, age, BMI, smoking, alcohol intake and folic acid supplementation during pregnancy, pregnancy complications, household income, parental education, child's birth weight, sex, breastfeeding, timing of introduction of fruit and vegetables, age at food-frequency questionnaire (FFQ), receiving dietary supplements, glycemic load, diet quality score, physical activity, screen time, and smoking in the household. [1] DF was analyzed as energy-adjusted DF using the residual method and models were additionally adjusted for energy intake. * p-value < 0.05. Abbreviations: BF%, body fat percentage; DBP, diastolic blood pressure; DF, dietary fiber; HDL-C, high-density lipoprotein cholesterol; SBP, systolic blood pressure; SDS, standard deviation score.

3.4. Additional Analyses

We observed no significant interaction of DF intake with child's sex or age at FFQ on any of the outcomes. Crude associations were comparable with those after adjustment for confounders (Supplementary Materials Table S2). When we restricted our analyses to children with complete data on all cardiometabolic factors, we observed similar results as obtained for the full sample (Supplementary Materials Table S3). When we analyzed the cardiometabolic risk factor score without triglycerides (TG) or without HDL-C in sensitivity analyses, effect estimates only slightly attenuated (Supplementary Materials Table S4). Finally, we observed no significant differences in DF intake, BF%, or blood pressure between children with or without blood samples (Supplementary Materials Table S5).

4. Discussion

This is the first study that investigated the association between DF intake, including DF from different sources, and cardiometabolic health in a large cohort of young children. Overall, a higher DF intake was associated with a lower cardiometabolic risk factor score. This was mainly determined by a better blood lipid profile. Furthermore, we observed that the association between DF intake and better cardiometabolic health was not explained by differences in energy intake and seemed to be primarily driven by intake of DF from potatoes, fruits, and vegetables. Although effect sizes were modest and without clinical implications on the individual level, small variations in cardiometabolic risk factors in childhood have been shown to predict health in later life [6,7], and a high DF intake already in early childhood may thereby contribute to a reduction in the cardiometabolic disease burden of a population.

Our observation that a higher DF intake was associated with better combined cardiometabolic health is in line with previous studies in adolescents and adults that showed that a higher DF intake was associated with a lower risk of metabolic syndrome [1,43]. Although associations with all individual cardiometabolic outcomes were in the expected direction, we observed that the association with overall cardiometabolic health in our population was mainly driven by higher HDL-C and lower triglyceride concentrations. In line with our results, Ludwig et al. [2] showed that a higher DF intake was associated with higher HDL-C and with lower triglyceride concentrations in adults. In contrast, two previous studies that examined these associations in children found no associations between DF intake and HDL-C or triglycerides [9,16]. However, these studies were small (n = 543 and n = 147) and may have been underpowered to detect such associations. A potential beneficial effect of DF intake on blood lipid levels could be explained by two mechanisms. First, DF decreases gastric emptying, which reduces the acute postprandial responses, and thereby controls glucose and lipid concentrations after a meal [24,44]. In the long-term, lower fluctuations of glucose and lipids can reduce the risk of cardiometabolic disorders. Second, absorption of lipid is affected by dietary fiber intake, which leads to a reduction in hepatic cholesterol. [45].

Although associations were all in the expected direction (i.e., improved cardiometabolic health), DF intake was not significantly associated with the individual cardiometabolic components BF%, insulin, DBP, or SBP in our population. Results from previous studies in children and adolescents are mixed, with studies reporting either null or beneficial associations for higher DF intake. Jenner et al. [15] reported associations between a higher DF intake and energy-adjusted DF intake with a lower DBP in boys, but not in girls, at the age of 9 years. Two studies observed no associations of DF with BF% in young children [11] or with BF% and insulin dynamics in adolescents [12], whereas three other studies reported that higher energy-adjusted DF intake was associated with lower BMI [8,10], lower visceral adiposity [13], and improved insulin-related outcomes [10] in children and adolescents. Since most of these studies were performed in older children [8,10,13] or in higher risk populations, such as obese teenagers [10,13], there may have been insufficient variability in our young and generally healthy population to observe a potential beneficial effect of DF intake on these individual cardiometabolic factors. Although very high DF intake has been hypothesized to have harmful effects on growth, studies do not support that high DF intake compromises growth of children in developed countries [18,20]. In line with this, we observed no associations of DF intake with repeatedly measured height or weight and we observed no indications for nonlinear associations of DF intake with any of the growth or cardiometabolic factors, suggesting that associations did not differ for low or high DF intakes in our study population with a generally high DF intake.

Considering that DF intake may result in satiation that could lead to a lower energy intake [24], associations between DF intake and cardiometabolic health were hypothesized to be explained by differences in energy intake. However, we observed no clear differences in associations for DF with or without energy adjustment. If any, the effect estimates became stronger after adjustment for energy intake, which is in line with results from two previous studies among children that showed larger effect estimates of DF on cardiometabolic outcomes after adjustment for energy [9,15]. This suggests that the effects of satiation may not play a major role among young children. In other words, a high DF intake does not necessarily displace energy intake [9] and a higher DF intake might be beneficial for cardiometabolic health via other mechanisms.

These other mechanisms may differ for different types and food sources of DF. In our study, we observed that associations of DF intake with blood lipids were mainly explained by intake of DF from fruits, vegetables, and potatoes, but not from cereals. Fruits and vegetables contain hemicellulose A, pectin, gums, and mucilage; and these types of DF may increase the viscosity that result in distension of the stomach [22]. Potatoes contain resistant starch, and in line with our results on blood lipids, Higgins et al. [23] reported that a replacement of 5.4% of dietary carbohydrates with resistant starch increased postprandial lipid oxidation. Resistant starch has also been associated with an increase in satiety in adults [46], and the mechanism behind lowering triglyceride concentrations probably involves increased intestinal viscosity [47]. Other studies showed that the solubility of DF could influence the associations [13,14]. Unfortunately, we were only able to make a division of DF by food sources, and not by type of DF. Therefore, there is still an overlap between intake of soluble and insoluble DF in our analyses. Finally, because of the low legume intake in our population, we might not have been able to detect associations for DF intake from legumes.

Our study was performed in a large population-based cohort with information available on many potential confounders. Although not all information on confounders was complete for all participants, we used multiple imputation of covariates to reduce attrition bias. Another strength is the availability of blood samples to measure detailed markers of cardiometabolic health. Blood samples were available in only 68.3% of the children, which may have led to selection bias. However, we observed no significant differences in DF intake, BF%, and blood pressure between children with or without blood samples [17] and results were similar when we restricted our analyses to the subjects with complete data on cardiometabolic health available, suggesting that bias due to missing blood samples may not be a large issue in the current analyses. A limitation is that blood lipids and insulin concentrations were measured in blood samples that were collected in non-fasting state. According to studies in adults, fasting time has little influence on cholesterol levels [48], but concentrations of triacylglycerol [48] and insulin [49] vary more substantially with differences in fasting time. Assuming that fasting time of the children when visiting our research center is randomly distributed, this measurement error would have led to non-differential misclassification of the outcomes and may therefore have resulted in an underestimation of our effect estimates for associations with insulin and blood lipids.

Regarding the nutritional assessment, an FFQ is an appropriate method because it reflects habitual diet. Furthermore, although FFQs are prone to measurement error, our validation study showed an intra-class correlation coefficient of 0.7 for DF intake [26,27], indicating a reasonably good validity. Unfortunately, we had no information available on intake of specific subtypes of DF, such as soluble and insoluble DF. A limitation is that this is an observational study, therefore, we cannot establish a causal relation. Although we had information available on many potential confounders, residual confounding from, for example, physical activity may still be an issue. Finally, we did not have cardiometabolic health data at the age of 1 year or dietary data at the age of 6 years, consequently, we were not able to perform longitudinal analyses for the cardiometabolic factors.

5. Conclusions

Results of this prospective cohort study suggest that a higher DF intake in infancy is associated with better combined cardiometabolic health, especially with a healthier blood lipid profile. These associations were not explained by differences in energy intake. Intake of DF from potatoes, fruits, and vegetables rather than cereals seemed to drive this association. Future studies should investigate the longitudinal association of DF intake, including different subtypes of DF, in early childhood with long-term cardiometabolic health.

Supplementary Materials:
Table S1: Population characteristics based on unimputed and imputed data; Table S2: Crude associations between DF intake and cardiometabolic outcomes; Table S3: Crude and covariate-adjusted associations between DF intake and cardiometabolic outcomes among children with complete data on cardiometabolic health (n = 1314); Table S4: Sensitivity analyses: associations between DF intake and the cardiometabolic risk factor score without TG or HDL-C; Table S5: Descriptives of children with and without blood samples available.

Acknowledgments: The Generation R Study was conducted by the Erasmus Medical Center in close collaboration with the School of Law and Faculty of Social Sciences of the Erasmus University Rotterdam, the Municipal Health Service-Rotterdam Metropolitan Area, the Rotterdam Homecare Foundation, and the Stichting Trombosedienst & Artsenlaboratorium Rijnmond, Rotterdam. The general design of the Generation R Study was made possible by financial support from the Erasmus Medical Center, Rotterdam; the Erasmus University, Rotterdam; the Dutch Ministry of Health, Welfare and Sport; and The Netherlands Organization for Health Research and Development (ZonMw). The authors Kim V. E. Braun, Jessica C. Kiefte-de Jong, Oscar H. Franco, and Trudy Voortman work in ErasmusAGE, a center for aging research across the life course funded by Nestle Nutrition (Nestec Ltd.), Metagenics Inc. and AXA. The funders had no role in design and conduct of the study; collection, management, analysis, and interpretation of the data; and preparation, review or approval of the manuscript.

Author Contributions: R.M.A.v.G., and K.V.E.B. designed the research project, conducted the analyses, and drafted the initial manuscript. J.C.K.-d.J., V.W.V.J., and O.H.F. were involved in the data collection and provided input regarding the interpretation of the results and writing of the manuscript. T.V. designed the research project and provided consultation regarding the data analysis, interpretation of results, and writing of the manuscript. All authors critically reviewed and approved the final manuscript as submitted and agree to be accountable for all aspects of the work.

Abbreviations

The following abbreviations have been used in the text:

BF%	Body Fat Percentage
BMI	Body Mass Index
DBP	Diastolic Blood Pressure
DF	Dietary Fiber
FFQ	Food Frequency Questionnaire
HDL-C	High Density Lipoprotein Cholesterol
LDL-C	Low Density Lipoprotein Cholesterol
SBP	Systolic Blood Pressure
SDS	Standard Deviation Score

References

1. Grooms, K.N.; Ommerborn, M.J.; Pham, D.Q.; Djousse, L.; Clark, C.R. Dietary fiber intake and cardiometabolic risks among us adults, nhanes 1999–2010. *Am. J. Med.* **2013**, *126*, 1059–1067. [CrossRef] [PubMed]
2. Ludwig, D.S.; Pereira, M.A.; Kroenke, C.H.; Hilner, J.E.; Van Horn, L.; Slattery, M.L.; Jacobs, D.R., Jr. Dietary fiber, weight gain, and cardiovascular disease risk factors in young adults. *JAMA* **1999**, *282*, 1539–1546. [CrossRef] [PubMed]
3. Satija, A.; Hu, F.B. Cardiovascular benefits of dietary fiber. *Curr. Atheroscler. Rep.* **2012**, *14*, 505–514. [CrossRef] [PubMed]

4. Dietz, W.H. Health consequences of obesity in youth: Childhood predictors of adult disease. *Pediatrics* **1998**, *101*, 518–525. [PubMed]
5. Juonala, M.; Magnussen, C.G.; Berenson, G.S.; Venn, A.; Burns, T.L.; Sabin, M.A.; Srinivasan, S.R.; Daniels, S.R.; Davis, P.H.; Chen, W.; et al. Childhood adiposity, adult adiposity, and cardiovascular risk factors. *N. Engl. J. Med.* **2011**, *365*, 1876–1885. [CrossRef] [PubMed]
6. Morrison, J.A.; Glueck, C.J.; Wang, P. Childhood risk factors predict cardiovascular disease, impaired fasting glucose plus type 2 diabetes mellitus, and high blood pressure 26 years later at a mean age of 38 years: The princeton-lipid research clinics follow-up study. *Metabolism* **2012**, *61*, 531–541. [CrossRef] [PubMed]
7. Morrison, J.A.; Glueck, C.J.; Woo, J.G.; Wang, P. Risk factors for cardiovascular disease and type 2 diabetes retained from childhood to adulthood predict adult outcomes: The princeton lrc follow-up study. *Int. J. Pediatr. Endocrinol.* **2012**. [CrossRef] [PubMed]
8. Cheng, G.; Karaolis-Danckert, N.; Libuda, L.; Bolzenius, K.; Remer, T.; Buyken, A.E. Relation of dietary glycemic index, glycemic load, and fiber and whole-grain intakes during puberty to the concurrent development of percent body fat and body mass index. *Am. J. Epidemiol.* **2009**, *169*, 667–677. [CrossRef] [PubMed]
9. Ruottinen, S.; Lagstrom, H.K.; Niinikoski, H.; Ronnemaa, T.; Saarinen, M.; Pahkala, K.A.; Hakanen, M.; Viikari, J.S.; Simell, O. Dietary fiber does not displace energy but is associated with decreased serum cholesterol concentrations in healthy children. *Am. J. Clin. Nutr.* **2010**, *91*, 651–661. [CrossRef] [PubMed]
10. Brauchla, M.; Juan, W.; Story, J.; Kranz, S. Sources of dietary fiber and the association of fiber intake with childhood obesity risk (in 2–18 year olds) and diabetes risk of adolescents 12–18 year olds: Nhanes 2003–2006. *J. Nutr. Metab.* **2012**. [CrossRef] [PubMed]
11. Buyken, A.E.; Cheng, G.; Gunther, A.L.; Liese, A.D.; Remer, T.; Karaolis-Danckert, N. Relation of dietary glycemic index, glycemic load, added sugar intake, or fiber intake to the development of body composition between ages 2 and 7 y. *Am. J. Clin. Nutr.* **2008**, *88*, 755–762. [PubMed]
12. Davis, J.N.; Alexander, K.E.; Ventura, E.E.; Kelly, L.A.; Lane, C.J.; Byrd-Williams, C.E.; Toledo-Corral, C.M.; Roberts, C.K.; Spruijt-Metz, D.; Weigensberg, M.J.; et al. Associations of dietary sugar and glycemic index with adiposity and insulin dynamics in overweight latino youth. *Am. J. Clin. Nutr.* **2007**, *86*, 1331–1338. [PubMed]
13. Davis, J.N.; Alexander, K.E.; Ventura, E.E.; Toledo-Corral, C.M.; Goran, M.I. Inverse relation between dietary fiber intake and visceral adiposity in overweight latino youth. *Am. J. Clin. Nutr.* **2009**, *90*, 1160–1166. [CrossRef] [PubMed]
14. Lin, Y.; Huybrechts, I.; Vereecken, C.; Mouratidou, T.; Valtuena, J.; Kersting, M.; Gonzalez-Gross, M.; Bolca, S.; Warnberg, J.; Cuenca-Garcia, M.; et al. Dietary fiber intake and its association with indicators of adiposity and serum biomarkers in european adolescents: The helena study. *Eur. J. Nutr.* **2015**, *54*, 771–782. [CrossRef] [PubMed]
15. Jenner, D.A.; English, D.R.; Vandongen, R.; Beilin, L.J.; Armstrong, B.K.; Miller, M.R.; Dunbar, D. Diet and blood pressure in 9-year-old australian children. *Am. J. Clin. Nutr.* **1988**, *47*, 1052–1059.
16. Rinaldi, A.E.; de Oliveira, E.P.; Moreto, F.; Gabriel, G.F.; Corrente, J.E.; Burini, R.C. Dietary intake and blood lipid profile in overweight and obese schoolchildren. *BMC Res. Notes* **2012**, *5*. [CrossRef] [PubMed]
17. Voortman, T.; van den Hooven, E.H.; Tielemans, M.J.; Hofman, A.; Kiefte-de Jong, J.C.; Jaddoe, V.W.; Franco, O.H. Protein intake in early childhood and cardiometabolic health at school age: The generation R study. *Eur. J. Nutr.* **2015**. [CrossRef] [PubMed]
18. Edwards, C.A.; Parrett, A.M. Dietary fibre in infancy and childhood. *Proc. Nutr. Soc.* **2003**, *62*, 17–23. [CrossRef] [PubMed]
19. Kranz, S.; Brauchla, M.; Slavin, J.L.; Miller, K.B. What do we know about dietary fiber intake in children and health? The effects of fiber intake on constipation, obesity, and diabetes in children. *Adv. Nutr.* **2012**, *3*, 47–53. [CrossRef] [PubMed]
20. Edwards, C.A.; Xie, C.; Garcia, A.L. Dietary fibre and health in children and adolescents. *Proc. Nutr. Soc.* **2015**, *74*, 292–302. [CrossRef] [PubMed]
21. Pereira, M.A.; O'Reilly, E.; Augustsson, K.; Fraser, G.E.; Goldbourt, U.; Heitmann, B.L.; Hallmans, G.; Knekt, P.; Liu, S.; Pietinen, P.; et al. Dietary fiber and risk of coronary heart disease: A pooled analysis of cohort studies. *Arch. Intern. Med.* **2004**, *164*, 370–376. [CrossRef] [PubMed]
22. Aggett, P.J.; Agostoni, C.; Axelsson, I.; Edwards, C.A.; Goulet, O.; Hernell, O.; Koletzko, B.; Lafeber, H.N.; Micheli, J.L.; Michaelsen, K.F.; et al. Nondigestible carbohydrates in the diets of infants and young children:

A commentary by the espghan committee on nutrition. *J. Pediatr. Gastroenterol. Nutr.* **2003**, *36*, 329–337. [CrossRef] [PubMed]

23. Higgins, J.A.; Higbee, D.R.; Donahoo, W.T.; Brown, I.L.; Bell, M.L.; Bessesen, D.H. Resistant starch consumption promotes lipid oxidation. *Nutr. Metab.* **2004**, *1*. [CrossRef] [PubMed]
24. Slavin, J.L. Dietary fiber and body weight. *Nutrition* **2005**, *21*, 411–418. [CrossRef] [PubMed]
25. Jaddoe, V.W.; van Duijn, C.M.; Franco, O.H.; van der Heijden, A.J.; van Iizendoorn, M.H.; de Jongste, J.C.; van der Lugt, A.; Mackenbach, J.P.; Moll, H.A.; Raat, H.; et al. The generation r study: Design and cohort update 2012. *Eur. J. Epidemiol.* **2012**, *27*, 739–756. [CrossRef] [PubMed]
26. Kiefte-de Jong, J.C.; de Vries, J.H.; Bleeker, S.E.; Jaddoe, V.W.; Hofman, A.; Raat, H.; Moll, H.A. Socio-demographic and lifestyle determinants of 'western-like' and 'health conscious' dietary patterns in toddlers. *Br. J. Nutr.* **2013**, *109*, 137–147. [CrossRef] [PubMed]
27. Voortman, T.; Kiefte-de Jong, J.C.; Geelen, A.; Villamor, E.; Moll, H.A.; de Jongste, J.C.; Raat, H.; Hofman, A.; Jaddoe, V.W.; Franco, O.H.; et al. The development of a diet quality score for preschool children and its validation and determinants in the generation R study. *J. Nutr.* **2015**, *145*, 306–314. [CrossRef] [PubMed]
28. Westenbrink, S.; Jansen-van der Vliet, M.; Brants, H.A.M.; van der Heijden, L.J.M.; Hulshof, K.F.A.M.; Langius, J.A.E.; van Oosten, H.M.; Pruissen-Boskaljon, J.C. *Nevo-Table 2006. Dutch Food Composition Table 2006*; The NEVO Foundation and the Dutch Nutrition Centre: The Hague, The Netherlands, 2006.
29. Bouchenak, M.; Lamri-Senhadji, M. Nutritional quality of legumes, and their role in cardiometabolic risk prevention: A review. *J. Med. Food* **2013**, *16*, 185–198. [CrossRef] [PubMed]
30. Braun, K.V.; Erler, N.S.; Kiefte-de Jong, J.C.; Jaddoe, V.W.; van den Hooven, E.H.; Franco, O.H.; Voortman, T. Dietary intake of protein in early childhood is associated with growth. *J. Nutr.* **2016**. in press.
31. Voortman, T.; Braun, K.V.; Kiefte-de Jong, J.C.; Jaddoe, V.W.; Franco, O.H.; van den Hooven, E.H. Protein intake in early childhood and body composition at the age of 6 years: The generation r study. *Int. J. Obes.* **2016**, *40*, 1018–1025. [CrossRef] [PubMed]
32. Kruithof, C.J.; Kooijman, M.N.; van Duijn, C.M.; Franco, O.H.; de Jongste, J.C.; Klaver, C.C.; Mackenbach, J.P.; Moll, H.A.; Raat, H.; Rings, E.H.; et al. The generation R study: Biobank update 2015. *Eur. J. Epidemiol.* **2014**, *29*, 911–927. [CrossRef] [PubMed]
33. Wong, S.N.; Tz Sung, R.Y.; Leung, L.C. Validation of three oscillometric blood pressure devices against auscultatory mercury sphygmomanometer in children. *Blood Press. Monit.* **2006**, *11*, 281–291. [CrossRef] [PubMed]
34. Field, A. *Discovering Statistics Using IBM SPSS Statistics*; SAGE Publications Ltd.: London, UK, 2013; pp. 176–180.
35. Eisenmann, J.C. On the use of a continuous metabolic syndrome score in pediatric research. *Cardiovasc. Diabetol.* **2008**, *7*. [CrossRef] [PubMed]
36. Statistics Netherlands. *Dutch Standard Classification of Education 2003 (Standaard Onderwijsindeling 2003)*; Statistics Netherlands (Centraal Bureau voor de Statistiek): Den Haag/Heerlen, The Netherlands, 2003.
37. Niklasson, A.; Ericson, A.; Fryer, J.G.; Karlberg, J.; Lawrence, C.; Karlberg, P. An update of the swedish reference standards for weight, length and head circumference at birth for given gestational age (1977–1981). *Acta Paediatr. Scand.* **1991**, *80*, 756–762. [CrossRef] [PubMed]
38. Kocevska, D.; Voortman, T.; Dashti, H.S.; van den Hooven, E.H.; Ghassabian, A.; Rijlaarsdam, J.; Schneider, N.; Feskens, E.J.; Jaddoe, V.W.; Tiemeier, H.; et al. Macronutrient intakes in infancy are associated with sleep duration in toddlerhood. *J. Nutr.* **2016**, *146*, 1250–1256. [CrossRef] [PubMed]
39. Willett, W.C.; Howe, G.R.; Kushi, L.H. Adjustment for total energy intake in epidemiologic studies. *Am. J. Clin. Nutr.* **1997**, *65*, 1220S–1228S. [PubMed]
40. Hastie, T.J. *Generalized Additive Models. Chapter 7 of Statistical Models in S*; Wadsworth & Brooks/Cole: Pacific Grove, CA, USA, 1992.
41. Sterne, J.A.; White, I.R.; Carlin, J.B.; Spratt, M.; Royston, P.; Kenward, M.G.; Wood, A.M.; Carpenter, J.R. Multiple imputation for missing data in epidemiological and clinical research: Potential and pitfalls. *BMJ* **2009**, *338*. [CrossRef] [PubMed]
42. Health Council of The Netherlands. *Guideline for Dietary Fiber Intake*; Health Council of The Netherlands: The Hague, The Netherlands, 2006; pp. 1–90.

43. Carlson, J.J.; Eisenmann, J.C.; Norman, G.J.; Ortiz, K.A.; Young, P.C. Dietary fiber and nutrient density are inversely associated with the metabolic syndrome in us adolescents. *J. Am. Diet. Assoc.* **2011**, *111*, 1688–1695. [CrossRef] [PubMed]
44. Heaton, K.W. Food fibre as an obstacle to energy intake. *Lancet* **1973**, *2*, 1418–1421. [CrossRef]
45. Fernandez, M.L. Soluble fiber and nondigestible carbohydrate effects on plasma lipids and cardiovascular risk. *Curr. Opin. Lipidol.* **2001**, *12*, 35–40. [CrossRef] [PubMed]
46. Willis, H.J.; Eldridge, A.L.; Beiseigel, J.; Thomas, W.; Slavin, J.L. Greater satiety response with resistant starch and corn bran in human subjects. *Nutr. Res.* **2009**, *29*, 100–105. [CrossRef] [PubMed]
47. Lattimer, J.M.; Haub, M.D. Effect of dietary fiber and its components on metabolic health. *Nutrients* **2010**, *2*, 1266–1289. [CrossRef] [PubMed]
48. Sidhu, D.; Naugler, C. Fasting time and lipid levels in a community-based population: A cross-sectional study. *Arch. Intern. Med.* **2012**, *172*, 1707–1710. [CrossRef] [PubMed]
49. Hancox, R.J.; Landhuis, C.E. Correlation between measures of insulin resistance in fasting and non-fasting blood. *Diabetol. Metab. Syndr.* **2011**, *3*, 23. [CrossRef] [PubMed]

10

Novel Combination of Prebiotics Galacto-Oligosaccharides and Inulin-Inhibited Aberrant Crypt Foci Formation and Biomarkers of Colon Cancer in Wistar Rats

Tahir Rasool Qamar [1], Fatima Syed [1], Muhammad Nasir [1], Habib Rehman [2], Muhammad Nauman Zahid [3], Rui Hai Liu [4] and Sanaullah Iqbal [1,*]

1 Department of Food Science and Human Nutrition, University of Veterinary & Animal Sciences, Lahore 54000, Punjab, Pakistan; tahirnutritionist@gmail.com (T.R.Q.); syed199146@gmail.com (F.S.); nasir@uvas.edu.pk (M.N.)
2 Department of Physiology, University of Veterinary & Animal Sciences, Lahore 54000, Punjab, Pakistan; habibrehman@uvas.edu.pk
3 Department of Population Medicine and Diagnostic Sciences, Cornell University, Ithaca, NY 14850, USA; mnz9@cornell.edu
4 Department of Food Science, Cornell University, Ithaca, NY 14850, USA; rl23@cornell.edu
* Correspondence: sanaullah.iqbal@uvas.edu.pk;

Abstract: The selectivity and beneficial effects of prebiotics are mainly dependent on composition and glycosidic linkage among monosaccharide units. This is the first study to use prebiotic galacto-oligosaccharides (GOS) that contains β-1,6 and β-1,3 glycosidic linkages and the novel combination of GOS and inulin in cancer prevention. The objective of the present study is to explore the role of novel GOS and inulin against various biomarkers of colorectal cancer (CRC) and the incidence of aberrant crypt foci (ACF) in a 1,2-dimethyl hydrazine dihydrochloride (DMH)-induced rodent model. Prebiotic treatments of combined GOS and inulin (57 mg each), as well as individual doses (GOS: 76–151 mg; inulin 114 mg), were given to DMH treated animals for 16 weeks. Our data reveal the significant preventive effect of the GOS and inulin combination against the development of CRC. It was observed that inhibition of ACF formation (55.8%) was significantly ($p \leqslant 0.05$) higher using the GOS and inulin combination than GOS (41.4%) and inulin (51.2%) treatments alone. This combination also rendered better results on short-chain fatty acids (SCFA) and bacterial enzymatic activities. Dose-dependent effects of prebiotic treatments were also observed on cecum and fecal bacterial enzymes and on SCFA. Thus, this study demonstrated that novel combination of GOS and inulin exhibited stronger preventive activity than their individual treatments alone, and can be a promising strategy for CRC chemoprevention.

Keywords: prebiotics; galacto-oligosaccharides; inulin; biomarkers; colon cancer

---

1. Introduction

Colorectal cancer (CRC) is one of the major causes of mortality in both genders among cancer-related deaths worldwide. Being quite a complex process, many factors contribute to the onset of colon cancer and the major risk factors include family history, age, pre-carcinogens present in the food chain and environment [1,2], inflammatory bowel diseases, low intake of vegetables, fruits and fibers, high consumption of red meat and processed meat [3,4], as well as hereditary genetic factors [5]. Epidemiological studies suggest that high intake of fruits and vegetables in human diets has been linked to a lower risk of colon cancer. Excessive scientific and public concerns have been shown in earlier studies to identify naturally-occurring substances in food for CRC chemoprevention [6,7]. In chemoprevention, those natural or synthetic bioactive compounds are used to prevent, delay, or reverse the formation of adenomas, as well as their progression into carcinomas through signal transduction pathways in tumor cells. Recently, prebiotics have gained much attention as natural dietary ingredients which have the potential to maintain a healthy environment in gastrointestinal tract to improve intestinal functions and to prevent colon cancer [8].

Prebiotics are emerging as bioactive ingredients in foods and can positively influence the gastrointestinal microbiota and metabolism [9]. The beneficial bacteria residing in the colon causes fermentation of prebiotics to produce short chain fatty acids (SCFA), including acetate, propionate, and butyrate, which are further involved in prevention of CRC [10,11]. Prebiotic galacto-oligosaccharides (GOS) are produced through transgalactosylation of lactose catalyzed by β-galactosidase (EC 3.2.1.23). During this process various products may be produced having β-1,3, β-1,4, or β-1,6 glycosidic linkages depending upon the source of the enzyme [12]. Previous studies have demonstrated that GOS having different glycosidic linkages have different health effects on the host [13], so glycosidic linkages used between monosaccharide residues is of high importance in imparting health benefits.

The current study was performed to assess, for the first time, the combined effects of prebiotics GOS and inulin, as well as their individual effect on the various biomarkers of the initiation process of rat colon carcinogenesis. Several previously-performed experimental studies have shown that administration of prebiotics, probiotics [14], and synbiotics [15] provide protective and preventive effects against early biomarkers and tumor development in the colon of carcinogen-induced rats [16–18]. Research on GOS' role in colon cancer prevention is very limited to date. GOS used in previous studies had β-1,4 as the primary glycosidic linkage [19,20] and no product with β-1,3 or β-1,6 linkages have yet been used against any cancer treatment. To the best of our knowledge, this is the first time to use prebiotic GOS that contains β-1,6 and β-1,3 glycosidic linkages in a cancer prevention study.

Inulin-type prebiotics have been extensively studied for their potential benefits, and a large number of experimental studies have shown anti-carcinogenic effects of inulin this is the reason we added inulin as the positive control in our experiment to compare GOS anti-carcinogenic effects with inulin, as very limited data is available for the efficacy of GOS against CRC. No study is available on the combined effect of GOS and inulin against CRC prevention. The objectives of the present study were to investigate the preventive effects of inulin and GOS supplementation separately and in combination against the incidence of aberrant crypt foci (ACF) in a 1,2-dimethyl hydrazine dihydrochloride (DMH)-induced rodent model and to evaluate their effects on various biomarkers of colon cancer. Our study suggests that GOS had a dose-dependent preventive effect on biomarkers of colon cancer and the combined effect of GOS and inulin exhibited stronger preventive activity than their individual treatments alone.

2. Materials and Methods

2.1. Chemicals

All chemicals and reagents were analytical grade and were purchased form Merck Chemicals (Darmstadt, Germany) unless otherwise stated. The DMH, m-nitrobenzoic acid, phenolphthalein-β-D-glucuronide, nitrophenyl-β-D-glucoside, and *ortho*-nitrophenyl-β-D-galactopyranoside (*o*NPG) were purchased from Sigma-Aldrich (St. Louis, MO, USA). The prebiotic inulin extracted from chicory roots was purchased from Cargill® (Minneapolis, MN, USA).

2.2. Animals

Six-week old male Wister rats were purchased from the University of Agriculture, Faisalabad-Pakistan and were housed in temperature and humidity control room (22 ± 2 °C and 55% ± 10%) under 12 h light and dark cycle. All rats received basal diet for one week acclimatization period before beginning the actual experiment. The experimental protocols used herein were approved by the University Ethics Committee for Animal Research.

2.3. Experimental Design

Rats were randomly divided into seven groups (12 per group); G1 was control group fed on AIN-93G/M as basal diet [21]. G2 (DMH alone) was DMH control group fed on basal diet, and Groups G3–G7 were treatment groups. Treatments with prebiotic GOS were given to Groups G3–G5. Group G6 was given inulin and Group G7 received combination of GOS and inulin along with basal diet. Dose was calculated using the human equivalent dose (HED) equation: HED = animal dose in mg/kg × (animal weight in kg/human weight in kg)$^{0.33}$ [22]. Groups G3, G4, and G5 received 76 mg (HED = 4 g), 114 mg (HED = 6 g), and 151 mg (HED = 8 g) GOS, respectively. Group G6 received 114 mg (HED = 6 g) of inulin and group G7 was given combination of GOS and inulin (GOS 57 mg + inulin 57 mg) 114 mg (HED = 6 g). The doses of prebiotics were given orally through tube feeding for a period of 16 weeks according to each group's mean body weight at beginning of experiment and were adjusted at the end of each week according to body weight changes. In order to make experimental conditions similar, groups G1 and G2 were administered the same amount of water orally. After 16 weeks, all animals were sacrificed by injection of 45 mg/kg body weight of sodium pentobarbital anesthesia.

2.4. Carcinogenic Injection

After acclimatization period of one week, respective groups were given prebiotics daily and after completion of four weeks of prebiotics doses, groups G2–G7 received four subcutaneous injections of DMH, 40 mg/kg body weight, twice a week for 2 weeks [23,24]. While G1, control group received similar subcutaneous injections of Ethylenediaminetetraacetic acid (EDTA) solution of pH 6.0 (DMH vehicle). All prebiotic doses were continued during DMH administration.

2.5. Preparation of Prebiotic GOS

The *Escherichia coli* BL21 (DE3) containing β-galactosidase (β-gal) gene from *Lactobacillus reuteri* L103 was courtesy of Dietmar Haltrich, Food Biotechnology Laboratory, University of Natural Resources and Life Sciences, Vienna Austria and was used for β-gal production. The enzyme, β-gal was produced by following the procedure explained by Iqbal et al. [25] and enzyme activity was measured for *o*NPG and lactose. The crude cell extract of β-gal was used for the production of prebiotic GOS through transgalactosylation of lactose (250 g/L) prepared in 50 mM sodium phosphate buffer, pH 6.5 at 37 °C. The reaction was carried out for 5 h and immediately stopped by heating at 95 °C for 5 min and stored at −20 °C for further analysis. The Megazyme assay kits (Wicklow, Ireland) were used to analyze glucose (GOPOD assay kit, K-GLUC), galactose and lactose (Lactose/Galactose assay kit, K-LACGAR) in the transgalactosylated mixture by following standard protocol given in the manual and GOS were calculated by subtraction method. The maximum GOS were produced at 75% lactose conversion after 5 h of reaction and the final mixture contained 30% GOS, 30% D-glucose, 15% D-galactose and 25% untransgalactosylated lactose. Furthermore, the mixture of GOS was composed of mainly disaccharide (allolactose) and tri-saccharides followed by tetra-saccharides. It was also observed that maximum GOS were produced at 5 h of lactose conversion and as the reaction continued, all GOS were converted to monosaccharides, glucose, and galactose.

2.6. Measurement of Body Weight Changes

The body weight changes of rats were recorded weekly on weighing scale (Model No. SCL66110 Olympia Plus Kent Scientific Corporation, Torrington, CT, USA).

2.7. *pH and Ammonia*

The pH of cecal and fecal digesta were measured using a microelectrode and a pH/ION meter (Model No. HI 111, Hanna Instruments, Ann Arbor, MI, USA). The ammonia concentration was determined by the method described by Lin and Visek [26].

2.8. *Aberrant Crypt Foci (ACF) Analysis*

After animals were sacrificed, the colon was carefully removed, opened longitudinally, and gently rinsed with saline to remove residual bowel contents followed by fixing flat in 10% buffered formalin for 24 h at room temperature. The colon was divided into proximal (near the cecum), middle, and distal colon (near the rectum). Methylene blue (0.2%) was used to stain all these three sections and ACF counting was performed under light microscope. The total number of ACF per rat were calculated as the sum of small, medium, and large ACF in colon [27].

2.9. *Samples Collection and Enzyme Analysis*

To ensure fresh fecal samples, before sacrificing animals fecal samples were collected by gently squeezing the rectal region of rats and cecum samples were collected after sacrificing each animal, which were processed immediately after collection. Azoreductase activity was determined according to the method described by Goldin and Gorbach [28] and for nitroreductase, β-glucuronidase, β-glucosidase, and azoreductase activities minor modifications were made in methods described by Goldin and Gorbach [28].

2.9.1. Nitroreductase Assay

Cold pre-reduced (0.2 M; pH 7.8) Tris-HCl buffer was used to suspend fresh cecum and fecal samples. Specimens were disrupted using spatula and were agitated by adding glass beads of 0.2-mm diameter in a tightly stoppered tube for several minutes on a vortex mixer. The supernatant was collected anaerobically by centrifuging the suspension at 500× *g* for 10 min. This supernatant was further processed for enzyme assay. The reaction was carried out anaerobically for 1 h at 30 °C (pH 7.8). The total volume of reaction mixture was 500 μL containing 0.08 M Tris-HCl buffer, 0.35 mM m-nitrobenzoic acid, 0.5 mM NADPH, 1 mM NADH and 200 μL fecal and cecum extracts. At the end of reaction 750 μL HCl of 1.2 N concentration was added in reaction mixture to stop chemical process. To measure the amount of m-aminobenzoic acid produced, readings were taken at 550 nm. A standard curve was prepared by using the Bratton-Marshall reaction on known concentrations of m-aminobenzoic acid.

2.9.2. β-Glucuronidase Assay

Fresh cecal and fecal samples were thawed in cold potassium phosphate buffer (0.1 M) having pH 7.0. The cecal and fecal suspensions were homogenized in a pre-chilled homogenizer. The filtrate was sonicated for 30 s (six times) bursts at 4 °C and then supernatant was collected by centrifuging at 500× *g* for 15 min. The enzyme reaction was carried out using supernatant at 37 °C (pH 6.8), 500 μL was the total volume of reaction mixture containing 0.02 M potassium phosphate buffer, 0.1 mM EDTA, 1 mM phenolphthalein-β-D-glucuronide, and 50 μL cecal and fecal extracts. At the end of reaction 2.5 mL glycine buffer (0.2 M) having pH 10.4 containing NaCl (0.2 M) was added to stop the reaction. A standard curve of phenolphthalein was prepared for comparison to determine the amount of phenolphthalein released, all readings were taken at 540 nm.

2.9.3. β-Glucosidase Assay

The samples for β-glucosidase assay were prepared as described for the β-glucuronidase assay. Reaction was carried out at 37 °C (pH 7.0), 500 μL was the total volume of reaction mixture containing 0.1 M potassium phosphate buffer, 1 mM nitrophenyl-β-D-glucoside and 100 μL cecal and fecal extracts.

At the end of reaction 2.5 mL sodium hydroxide of 0.01 M concentration was added in reaction mixture to stop chemical process. A standard curve of nitrophenol was prepared for comparison to determine the amount of nitrophenol released, all readings were taken at 420 nm.

2.10. Short Chain Fatty Acids

After collection, cecal and fecal contents were stored at −80 °C until analysis of SCFAs using gas chromatography (Agilent 6890 Plus gas chromatograph, Santa Clara, CA, USA) and expressed as μmol/g of cecal/fecal material [29]. One gram of cecal/fecal sample was thawed and suspended in 5 mL of distilled water followed by homogenization (UltraTurrax T 25, Staufen, Germany) for 3 min, resulting in a 20% (*w*/*v*) cecal/fecal suspension. The HCl (5 M) was used to adjust the pH of suspension to 2–3 and was placed on shaker for 10 min at room temperature followed by centrifugation (5000 rpm) for 20 min and the clear supernatant was separated. 2-ethylbutyric acid solution was added in supernatant as internal standard having final concentration of 1 mM and this prepared supernatant was used for the quantification of acetic, propionic, and butyric acids using standards of these fatty acids.

2.11. Statistical Analysis

All of the results were expressed as mean ± standard error (SE). The inter group variation was assessed by one way analysis of variance (ANOVA) using SPSS software (ver. 18). In all significant results, post hoc comparison was performed using the Duncan Multiple Range test (DMRt). Differences were considered significant at $p < 0.05$.

3. Results

3.1. Body Weight and Food Intake

All groups were provided with a basal diet, along with DMH and different treatments of prebiotics, GOS, and inulin, except group G1 (fed only on basal diet) and G2 (basal diet and DMH without prebiotics). There were no significant differences in food intake among all groups (Table 1).

Table 1. Average food intake in different groups of animals throughout the experiment.

Groups	Food Intake (g/Rat/Day)
G1 (Basal Diet Control Group)	20.0 ± 0.5 [a]
G2 (DMH Control Group)	20.6 ± 0.6 [a]
G3 (DMH + GOS 76 mg)	21.0 ± 0.6 [a]
G4 (DMH + GOS 114 mg)	20.3 ± 0.5 [a]
G5 (DMH + GOS 151 mg)	20.1 ± 0.5 [a]
G6 (DMH + Inulin 114 mg)	21.0 ± 0.6 [a]
G7 (DMH + GOS 57 mg + Inulin 57 mg)	20.7 ± 0.6 [a]

Note: Values are expressed as mean ± SE. Means with the same letters are not significantly different ($p \leqslant 0.05$).

Group G1 gained significant body weight ($p \leqslant 0.05$) as compared to all other groups. DMH administration significantly reduced the body weight compared to group G1 as shown in Figure 1 (Body weight gain = final body wt. − initial body wt.). Group G2 gained the lowest body weight as compared to all other groups. Groups G3–G5, given GOS treatments, showed resistance to DMH-induced body weight loss and manifested dose-dependent alleviation of their body weights ($p \leqslant 0.05$) as compared to Group G2. Moreover, inulin, at a dose of 114 mg, exerted a better effect on body weight recovery than GOS treatment at the same dose. Interestingly, the combination of GOS and inulin achieved the best results in preventing DMH-induced body weight loss (Figure 1).

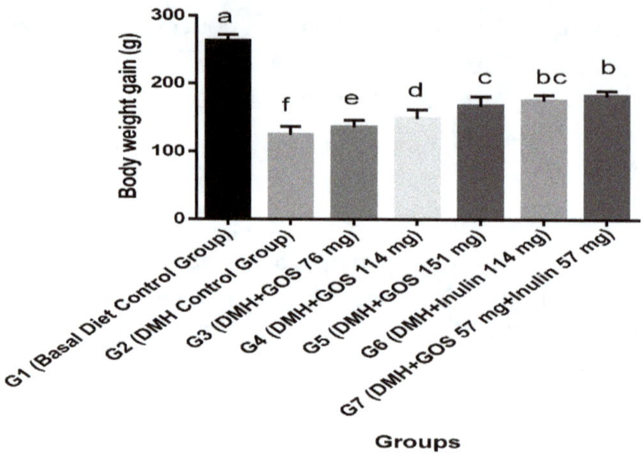

Figure 1. Change in body weights in DMH-initiated and non-initiated animals. Among DMH-treated animals, group G7 attained highest body weight. Body weight loss was maximum in the DMH control group. Values are expressed as mean ± SE. Bars with no letters in common are significantly different ($p \leqslant 0.05$).

3.2. *Individual Effect of GOS and Inulin on Aberrant Crypt Foci (ACF)*

ACF analysis was carried out at the end of 16 weeks and results are shown in Table 2 and Figure 2. The effect of prebiotics on the occurrence and distribution of ACF among different parts of the colon is shown in Table 2. There was no ACF detected in basal diet control group (G1). With DMH treatment, total numbers of ACF in the colon in Group G2 were 170.4 ± 7.34. A prominent reduction in the numbers of ACF was observed in DMH + prebiotic treated animals as compared to Group G2. Groups G4 and G5, given GOS, showed significant ($p \leqslant 0.05$) reductions in total ACF as compared to G2. Group G5 saw a significant ($p \leqslant 0.05$) reduction of total ACF as compared to other GOS groups (G3 and G4). Group G6 also showed a significant ($p \leqslant 0.05$) reduction of total ACF as compared to G2, G3, and G4, however, it was statistically similar to G5. The maximum percentage of total ACF inhibition was achieved in G6 (51.2%) in case of individual effects of prebiotics, followed by G5 (41.4%) and G4 (22.8%).

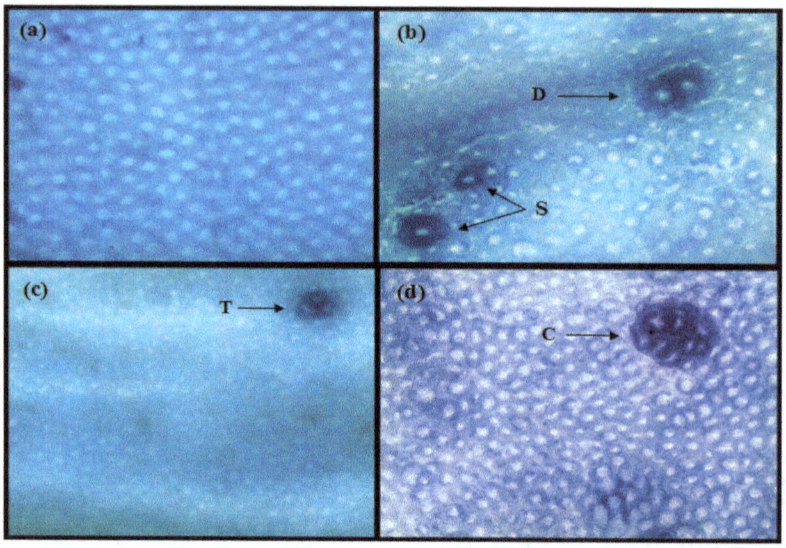

Figure 2. Histological examination of colon for ACF. (**a**) Normal crypts of control group animals; (**b**–**d**) DMH-treated animals showing aberrant crypt foci. Arrows indicate ACF: singlet (S); doublet (D); triplet (T); and cluster (C).

Table 2. Effect of prebiotic treatments on aberrant crypt foci (ACF) in proximal, middle, and distal colon in DMH-initiated and non-initiated animals (n = 12).

ACF	G1 (Basal Diet Control Group)	G2 (DMH Control Group)	G3 (DMH + GOS 76 mg)	G4 (DMH + GOS 114 mg)	G5 (DMH + GOS 151 mg)	G6 (DMH + Inulin 114 mg)	G7 (DMH + GOS 57 mg + Inulin 57 mg)
ACF/proximal colon	ND	24.6 ± 2.73^{a}	23.8 ± 2.87^{a}	12.6 ± 2.13^{b}	$8.7 \pm 1.47^{b,c}$	$7.5 \pm 1.05^{b,c}$	5.3 ± 0.63^{c}
ACF/middle colon	ND	39.6 ± 4.03^{a}	33.3 ± 3.09^{a}	23.8 ± 2.82^{b}	15.2 ± 1.86^{c}	$16.2 \pm 1.92^{b,c}$	$18.8 \pm 2.72^{b,c}$
ACF/distal colon	ND	106.3 ± 5.77^{a}	92.3 ± 5.50^{a}	95.2 ± 5.63^{a}	76.0 ± 5.32^{b}	59.6 ± 4.98^{c}	51.2 ± 4.14^{c}
Total ACF/colon	ND	170.4 ± 7.34^{a}	153.1 ± 9.23^{a}	131.6 ± 9.77^{b}	99.8 ± 8.93^{c}	$83.3 \pm 5.52^{c,d}$	75.3 ± 6.95^{d}
% of total ACF inhibition	-	-	10.2	22.8	41.4	51.2	55.8

Note: Values are expressed as m ± SE. Means in the same row with different superscript letters are significantly different ($p \leqslant 0.05$); DMH = 1,2 dimethylhydrazine dihydrochloride (4 × 40 mg/kg body weight, subcutaneous); ND = Not detected.

3.3. Combined Effect of Inulin and GOS on ACF

The combined effects of GOS and inulin showed much better results in ACF inhibition than their individual treatments. Group G7 showed a significant ($p \leqslant 0.05$) reduction of ACF in all parts of colon (proximal, middle and distal). The combination of GOS and inulin treatment showed 55.8% inhibition of ACF formation in animals, which is significantly ($p \leqslant 0.05$) higher than the GOS treatment alone.

3.4. SCFA, pH, and Ammonia

Groups G3–G5, which were receiving GOS, showed significant ($p \leqslant 0.05$) increases in cecum acetate levels as compared to Group G2, while groups G4 and G5 were higher ($p \leqslant 0.05$) in cecum 0.05) butyrate, fecal acetate, and propionate levels, only G5 among GOS groups showed significant ($p \leqslant$ higher concentrations of fecal butyrate compared to the DMH control (G2) group, as shown in Table 3. Inulin (G6) treatment showed significantly higher levels ($p \leqslant 0.05$) of cecum and fecal acetate, propionate, and butyrate concentrations when compared with the DMH control group (G2). Interestingly, the combination of GOS and inulin treatment (G7) exhibited the highest cecum and fecal levels of acetate, propionate, and butyrate among all of the treatment groups. In addition to SCFA, pH and ammonia levels are also indicators of fermentation status. The fecal and cecal pH was not significantly altered among all groups (Table 3). Nevertheless, prebiotic treatments significantly reduced ($p \leqslant 0.05$) the ammonia levels in cecum and fecal overall. The combination of GOS and inulin significantly ($p \leqslant 0.05$) reduced the levels of cecal and fecal ammonia than GOS groups alone at doses of 114 mg and 76 mg, respectively.

3.5. Bacterial Enzymes

Overall, Group G2 showed higher levels of enzyme activities in cecum and fecal contents. Among those groups which were given GOS as treatments, G5 showed significantly ($p \leqslant 0.05$) lower concentrations of β-glucoronidase, and both G4 and G5 showed significantly ($p \leqslant 0.05$) lower concentrations of nitroreductase and azoreductase in cecum contents compared to G2. Regarding fecal content, G4 and G5 were able to significantly ($p \leqslant 0.05$) reduce the concentrations of β-glucoronidase, nitroreductase, and azoreductase, while only G5 was able to reduce ($p \leqslant 0.05$) the concentration of β-glucosidase compared to G2. Group G6, which was given inulin, also showed significantly ($p \leqslant 0.05$) lower concentrations of all enzymes in cecum and fecal contents as compared to DMH control group (G2). We observed that combination treatment of GOS and inulin (G7) resulted in the lowest concentrations of all enzymes in cecal and fecal samples, as shown in Table 4. Specifically, addition of a GOS and inulin mixture in both cecum and feces reduced the activity of all enzymes more efficiently, compared to individual treatments of GOS and inulin.

Table 3. Effect of prebiotic treatments on SCFA, pH, and ammonia concentrations of cecal and fecal contents in DMH-initiated and non-initiated animals ($n = 12$).

Parameters		G1 (Basal Diet Control Group)	G2 (DMH Control Group)	G3 (DMH + GOS 76 mg)	G4 (DMH + GOS 114 mg)	G5 (DMH + GOS 151 mg)	G6 (DMH + Inulin 114 mg)	G7 (DMH + GOS 57 mg + Inulin 57 mg)
CECUM	Acetate	$82.6 \pm 2.73^{c,d}$	80.5 ± 3.30^{e}	$86.3 \pm 3.66^{c,d}$	$91.4 \pm 3.08^{b,c}$	$97.1 \pm 2.89^{a,b}$	$99.3 \pm 3.55^{a,b}$	104.0 ± 3.95^{a}
	Propionate	23.3 ± 1.89^{c}	22.7 ± 1.96^{c}	$24.7 \pm 2.21^{b,c}$	$27.8 \pm 1.41^{b,c}$	$28.2 \pm 1.54^{b,c}$	$29.3 \pm 1.58^{a,b}$	33.6 ± 1.79^{a}
	Butyrate	$15.7 \pm 0.79^{c,d}$	15.4 ± 1.08^{d}	$16.3 \pm 1.13^{c,d}$	$18.8 \pm 1.08^{b,c}$	$19.7 \pm 1.19^{a,b}$	$20.2 \pm 0.99^{a,b}$	22.7 ± 1.44^{a}
	pH	6.6 ± 0.15	6.7 ± 0.14	6.5 ± 0.12	6.5 ± 0.07	6.4 ± 0.11	6.4 ± 0.13	6.3 ± 0.18
	Ammonia	15.3 ± 1.48^{a}	15.6 ± 1.69^{a}	14.9 ± 2.05^{a}	$12.8 \pm 1.62^{a,b}$	$11.1 \pm 1.06^{a,b,c}$	$10.3 \pm 1.15^{b,c}$	7.7 ± 0.64^{c}
FECAL	Acetate	55.4 ± 2.60^{c}	53.8 ± 2.84^{c}	$57.5 \pm 3.08^{b,c}$	$63.7 \pm 2.38^{a,b}$	67.1 ± 3.16^{a}	69.6 ± 2.58^{a}	70.4 ± 2.64^{a}
	Propionate	$15.4 \pm 0.83^{b,c}$	15.3 ± 0.78^{c}	$16.8 \pm 0.98^{b,c}$	18.4 ± 1.05^{b}	21.3 ± 1.04^{a}	22.3 ± 1.07^{a}	24.3 ± 1.27^{a}
	Butyrate	5.5 ± 0.51^{c}	5.3 ± 0.53^{c}	6.2 ± 0.67^{c}	$7.3 \pm 0.66^{b,c}$	$8.4 \pm 0.73^{a,b}$	$8.8 \pm 0.73^{a,b}$	9.8 ± 0.94^{a}
	pH	6.6 ± 0.16	6.6 ± 0.14	5.5 ± 0.10	6.4 ± 0.08	6.4 ± 0.11	6.4 ± 0.13	6.3 ± 0.11
	Ammonia	10.1 ± 1.13^{a}	10.6 ± 1.34^{a}	$8.8 \pm 0.84^{a,b}$	$6.8 \pm 0.87^{b,c}$	$5.9 \pm 0.95^{b,c}$	5.5 ± 0.92^{c}	4.2 ± 0.37^{c}

Note: Values are expressed as mean ± SE. Means in the same row with different letters are significantly different ($p \leqslant 0.05$); DMH = 1,2 dimethylhydrazine dihydrochloride (4 × 40 mg/kg body weight, subcutaneous); SCFAs = μmol/g; ammonia = mM.

Table 4. Effect of prebiotic treatments on cecal and fecal enzyme activities in DMH-initiated and non-initiated animals ($n = 12$).

Enzymes		G1 (Basal Diet Control Group)	G2 (DMH Control Group)	G3 (DMH + GOS 76 mg)	G4 (DMH + GOS 114 mg)	G5 (DMH + GOS 151 mg)	G6 (DMH + Inulin 114 mg)	G7 (DMH + GOS 57 mg + Inulin 57 mg)
CECUM	β-Glucosidase	$0.97 \pm 0.12^{a,b}$	1.13 ± 0.21^{a}	1.09 ± 0.11^{a}	$0.83 \pm 0.11^{a,b,c}$	$0.77 \pm 0.11^{a,b,c}$	$0.64 \pm 0.12^{b,c}$	0.52 ± 0.13^{c}
	β-Glucoronidase	3.15 ± 0.19^{a}	3.19 ± 0.19^{a}	2.94 ± 0.18^{a}	$2.57 \pm 0.18^{a,b}$	2.19 ± 0.27^{b}	2.27 ± 0.25^{b}	1.94 ± 0.19^{b}
	Nitroreductase	4.17 ± 0.65^{a}	4.33 ± 0.53^{a}	4.16 ± 0.82^{a}	2.58 ± 0.54^{b}	2.17 ± 0.27^{b}	2.02 ± 0.21^{b}	1.68 ± 0.19^{b}
	Azoreductase	10.75 ± 1.14^{a}	10.58 ± 1.06^{a}	$8.42 \pm 0.97^{a,b}$	7.25 ± 0.93^{b}	$5.67 \pm 0.69^{b,c}$	$6.08 \pm 0.86^{b,c}$	4.33 ± 0.58^{c}
FECAL	β-Glucosidase	$0.80 \pm 0.12^{a,b}$	1.12 ± 0.13^{a}	$0.73 \pm 0.08^{b,c}$	$0.81 \pm 0.10^{a,b}$	$0.57 \pm 0.10^{b,c}$	$0.47 \pm 0.10^{b,c}$	0.43 ± 0.11^{c}
	β-Glucoronidase	2.56 ± 0.33^{a}	2.64 ± 0.35^{a}	$2.14 \pm 0.26^{a,b}$	$1.71 \pm 0.19^{b,c}$	$1.50 \pm 0.25^{b,c}$	1.37 ± 0.12^{c}	1.17 ± 0.11^{c}
	Nitroreductase	$2.67 \pm 0.36^{a,b}$	2.92 ± 0.45^{a}	$2.66 \pm 0.62^{a,b}$	$1.75 \pm 0.18^{b,c}$	1.27 ± 0.16^{c}	1.14 ± 0.17^{c}	0.97 ± 0.16^{c}
	Azoreductase	6.58 ± 0.85^{a}	6.83 ± 0.81^{a}	$5.75 \pm 0.79^{a,b}$	$4.33 \pm 0.54^{b,c}$	$3.67 \pm 0.33^{c,d}$	$3.42 \pm 0.23^{c,d}$	2.17 ± 0.28^{d}

Note: Values are expressed as mean ± SE. Means in the same row with different letters are significantly different ($p \leqslant 0.05$); DMH = 1,2 dimethylhydrazine dihydrochloride (4 × 40 mg/kg body weight, subcutaneous); β-Glucosidase = μg/min/mg cecal or fecal protein; β-Glucoronidase = μg/min/mg cecal or fecal protein; Nitroreductase = μg/h/mg cecal or fecal protein; Azoreductase = μg/h/mg cecal or fecal protein.

4. Discussion

CRC is one of the most common cancers and is the leading cause for morbidity and mortality, even in developed countries. Scientists have focused on various bioactive components in foods to evaluate their role in prevention of CRC. Our data demonstrate that the combination of GOS and inulin provided a significant preventive effect against the development of CRC. Furthermore, the inhibition of ACF formation was significantly higher using this novel combination than inulin and GOS treatments alone. The results of current study also suggest that, in comparison to GOS or inulin individually in different doses, the combination of GOS and inulin rendered better resistance against DMH-induced body weight loss and showed higher levels of cecal and fecal SCFA (acetate, propionate, and butyrate).

ACF are pre-adenomatous morphological putative lesions within the colonic mucosa that may lead to progression to colon cancer. In the present study colon samples were collected after 16 weeks for ACF analysis and, as reported in previous literature, this time period is sufficient for the development of ACF and to observe the effects of treatments. Our results indicated that various doses of prebiotics significantly ($p > 0.05$) inhibited DMH-induced colonic ACF formation in rats. We also showed that GOS inhibited ACF formation in rats in a dose-dependent manner; among all GOS groups, G5 had the maximum effect on ACF inhibition (55.8%), followed by G4 (41.4%) and G3 (22.8%) when compared to the G2 group. Only one previous study [20] reported a high dose of commercial GOS (β-1,4 linkage), at 20% concentration in the diet, inhibited ACF formation. Interestingly, our results showed that the combination of prebiotics with both GOS and inulin (G7) had not only reduced the number of ACF in the proximal, middle, and distal colon, but also altered the distribution of ACF in the entire colon (Table 2). This suggests that administration of prebiotics in combination is able to exert a pronounced chemopreventive effect on preneoplastic ACF formation. Previous experimental studies also support our findings and suggest that prebiotics are effective enough to inhibit total ACF counts chemically-induced in the colon [8,20,30–32]. As it is observed that inulin was better than GOS in reducing ACF counts, it might be due to inulin being slowly degraded and passing further along the colon before being completely degraded in the upper parts of intestine [33]. Another reason might be the monosaccharides in GOS which promote the growth of microbes without discriminating beneficial and harmful microbes. A previous study reported that inulin was able to inhibit 78.8% ACF formation in rats [30]. The reduced ACF counts in prebiotic-treated animals may be due to the modulation of microbiota and increased concentrations of SCFAs, as these are important for normal development of colonic epithelial cells [16,31].

Those groups which were receiving prebiotics, particularly G5–G7, showed higher levels of SCFA production and reductions in ammonia in cecal and fecal contents of rats (Table 3). The SCFA, especially acetate, propionate, and butyrate, are the major products of prebiotic anaerobic fermentation, which results in the lowering of colon pH and increasing the growth of beneficial bacteria, and ultimately attribute to the health benefits of prebiotics [34]. Among these SCFA, butyrate has received much attention in colon cancer prevention with multiple roles, including intestinal barrier function, minerals absorption, cell growth and differentiation [35], as well as its immuno-modulatory activity through its histone deacetylase (HDAC) inhibitory activity on nuclear factor κB (NF-κB) and its expression in colon carcinoma cells [36]. The butyrigenic effect of prebiotic GOS and inulin is very much desirable and has been suggested to be a major contributor to prevent/inhibit colon carcinogenesis [37]. Higher dietary protein can raise ammonia levels in the colon [38] and increase CRC risk through enhancing colonocyte proliferation [26]. Prebiotic supplementation or increased levels of butyrate in the colon may reduce ammonia-mediated toxicity [39,40]. In the present study, significant ($p > 0.05$) reduction in ammonia and increase in SCFA's production in cecum and fecal samples (Table 3) during prebiotic treatments indicated a degree of shift from proteolytic activity to saccharolytic fermentation. This is particularly important in the distal colon where proteolytic fermentation predominates, leading to the accumulation of toxic metabolites. A previous study using prebiotic fructans was consistent with our results with lower levels of ammonia in the prebiotic-treated groups [8,40]. In our findings, high concentrations of dietary GOS (G5 151 mg, HED 8 g), inulin (G6 114 mg, HED 6 g), and GOS + inulin (G7, 57 mg each, HED 6 g) significantly ($p > 0.05$) enhanced the production of SCFA with reduction of ammonia and, interestingly, without a change in pH. Similar findings have been observed in earlier studies using prebiotics and probiotics in combination and ITF against CRC [8,16,32].

The gastrointestinal tract (GIT), particularly the colon, is considered a complex natural ecosystem occupied by large number of micro-organisms. This microbiota is known to play a key role in the well-being and health of the host [41]. The substances produced by colonic microflora have different effects on the host, such as carcinogenic, genotoxic, tumor-promoting, and anti-carcinogenic activities [15]. Enzymes, particularly β-glucuronidase, β-glucosidase, azoreductase, nitroreductase, 7-β-dehydrogenase, and 7-β-dehydrolase, are involved in conversions of endogenous toxins and genotoxic compounds [34]. It is proven that changes in concentrations of these bacterial enzymes is an indication of change in GIT microbiota [42] In our findings, the levels of enzymes (β-glucuronidase, β-glucosidase, azoreductase and nitroreductase) in cecal and fecal contents were lower in treatment groups. It is well documented that the higher levels of β-glucuronidase and β-glucosidase are considered as biomarkers of colon cancer playing a significant role in colon carcinogenesis and are involved in the carcinogenesis of neoplasms [28], as β-glucuronidase is involved in restoration of the toxic properties of some xenobiotics in colon, its reduced level is taken as a positive effect for colon cancer prevention [43]. Higher levels of bacterial nitroreductase are considered harmful as it is involved in the synthesis of nitrosamines in the colon produced by the interaction of amines with the product of nitrate/nitrite reduction [43]. The decreased activity of β-glucosidase and β-glucuronidase in the present study with prebiotic treatment may be due to the improved intestinal microbiota and many other in vivo factors like pH, ammonia production and substrate availability. Moreover, earlier in vivo studies have also documented that inulin and oligofructose supplementation in fecal bacterial cultures led to enhanced growth of bifidobacterium, having low β-glucuronidase and β-glucosidase activity, and reduced growth of *Escherichia coli* and *Clostridium* sp. that are known to have higher β-glucuronidase activity [30]. The previous study [30] using inulin and lactulose prebiotics also found significantly ($p \leqslant 0.05$) decreased activity of β-glucuronidase and β-glucosidase in animals belonging to the inulin + DMH group compared with the lactulose + DMH-treated group strengthens our findings.

5. Conclusions

In conclusion, this study reveals that GOS prebiotic treatment has a dose-dependent chemo-preventive effect against DMH-induced ACF formation and CRC-related bio-markers. A GOS dose of 8 g (HED) per day is more effective at producing these outcomes than lower doses of 4 and 6 g per day. Novelty of the present study is utilization of GOS containing β-1,6 and β-1,3 glycosidic linkages, which have never been used before in any cancer prevention study. A novel combination of GOS and inulin exhibited stronger preventive activity than their individual treatments alone. As epidemiological data indicates increasing prevalence of CRC throughout the world, and dietary patterns are considered one of major risk factors, it time to focus on dietary strategies for chemoprevention of CRC. Results of the present study encourage inclusion of prebiotic combinations in routine diet and can be a promising strategy for CRC chemoprevention. Further studies are needed to understand the mechanisms of action of different prebiotics containing a variety of linkages in CRC prevention.

Acknowledgments: We are really thankful to Dietmar Haltrich, Food Biotechnology Laboratory, University of Natural Resources and Life Sciences, Vienna-Austria for providing us *E. coli* BL21 (DE3) containing β-galactosidase (β-gal) gene from *Lactobacillus reuteri* L103. Authors are very much thankful to Higher Education Commission, Islamabad—Pakistan for funding this study under project (112-25974-2AV1-346).

Author Contributions: Tahir Rasool Qamar conceptualized, designed, and conducted all analyses. Fatima Syed helped in performing efficacy study. Muhammad Nasir assisted in data collecting management. Habib-ur-Rehman contributed to analysis design. Muhammad Nauman Zahid contributed to the study concept and design and interpretation of the data. Rui Hai Liu helped in statistical analysis, and manuscript writing and Sanaullah Iqbal supervised the study and helped in manuscript writing.

References

1. Benson, A.L. Epidemiology, disease progression, and economic burden of colorectal cancer. *J. Manag. Care Pharm.* **2007**, *13*, S5–S18. [CrossRef] [PubMed]
2. Watson, A.J.; Collins, P.D. Colon cancer: A civilization disorder. *Dig. Dis.* **2011**, *29*, 222–228. [CrossRef] [PubMed]
3. Bastide, N.M.; Pierre, F.H.; Corpet, D.E. Heme iron from meat and risk of colorectal cancer: A meta-analysis and a review of the mechanisms involved. *Cancer Prev. Res.* **2011**, *4*, 177–184. [CrossRef] [PubMed]
4. Khan, N.; Afaq, F.; Mukhtar, H. Lifestyle as risk factor for cancer: Evidence from human studies. *Cancer Lett.* **2010**, *293*, 133–143. [CrossRef] [PubMed]
5. Van Engeland, M.; Derks, S.; Smits, K.M.; Meijer, G.A.; Herman, J.G. Colorectal cancer epigenetics: Complex simplicity. *J. Clin. Oncol.* **2011**, *29*, 1382–1391. [CrossRef] [PubMed]
6. Poulsen, M.; Mortensen, A.; Binderup, M.L.; Langkilde, S.; Markowski, J.; Dragsted, L.O. The effect of apple feeding on markers of colon carcinogenesis. *Nutr. Cancer* **2011**, *63*, 402–409. [CrossRef] [PubMed]
7. Tarapore, R.S.; Siddiqui, I.A.; Mukhtar, H. Modulation of wnt/beta-catenin signaling pathway by bioactive food components. *Carcinogenesis* **2012**, *33*, 483–491. [CrossRef] [PubMed]
8. Fotiadis, C.I.; Stoidis, C.N.; Spyropoulos, B.G.; Zografos, E.D. Role of probiotics, prebiotics and synbiotics in chemoprevention for colorectal cancer. *World J. Gastroenterol.* **2008**, *14*, 6453–6457. [CrossRef] [PubMed]
9. Macfarlane, G.T.; Macfarlane, S. Fermentation in the human large intestine: Its physiologic consequences and the potential contribution of prebiotics. *J. Clin. Gastroenterol.* **2011**, *45*, S120–S127. [CrossRef] [PubMed]
10. Campbell, J.M.; Fahey, G.C., Jr.; Wolf, B.W. Selected indigestible oligosaccharides affect large bowel mass, cecal and fecal short-chain fatty acids, pH and microflora in rats. *J. Nutr.* **1997**, *127*, 130–136. [PubMed]
11. Ebert, M.N.; Beyer-Sehlmeyer, G.; Liegibel, U.M.; Kautenburger, T.; Becker, T.W.; Pool-Zobel, B.L. Butyrate induces glutathione s-transferase in human colon cells and protects from genetic damage by 4-hydroxy-2-nonenal. *Nutr. Cancer* **2001**, *41*, 156–164. [CrossRef] [PubMed]
12. Torres, D.P.M.; Gonçalves, M.d.P.F.; Teixeira, J.A.; Rodrigues, L.R. Galacto-oligosaccharides: Production, properties, applications, and significance as prebiotics. *Compr. Rev. Food Sci. Food Saf.* **2010**, *9*, 438–454. [CrossRef]
13. Laparra, J.M.; Diez-Municio, M.; Herrero, M.; Moreno, F.J. Structural differences of prebiotic oligosaccharides influence their capability to enhance iron absorption in deficient rats. *Food Funct.* **2014**, *5*, 2430–2437. [CrossRef] [PubMed]
14. Sivieri, K.; Spinardi-Barbisan, A.L.T.; Barbisan, L.F.; Bedani, R.; Pauly, N.D.; Carlos, I.Z.; Benzatti, F.; Vendramini, R.C.; Rossi, E.A. Probiotic *Enterococcus faecium* CRL 183 inhibit chemically induced colon cancer in male Wistar rats. *Eur. Food Res. Technol.* **2008**, *228*, 231–237. [CrossRef]
15. Gallaher, D.D.; Khil, J. The effect of synbiotics on colon carcinogenesis in rats. *J. Nutr.* **1999**, *129*, 1483S–1487S. [PubMed]
16. Femia, A.P.; Luceri, C.; Dolara, P.; Giannini, A.; Biggeri, A.; Salvadori, M.; Clune, Y.; Collins, K.J.; Paglierani, M.; Caderni, G. Antitumorigenic activity of the prebiotic inulin enriched with oligofructose in combination with the probiotics lactobacillus rhamnosus and bifidobacterium lactis on azoxymethane-induced colon carcinogenesis in rats. *Carcinogenesis* **2002**, *23*, 1953–1960. [CrossRef] [PubMed]
17. Pool-Zobel, B.; van Loo, J.; Rowland, I.; Roberfroid, M.B. Experimental evidences on the potential of prebiotic fructans to reduce the risk of colon cancer. *Br. J. Nutr.* **2002**, *87* (Suppl. S2), S273–S281. [CrossRef] [PubMed]
18. Reddy, B.S. Prevention of colon cancer by pre- and probiotics: Evidence from laboratory studies. *Br. J. Nutr.* **1998**, *80*, S219–S223. [PubMed]
19. Wijnands, M.V.; Appel, M.J.; Hollanders, V.M.; Woutersen, R.A. A comparison of the effects of dietary cellulose and fermentable galacto-oligosaccharide, in a rat model of colorectal carcinogenesis: Fermentable

fibre confers greater protection than non-fermentable fibre in both high and low fat backgrounds. *Carcinogenesis* **1999**, *20*, 651–656. [CrossRef] [PubMed]

20. Wijnands, M.V.; Schoterman, H.C.; Bruijntjes, J.B.; Hollanders, V.M.; Woutersen, R.A. Effect of dietary galacto-oligosaccharides on azoxymethane-induced aberrant crypt foci and colorectal cancer in fischer 344 rats. *Carcinogenesis* **2001**, *22*, 127–132. [CrossRef] [PubMed]
21. Reeves, P.G.; Rossow, K.L.; Lindlauf, J. Development and testing of the ain-93 purified diets for rodents: Results on growth, kidney calcification and bone mineralization in rats and mice. *J. Nutr.* **1993**, *123*, 1923–1931. [PubMed]
22. Reagan-Shaw, S.; Nihal, M.; Ahmad, N. Dose translation from animal to human studies revisited. *FASEB J.* **2008**, *22*, 659–661. [CrossRef] [PubMed]
23. Dias, M.C.; Spinardi-Barbisan, A.L.; Rodrigues, M.A.; de Camargo, J.L.; Teran, E.; Barbisan, L.F. Lack of chemopreventive effects of ginger on colon carcinogenesis induced by 1,2-dimethylhydrazine in rats. *Food Chem. Toxicol.* **2006**, *44*, 877–884. [CrossRef] [PubMed]
24. Dias, M.C.; Vieiralves, N.F.; Gomes, M.I.; Salvadori, D.M.; Rodrigues, M.A.; Barbisan, L.F. Effects of lycopene, synbiotic and their association on early biomarkers of rat colon carcinogenesis. *Food Chem. Toxicol.* **2010**, *48*, 772–780. [CrossRef] [PubMed]
25. Iqbal, S.; Nguyen, T.H.; Nguyen, T.T.; Maischberger, T.; Haltrich, D. Beta-galactosidase from *Lactobacillus plantarum* WCFS1: Biochemical characterization and formation of prebiotic galacto-oligosaccharides. *Carbohydr. Res.* **2010**, *345*, 1408–1416. [CrossRef] [PubMed]
26. Lin, H.C.; Visek, W.J. Large intestinal ph and ammonia in rats: Dietary fat and protein interactions. *J. Nutr.* **1991**, *121*, 832–843. [PubMed]
27. Bird, R.P. Role of aberrant crypt foci in understanding the pathogenesis of colon cancer. *Cancer Lett.* **1995**, *93*, 55–71. [CrossRef]
28. Goldin, B.R.; Gorbach, S.L. The relationship between diet and rat fecal bacterial enzymes implicated in colon cancer. *J. Natl. Cancer Inst.* **1976**, *57*, 371–375. [PubMed]
29. Zhao, G.; Nyman, M.; Åke Jönsson, J. Rapid determination of short-chain fatty acids in colonic contents and faeces of humans and rats by acidified water-extraction and direct-injection gas chromatography. *Biomed. Chromatogr.* **2006**, *20*, 674–682. [CrossRef] [PubMed]
30. Verma, A.; Shukla, G. Administration of prebiotic inulin suppresses 1,2 dimethylhydrazine dihydrochloride induced procarcinogenic biomarkers fecal enzymes and preneoplastic lesions in early colon carcinogenesis in sprague dawley rats. *J. Funct. Foods* **2013**, *5*, 991–996. [CrossRef]
31. Aachary, A.A.; Gobinath, D.; Srinivasan, K.; Prapulla, S.G. Protective effect of xylooligosaccharides from corncob on 1,2-dimethylhydrazine induced colon cancer in rats. *Bioact. Carbohydr. Diet. Fibre* **2015**, *5*, 146–152. [CrossRef]
32. Pool-Zobel, B.L.; Sauer, J. Overview of experimental data on reduction of colorectal cancer risk by inulin-type fructans. *J. Nutr.* **2007**, *137*, 2580S–2584S. [PubMed]
33. Van de Wiele, T.; Boon, N.; Possemiers, S.; Jacobs, H.; Verstraete, W. Inulin-type fructans of longer degree of polymerization exert more pronounced in vitro prebiotic effects. *J. Appl. Microbiol.* **2007**, *102*, 452–460. [CrossRef] [PubMed]
34. Macfarlane, G.T.; Macfarlane, S. Bacteria, colonic fermentation, and gastrointestinal health. *J. AOAC Int.* **2012**, *95*, 50–60. [CrossRef] [PubMed]
35. Daly, K.; Cuff, M.A.; Fung, F.; Shirazi-Beechey, S.P. The importance of colonic butyrate transport to the regulation of genes associated with colonic tissue homoeostasis. *Biochem. Soc. Trans.* **2005**, *33*, 733–735. [CrossRef] [PubMed]
36. Vinolo, M.A.; Rodrigues, H.G.; Nachbar, R.T.; Curi, R. Regulation of inflammation by short chain fatty acids. *Nutrients* **2011**, *3*, 858–876. [CrossRef] [PubMed]
37. Fung, K.Y.; Cosgrove, L.; Lockett, T.; Head, R.; Topping, D.L. A review of the potential mechanisms for the lowering of colorectal oncogenesis by butyrate. *Br. J. Nutr.* **2012**, *108*, 820–831. [CrossRef] [PubMed]
38. Lupton, J.R.; Marchant, L.J. Independent effects of fiber and protein on colonic luminal ammonia concentration. *J. Nutr.* **1989**, *119*, 235–241. [PubMed]
39. De Preter, V.; Vanhoutte, T.; Huys, G.; Swings, J.; de Vuyst, L.; Rutgeerts, P.; Verbeke, K. Effects of *Lactobacillus casei* shirota, *Bifidobacterium breve*, and oligofructose-enriched inulin on colonic nitrogen-protein

metabolism in healthy humans. *Am. J. Physiol. Gastrointest. Liver Physiol.* **2007**, *292*, G358–G368. [CrossRef] [PubMed]

40. Geboes, K.P.; de Hertogh, G.; de Preter, V.; Luypaerts, A.; Bammens, B.; Evenepoel, P.; Ghoos, Y.; Geboes, K.; Rutgeerts, P.; Verbeke, K. The influence of inulin on the absorption of nitrogen and the production of metabolites of protein fermentation in the colon. *Br. J. Nutr.* **2006**, *96*, 1078–1086. [CrossRef] [PubMed]
41. Tappenden, K.A.; Deutsch, A.S. The physiological relevance of the intestinal microbiota—Contributions to human health. *J. Am. Coll. Nutr.* **2007**, *26*, 679S–683S. [CrossRef] [PubMed]
42. Klewicka, E.; Zduńczyk, Z.; Juśkiewicz, J. Effect of lactobacillus fermented beetroot juice on composition and activity of cecal microflora of rats. *Eur. Food Res. Technol.* **2009**, *229*, 153–157. [CrossRef]
43. Ayesh, R.; Weststrate, J.A.; Drewitt, P.N.; Hepburn, P.A. Safety evaluation of phytosterol esters. Part 5. Faecal short-chain fatty acid and microflora content, faecal bacterial enzyme activity and serum female sex hormones in healthy normolipidaemic volunteers consuming a controlled diet either with or without a phytosterol ester-enriched margarine. *Food Chem. Toxicol.* **1999**, *37*, 1127–1138. [PubMed]

11

Whole Grains Contribute Only a Small Proportion of Dietary Fiber to the U.S. Diet

Sibylle Kranz [1,*], Kevin W. Dodd [2], Wen Yen Juan [3], LuAnn K. Johnson [4] and Lisa Jahns [4]

1 Department of Kinesiology, University of Virginia, Charlottesville, VA 22904, USA
2 National Cancer Institute, Bethesda, MD 20892, USA; doddk@mail.nih.gov
3 Nutrition Assessment and Evaluation, Office of Nutrition and Food Labeling, Center for Food and Applied Nutrition, United States Food and Drug Administration, College Park, MD 20740, USA; wenyen.juan@fda.hhs.gov
4 United States Department of Agriculture, Agricultural Research Service, Grand Forks Human Nutrition Research Center, Grand Forks, ND 58203, USA; luann.johnson@ars.usda.gov (L.K.J.); lisa.jahns@ars.usda.gov (L.J.)
* Correspondence: sibylle.kranz@virginia.edu;

Abstract: Dietary fiber (DF), found in whole fruits, vegetables, and whole grains (WG), is considered a nutrient of concern in the US diet and increased consumption is recommended. The present study was designed to highlight this critical importance of the difference between WG, high-fiber WG, and sources of fiber that are not from WG. The study is based on the two-day diets reported consumed by the nationally representative sample of Americans participating in What We Eat In America, the dietary component of the National Health and Nutrition Examination Survey from 2003–2010. Foods consumed were classified into tertiles of DF and WG and the contribution of fiber by differing levels of WG content were examined. Foods containing high amounts of WG and DF only contributed about 7% of total fiber intake. Overall, grain-based foods contributed 54.5% of all DF consumed. Approximately 39% of DF came from grain foods that contained no WG, rather these foods contained refined grains, which contain only small amounts of DF but are consumed in large quantities. All WG-containing foods combined contributed a total of 15.3% of DF in the American diet. Thus, public health messaging needs to be changed to specifically encourage consumption of WG foods with high levels of DF to address both recommendations.

Keywords: whole grain intake; dietary fiber; nutrition monitoring; Dietary Guidelines for Americans; healthy diet; sources of dietary fiber

---

1. Introduction

1.1. Dietary Fiber

Dietary fiber (DF), which occurs in whole fruits, vegetables, and whole grains (WG), is considered a nutrient of concern in the US diet and increased consumption is recommended. [1] In the UK, recommendations are 30 g/day for adults [2]. The recommended DF intake in the US is at least 14 g of fiber per 1000 kcal of total energy consumed, which translates to roughly 19 g per day for children 1–3 years old to between 25–35 g per day for adults [3]. Although intake increased slightly among some Americans over a 10-year period [4], fiber intake is low in the American diet with less than 3% of the population meeting recommendations [5,6]; most Americans consume very low amounts [7]. As fiber intake is inversely associated with body weight [8–12], cardiovascular disease (CVD) risk factors [13–15], some cancers, and potentially type 2 diabetes and other chronic diseases [16,17], it is important to increase consumption to improve population health. The greatest source of fiber in the diet is vegetables (22%), followed by mixed dishes (12%), yeast breads (12%), and fruits (11%) [4].

1.2. Whole Grains

One of the sources of dietary fiber, WG, has also been associated with decreased risks of obesity, type 2 diabetes, and CVD [18–20]. The World Health Organization recommends consuming WG as part of a healthy diet [21]. Many countries and organizations also have recommendations for WG intake, although intake guidelines vary substantially [22]. WG were first introduced as a food group for recommended intake in the Dietary Guidelines for Americans (DGA) 2005 and have been maintained as part of the USDA Healthy US-Style Food Patterns as a food group to be recommended in the 2015–2020 DGA [23,24]. The 2015–2020 DGA provides food-based guidance and recommends that Americans consume at least one-half of their daily suggested total grains as WG, which is equivalent to at least 3 oz. equivalents per day for many individuals consuming more than 1600 calories per day. However, nationally representative intake data suggest that only 2%–7% of Americans meet this recommendation [25,26]. The greatest sources of WG in the diet of adults are yeast breads (27%), ready-to-eat (RTE) cereals (23%), and pastas, cooked cereal and rice (21%) [4]. However, those food sources are not generally 100% WG. The American diet does not include many foods that are 100% WG, but rather foods that contain some small proportion of WG, such as breads, cereals, or pastry made with some WG flour. The US Food and Drug Administration classification of WG is limited to those products which retain all of the main biological components of the grain (germ, endosperm, and bran) in the same relative proportion as in the intact grain [27], which is not necessary related to the amount of dietary fiber. Therefore, the "whole grain"-containing foods recommended by the DGA encompass a wide variety of foods, ranging from those with proportionally low to those with very high amounts of dietary fiber, depending upon the type of grain.

1.3. Significance

DGA recommendations focus on increasing the consumption of WG [28,29] to half of all consumed grains, however, due to the large variation of dietary fiber content in WG foods (g/100 g), it is important to differentiate between high fiber and low fiber WG foods. The present study was designed to highlight this critical importance of the difference between WG, high-fiber WG, and sources of fiber that are not from WG. A previous analysis using the 2009–2010 National Health and Nutrition Examination Survey (NHANES) found that fiber consumption was related to WG consumption [30]; however, the sample was small (only one NHANES wave), which limited the amounts of food that were included in the analysis. Due to the high number of foods in the US food supply that use the words "whole grain" in several locations on food packaging for marketing purposes, a timely research question is: "what are the food sources of DF consumed by the American population, and what proportion of dietary fiber is contributed by WG?" To answer this question, we pooled data from 8 years of NHANES surveys in the US, from 2003–2004 to 2009–2010 and examined the relationships between WG foods and DF from these foods.

2. Materials and Methods

2.1. Data Set

The study is based on the two-day diets reported consumed by the nationally representative sample of Americans participating in What We Eat In America (WWEIA), the dietary component of NHANES, and is reflected in oz. equivalent of the MyPlate "whole grains" food group [31]. NHANES is a nationally representative, cross-sectional survey of the non-institutionalized civilian U.S. population and is conducted by the National Center for Health Statistics, Centers for Diseases Control and Prevention. Details of both WWEIA and NHANES can be found elsewhere [32]. In short, participants completed two interviewer-assisted 24-h recalls; day one recalls were administered in-person and day two recalls were conducted over the phone. Primary caregivers reported proxy intake for children less than six years old and assisted children ages 6–11 years; individuals age 12 and older self-reported their previous day's food intake. All dietary interviews were conducted by trained interviewers using the U.S. Department of Agriculture's Automated Multiple-Pass Method [33].

For this study, total grain, WG, and DF intakes were estimated using day one dietary intake data collected from 34,391 individuals aged 2 years and older participating in the WWEIA, NHANES 2003–2004, 2005–2006, 2007–2008, and 2009–2010 continuing surveys.

WG were defined as grains that include the entire grain kernel—the bran, germ, and endosperm. WG values were obtained for all reported foods in all survey years using the MyPyramid Equivalents Database (MPED), 2.0 for USDA Survey Food Codes, 2003–2004 (MPED 2.0) and the Center for Nutrition Policy and Promotion Addendum to MPED 2.0 [34,35]. At the time of analysis, the new MPED including the Equivalents database for NHANES 2009–2010 was not available, thus the authors generated a proxy food list to identify the food codes containing WG. Since only a small proportion of Americans meet the WG or the DF dietary guidance, consumption patterns were not based on the intake level of the individuals but conducted on the food level, to help explain why so many Americans have insufficient amounts of WG and DF in their diets. Foods containing WG were categorized as described below. Dietary fiber intake values were obtained from the USDA Food and Nutrition Database for Dietary Studies (FNDDS) version 2.0 and version 4.1 [36].

2.2. *Study Variables*

Four categories of dietary fiber density food (no, low, medium, or high dietary fiber) and five categories of WG food (not a grain food, a grain food with no WG, a grain food with low amounts of WG, a grain food with medium amounts of WG, and a grain food with high amounts of WG) were established. The dietary fiber and WG categories "low, medium, and high" were established based on unweighted tertiles of dietary fiber density (g/100 g of food) and of WG density (oz. equivalents /100 g of food) of all food codes in the FNDDS that were reported consumed at least once in day one dietary intake data. As this research focuses on WG and fiber intake, foods not containing grains were not included in analysis beyond the description of their contribution to total fiber intake.

To maintain the nationally representative character of the data, the calculation of the proportion of foods consumed in each of the fiber (low, medium, high) and WG (no grains, no WG, low WG, medium WG, and high WG) categories in the total population and the male and female population of 2–18 years old and 19–85 years old were computed using survey sample weights. All analyses were performed using SAS, version 9.3 (SAS Institute, Cary, NC, USA). It is important to point out that this analysis was conducted to identify the foods available to the consumer based on their WG and DF content and their contribution to average usual intake, not to any particular individual's dietary intake. This approach was chosen to highlight the complexity of access to high-fiber foods in the US food supply.

3. Results

The number of survey respondents and their socio-economic characteristics are reflected in Table 1. Approximately 50% of the sample were males, more individuals were Non-Hispanic white and more had higher than high school education, which is reflective of the US census data. The educational levels of individuals 18 years and younger are not reported here, as they are likely still in school and their terminal degrees are not known. A greater proportion of younger individuals was from low-income families while the majority of the adult population was from medium or high income households.

Table 1. Characteristics of study population, 2003–2010.

Participant Characteristic	Children 2–18		Adults 19 & Older	
	Males	Females	Males	Females
Unweighted sample size (*N*)	6775	6646	10,181	10,789
Gender (%)	50.7	49.3	47.9	52.1
Race-ethnicity (%)				
Non-Hispanic white	30.9	29.3	34.0	36.8
Non-Hispanic black	7.0	7.4	5.1	6.3
Mexican American	9.5	9.1	6.1	6.1
Other	3.3	3.4	2.6	2.8
Poverty Income Ratio (PIR) (%)				
<1.3	15.5	16.4	9.0	12.0
1.3–1.84	5.8	5.4	4.6	5.8
1.85–3.4	12.8	11.4	11.5	12.5
>3.4	17.1	15.7	22.8	21.8
Education (%)				
No high school diploma	N/A	N/A	8.9	9.8
High school graduate	N/A	N/A	12.3	13.0
More than high school	N/A	N/A	26.6	29.2

All foods analyzed were reported as consumed by the population. As shown in Table 2, foods containing high amounts of WG and DF only contributed about 7% of total fiber intake. Overall, all grain-based foods consumed only contributed 54.5% of all DF consumed—the remaining 45.5% of DF was supplied from non-grain foods. Approximately 39% of DF came from grain foods that contained no WG, rather these foods contained refined grains, which contain only small amounts of DF but are consumed in large quantities. All WG-containing foods combined contributed a total of 15.3% of DF in the American diet.

Table 2. Percent of whole grain and fiber consumed by tertiles of WG (oz. equivalents/100 g food) and dietary fiber (g/100 g food) in diets of Americans ages 2–85 years, 2003–2010.

Whole Grain (Tertiles)	Fiber (Tertiles)	WG %	Fiber %	% Reporting
High WG (WG $\geq$ 1.33)	High Fiber (DF $\geq$ 1.7)	50.4	6.6	7.9
Medium WG (0.71 < WG < 1.33)	High Fiber (DF $\geq$ 1.7)	29.9	4.7	7.9
	Medium Fiber (0.9 < DF < 1.7)	10.5	0.8	1.1
	Low Fiber (0 < DF $\leq$ 0.9)	0.2	0.01	0.02
Low WG (0 < WG $\leq$ 0.71)	High Fiber (DF $\geq$ 1.7)	8.1	3.0	6.8
	Medium Fiber (0.9 < DF < 1.7)	0.1	0.1	0.2
	Low Fiber (0 < DF $\leq$ 0.9)	0.9	0.1	0.6
No WG	Any Fiber (DF > 0)	0.0	39.2	33.1
Total		100.0	54.5	

The distribution of total DF contributed by each of the five WG categories is reflected in Figure 1. The distribution did not differ between the total population and the age and gender subgroups, thus, results from the subgroups are not included but are available upon request. As the pie charts show, low DF consumers obtained approximately 2/3 of their daily average DF from food sources that were not grains. The proportional contribution of non-grains decreased with increasing level of total DF in the diet, in that the high DF diets were characterized by having only approximately 35% from non-grain food sources but approximately 25% were from medium or high WG foods.

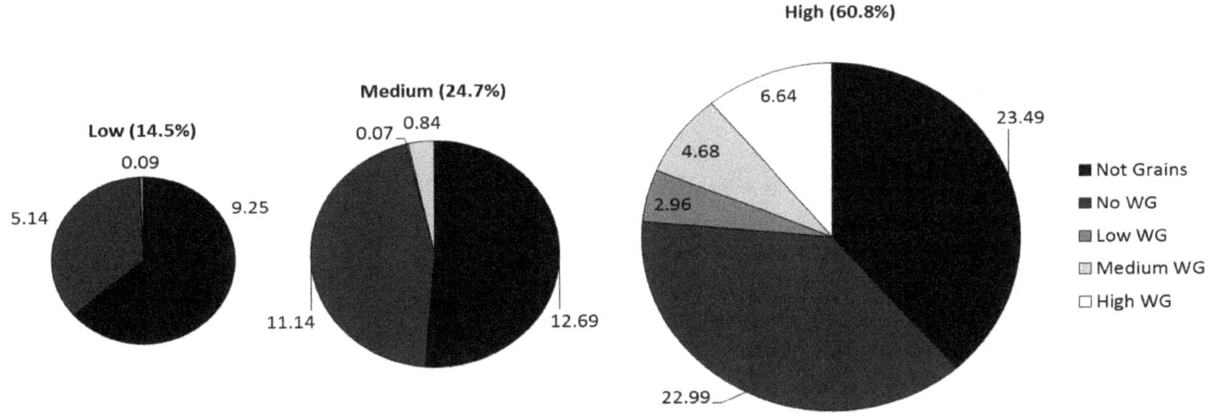

Figure 1. Percent of total dietary fiber intake provided by low, medium, and high fiber foods (defined by g fiber/100 g food) in the diets of Americans ages 2–85 years old.

4. Discussion

Sixty percent of Americans report trying to consume more fiber and WG; however, 35% believe that they are already getting enough WG [37]. Recent discussions on venues to improve the American diet have concluded that while WG foods are a good source of several essential nutrients and should be continued to be emphasized as part of a healthy diet, efforts to improve DF intake will fail if they are based solely on the recommendation to increase WG foods [38]. Therefore, such efforts should specifically encourage the consumption of high-fiber foods, including high-fiber WG foods such as multigrain bread, popcorn, or high-fiber ready-to-eat cereal.

Results from the present study are in concordance with these findings. Data indicate that the WG foods consumed by Americans contribute very little to total DF intake. Estimates show that more than three-fourths of DF consumed by adults and children were provided by foods that are not grains or are refined grains but do not contain WG. It is noteworthy to point out that the proportion of DF from WG products might be higher if individuals would consume the recommended amount of WG. However, since only a very small proportion of the American population falls into that category, no generalizable models to predict potential DF from WG foods can be established [28,38].

In previous research, we showed that the majority of DF in children's diets was provided by high consumption of low-fiber foods, and that healthy-weight children were more likely to consume high-fiber foods than overweight/obese children [39]. Thus, in an effort to address overweight/obesity in American children the relationship between WG and DF has to be clarified to motivate the population to seek foods that are high in DF and WG. Currently, this differentiation is not clear, which is due in part to the fact that WG consumption is encouraged by the DGA in terms of "servings of WG-containing foods" while the recommendation for DF expressed in the DRI as 14 g/1000 kcal consumed is not as widely distributed. DF consumers had diets that were disproportionately high in non-grain or non-WG foods; only a very small proportion of the fiber consumed originated from low WG food. In the medium and high DF diets, however, the diversity of the sources of fiber increased and included at least some amounts of medium or high WG foods. One could assume that even low DF consumers would have some portion of the DF they consume from medium or high WG foods but the data indicate individuals with low DF select an intake pattern in which those foods are avoided. Future research is needed to understand (a) if consumers are aware that their diets are low in DF and (b) the factors leading to this pattern of low WG and low DF diets. Once this information has been generated, potential intervention points to move consumers to a diet that contains at least some medium and high WG foods can be developed and implemented.

It is noteworthy to point out that some of the consumer's misconceptions about their DF intake are likely based on the use of two different metrics: front-of package labeling about the food being a "good" source of WG, while food's content of DF can be labeled using the CODEX definitions for nutrient claims ("high" in fiber (must contain 6 g DF/100 g of food, or 3 g DF per 100 kcal from the food, or 20% of dietary reference values delivered in one serving). To eliminate this confusion, packages would have to be labeled with two statements: one concerning the level of WG in the product and another to address the amount of DF in the food.

As all studies based on the NHANES, this study too has several limitations. First, our analysis was based on self-reported dietary intake records, which may include biased reporting and may not be reflective of the rapidly changing U.S. food supply. Many more high-fiber foods may be available in the American food supply but if they were not reported by the participants of NHANES, they were not included in this analysis. Our approach, therefore, may well underestimate the number of high WG, high-fiber foods in the marketplace. Also, the food industry has responded to the recommendation to consume more dietary fiber by reformulating food products and adding WG, fiber, or both. Currently it is not possible to differentiate between naturally occurring fibers and fiber added to products, such as wheat bran added to breads. Furthermore, the food supply now also includes different, new, types of fiber, which are found in foods in varying proportions and which may have disparate health effects.

Despite the limitations, the strengths of this study include the large, nationally representative sample and the use of four NHANES waves, which increases the variety and number of foods included in the analysis. Also, unlike other researchers who categorize consumers by their level of WG or DF intake, we focused on a food-based analysis to help explain the high proportion of Americans not meeting the intake guidelines. Although this effort requires the establishing of a different set of cut points, it allows the data-driven analysis, thus enhancing our understanding of the population intake patterns. In this particular instance, the methodology specifically developed for this project to optimally estimate WG and DF intake sources moves the field beyond other studies, which were limited by describing intakes in pre-established groups of people who meet or fail to meet the intake recommendations [40]. Based on the study presented here, public health efforts to change the intake behavior of those who do not meet the WG and DF intake recommendations can be developed.

5. Conclusions

The Dietary Guidelines for Americans include the recommendation to consume at least 50% of grains from WG and the DRI stipulate that a healthy diet contain 14 g of DF per 1000 kcal consumed. Most Americans don't meet either recommendation. The data presented here show that the WG products consumed by Americans are very low in dietary fiber, thus, public health messaging needs to be changed to encourage consumption of WG foods with high levels of DF to address both recommendations.

Acknowledgments: Financial support was provided by the USDA/Agricultural Research Service, (USDA 3062-51000-051-00D) and The Kellogg Citizenship Fund.

Author Contributions: S.K. conceived of this study and led all analysis and the writing of publications and presentation materials, L.J. and W.J. significantly contributed to the conceptualization of the design, K.D. led the statistical analysis, and L.K.J. conducted all programming involved in this study. All authors have read and agreed to the final version of this manuscript.

References

1. U.S. Department of Health and Human Services; U.S. Department of Agriculture. *2015–2020 Dietary Guidelines for Americans*, 8th ed.2015. Available online: https://health.gov/dietaryguidelines/2015/guidelines/ (accessed on 13 December 2016).
2. NHS. How to Get More Fibre into Your Diet. Available online: http://www.nhs.uk/Livewell/Goodfood/Pages/how-to-get-more-fibre-into-your-diet.aspx/ (accessed on 13 January 2017).

3. Institute of Medicine of the National Academy of Sciences. *Dietary Reference Intakes for Energy, Carbohydrate, Fiber, Fat, Fatty Acids, Cholesterol, Protein, and Amino Acids (Macronutrients)*; National Academy Press: Washington, DC, USA, 2002.
4. McGill, C.; Fulgoni, V.L., III; Devareddy, L. Ten-year trends in fiber and whole grain intakes and food sources for the United States population: National Health and Nutrition Examination Survey 2001–2010. *Nutrients* **2015**, *7*, 1119. [CrossRef] [PubMed]
5. Keast, D.R.; Fulgoni, V.L.; Nicklas, T.A.; O'Neil, C.E. Food sources of energy and nutrients among children in the United States: National Health and Nutrition Examination Survey 2003–2006. *Nutrients* **2013**, *5*, 283–301. [CrossRef] [PubMed]
6. O'Neil, C.E.; Keast, D.R.; Fulgoni, V.L.; Nicklas, T.A. Food sources of energy and nutrients among adults in the US: NHANES 2003–2006. *Nutrients* **2012**, *4*, 2097–2120. [CrossRef] [PubMed]
7. Lin, B.H.; Yen, S.T. The U.S. Grain Consumption Landscape: Who Eats Grain, in What Form, Where, and How Much? Economic Research Report Number 50. United States Department of Agriculture, Department of Economic Research Service, 2007–2011. Available online: http://purl.umn.edu/55967 (accessed on 13 December 2016).
8. Gropper, S.S.; Acosta, P.B. The therapeutic effect of fiber in treating obesity. *J. Am. Coll. Nutr.* **1987**, *6*, 533–535. [CrossRef] [PubMed]
9. Johnson, L.; Mander, A.P.; Jones, L.R.; Emmett, P.M.; Jebb, S.A. Energy-dense, low-fiber, high-fat dietary pattern is associated with increased fatness in childhood. *Am. J. Clin. Nutr.* **2008**, *87*, 846–854. [PubMed]
10. Slavin, J.L. Dietary fiber and body weight. *Nutrition* **2005**, *21*, 411–418. [CrossRef] [PubMed]
11. Howarth, N.C.; Huang, T.T.; Roberts, S.B.; McCrory, M.A. Dietary fiber and fat are associated with excess weight in young and middle-aged US adults. *J. Am. Diet. Assoc.* **2005**, *105*, 1365–1372. [CrossRef] [PubMed]
12. Du, H.; van der, A.D.; Boshuizen, H.C.; Forouhi, N.G.; Wareham, N.J.; Halkjaer, J.; Tjonneland, A.; Overvad, K.; Jakobsen, M.U.; Boeing, H.; et al. Dietary fiber and subsequent changes in body weight and waist circumference in European men and women. *Am. J. Clin. Nutr.* **2010**, *91*, 329–336. [CrossRef] [PubMed]
13. Overby, N.C.; Sonestedt, E.; Laaksonen, D.E.; Birgisdottir, B.E. Dietary fiber and the glycemic index: A background paper for the Nordic nutrition recommendations 2012. *Food. Nutr. Res.* **2013**, *57*. [CrossRef] [PubMed]
14. Johansson-Persson, A.; Ulmius, M.; Cloetens, L.; Karhu, T.; Herzig, K.H.; Onning, G. A high intake of dietary fiber influences C-reactive protein and fibrinogen, but not glucose and lipid metabolism, in mildly hypercholesterolemic subjects. *Eur. J. Nutr.* **2014**, *53*, 39–48. [CrossRef] [PubMed]
15. Slavin, J. Fiber and prebiotics: Mechanisms and health benefits. *Nutrients* **2013**, *5*, 1417–1435. [CrossRef] [PubMed]
16. Kranz, S.; Brauchla, M.; Slavin, J.L.; Miller, K.B. What do we know about dietary fiber intake in children and health? The effects of fiber intake on constipation, obesity, and diabetes in children. *Adv. Nutr.* **2012**, *3*, 47–53. [CrossRef] [PubMed]
17. Kaczmarczyk, M.M.; Miller, M.J.; Freund, G.G. The health benefits of dietary fiber: Beyond the usual suspects of type 2 diabetes mellitus, cardiovascular disease and colon cancer. *Metabolism* **2012**, *61*, 1058–1066. [CrossRef] [PubMed]
18. Anderson, J.W.; Baird, P.; Davis, R.H., Jr.; Ferreri, S.; Knudtson, M.; Koraym, A.; Waters, V.; Williams, C.L. Health benefits of dietary fiber. *Nutr. Rev.* **2009**, *67*, 188–205. [CrossRef] [PubMed]
19. Jonnalagadda, S.S.; Harnack, L.; Hai Liu, R.; McKeown, N.; Seal, C.; Liu, S.; Fahey, G.C. Putting the whole grain puzzle together: Health benefits associated with whole grains—Summary of American society for nutrition 2010 satellite symposium. *J. Nutr.* **2011**, *141*, 1011S–1022S. [CrossRef] [PubMed]
20. Cho, S.S.; Qi, L.; Fahey, G.C.; Klurfeld, D.M. Consumption of cereal fiber, mixtures of whole grain and bran, and whole grains and risk reduction in type 2 diabetes, obesity, and cardiovascular disease. *Am. J. Clin. Nutr.* **2013**, *98*, 594–619. [CrossRef] [PubMed]
21. World Health Organization. Healthy Diet Fact Sheet n°394. Available online: http://www.who.int/mediacentre/factsheets/fs394/en/ (accessed on 13 January 2017).
22. Oldways Trust. Whole Grain Guidelines Worldwide. Available online: http://wholegrainscouncil.org/whole-grains-101/how-much-enough/whole-grain-guidelines-worldwide (accessed on 13 January 2017).

23. U.S. Department of Health and Human Services; U.S. Department of Agriculture. *Dietary Guidelines for Americans 2005*. Available online: https://www.cnpp.usda.gov/dietary-guidelines-2005 (accessed on 13 December 2016).
24. U.S. Department of Agriculture; U.S. Department of Health and Human Services. Dietary Guidelines for Americans 2010. Available online: https://www.cnpp.usda.gov/dietary-guidelines-2010 (accessed on 13 December 2016).
25. Krebs-Smith, S.M.; Guenther, P.M.; Subar, A.F.; Kirkpatrick, S.I.; Dodd, K.W. Americans do not meet federal dietary recommendations. *J. Nutr.* **2010**, *140*, 1832–1838. [CrossRef] [PubMed]
26. O'Neil, C.E.; Nicklas, T.A.; Zanovec, M.; Cho, S. Whole-grain consumption is associated with diet quality and nutrient intake in adults: The National Health and Nutrition Examination Survey, 1999–2004. *J. Am. Diet. Assoc.* **2010**, *110*, 1461–1468. [CrossRef] [PubMed]
27. Food and Drug Administration. *Draft Guideline: Whole Grains Label Statements, Guidance for Industry and FDA Staff*; Food and Drug Administration: College Park, MD, USA, 2006.
28. Clemens, R.; Kranz, S.; Mobley, A.R.; Nicklas, T.A.; Raimondi, M.P.; Rodriguez, J.C.; Slavin, J.L.; Warshaw, H. Filling America's fiber intake gap: Summary of a roundtable to probe realistic solutions with a focus on grain-based foods. *J. Nutr.* **2012**, *142*, 1390s–1401s. [CrossRef] [PubMed]
29. Nicklas, T.A.; O'Neil, C.E.; Liska, D.J.; Almeida, N.G.; Fulgoni, V.L., III. Modeling dietary fiber intakes in US adults: Implications for public policy. *Food Nutr. Sci.* **2011**, *2*, 925–931. [CrossRef]
30. Reicks, M.; Jonnalagadda, S.; Albertson, A.M.; Joshi, N. Total dietary fiber intakes in the US population are related to whole grain consumption: Results from the national health and nutrition examination survey 2009 to 2010. *Nutr. Res.* **2014**, *34*, 226–234. [CrossRef] [PubMed]
31. U.S. Department of Agriculture. ChooseMyPlate.gov. Available online: https://www.choosemyplate.gov/ (accessed on 13 December 2016).
32. Centers for Disease Control and Prevention; National Center for Health Statistics. National Health and Nutrition Examination Survey (NHANES). Available online: https://www.cdc.gov/nchs/nhanes/ (accessed on 13 December 2016).
33. Moshfegh, A.J.; Rhodes, D.G.; Baer, D.J.; Murayi, T.; Clemens, J.C.; Rumpler, W.V.; Paul, D.R.; Sebastian, R.S.; Kuczynski, K.J.; Ingwersen, L.A.; et al. The US Department of Agriculture Automated Multiple-Pass Method reduces bias in the collection of energy intakes. *Am. J. Clin. Nutr.* **2008**, *88*, 324–332. [PubMed]
34. Bowman, S.A.; Friday, J.E.; Moshfegh, A. MyPyramid Equivalents Database, 2.0 for USDA Survey Foods 2003–2004. Available online: https://www.ars.usda.gov/northeast-area/beltsville-md/beltsville-human-nutrition-research-center/food-surveys-research-group/docs/mped-databases-for-downloading/ (accessed on 26 February 2017).
35. Center for Nutrition Policy and Promotion. CNPP 03-04 Fruit Database. Available online: https://www.cnpp.usda.gov/healthy-eating-index-support-files-03-04 (accessed on 16 February 2017).
36. Food and Nutrient Database for Dietary Studies. Available online: https://www.ars.usda.gov/northeast-area/beltsville-md/beltsville-human-nutrition-research-center/food-surveys-research-group/docs/fndds/ (accessed on 16 February 2017).
37. International Food Information Council. 2016 Food and Health Survey. Available online: http://www.foodinsight.org/sites/default/files/2016-Food-and-Health-Survey-Report_%20FINAL_0.pdf (accessed on 13 December 2016).
38. Mobley, A.R.; Slavin, J.L.; Hornick, B.A. The future of grain foods recommendations in dietary guidance. *J. Nutr.* **2013**, *143*, 1527S–1532S. [CrossRef] [PubMed]
39. Brauchla, M.; Juan, W.; Story, J.; Kranz, S. Sources of dietary fiber and the association of fiber intake with childhood obesity risk (in 2–18 years old) and diabetes risk of adolescents 12–18 years old: NHANES 2003–2006. *J. Nutr. Metab.* **2012**, *2012*. [CrossRef] [PubMed]
40. Hur, I.Y.; Reicks, M. Relationship between whole-grain intake, chronic disease risk indicators, and weight status among adolescents in the National Health and Nutrition Examination Survey, 1999–2004. *J. Am. Diet. Assoc.* **2012**, *112*, 46–55. [CrossRef] [PubMed]

12

A High Fiber Cookie Made with Resistant Starch Type 4 Reduces Post-Prandial Glucose and Insulin Responses in Healthy Adults

Maria L. Stewart * and J. Paul Zimmer

Global Nutrition R & D, Ingredion Incorporated, 10 Finderne Ave, Bridgewater, NJ 08807, USA; paul.zimmer@ingredion.com
* Correspondence: maria.stewart@ingredion.com;

Abstract: Distarch phosphate is a resistant starch type 4 (RS4) containing phosphodiester cross-links within and between starch molecules. This study examined the glycemic effects of VERSAFIBE 1490™ resistant starch, a distarch phosphate derived from potato, containing 90% total dietary fiber (TDF, AOAC 991.43 method). In this double-blind, randomized, placebo-controlled, cross-over study, 28 healthy adults consumed a cookie containing 24 g fiber from distarch phosphate (fiber cookie) or a control cookie containing 0.5 g fiber that was matched for fat, protein, and total carbohydrate content. Intravenous blood glucose, intravenous blood insulin, and capillary glucose were measured for two hours after cookie consumption. The fiber cookie reduced the post-prandial blood glucose incremental area under the curve from 0 to 120 minutes ($iAUC_{0\text{-}120min}$) by 44% ($p = 0.004$) and reduced the maximum glucose concentration ($C_{max0\text{-}120min}$) by 8% ($p = 0.001$) versus the control cookie. Consumption of the fiber cookie resulted in a significant 46% reduction of the post-prandial serum insulin $iAUC_{0\text{-}120min}$ ($p < 0.001$) and a 23% reduction in $Cmax_{0\text{-}120min}$ ($p = 0.007$) versus the control cookie. This study shows that distarch phosphate RS4 can be incorporated into a cookie and significantly reduce post-prandial glucose and insulin responses in healthy adults.

Keywords: resistant starch type 4; dietary fiber; post-prandial; blood glucose; insulin; capillary glucose; glycemic response

1. Introduction

Resistant starch (RS) is a complex carbohydrate (glucose polymer) that resists digestion and absorption in the small intestine. Resistant starches are classified into five types: RS1 (physically inaccessible starches), RS2 (granular starches with B- or C-polymorph), RS3 (retrograded starches), RS4 (chemically modified starches), and RS5 (amylose-lipid complexes) [1]. Resistant starch type 4 is a unique class of resistant starch due to the diversity of chemical modifications that decrease digestibility. Common chemical modifications include cross-linking, substitution, and pyrodextrinization [2].

Resistant starch, in general, is known for improving physiological endpoints such as improving bowel function [3] and controlling glycemia [4]. In these reviews, all sources of RS are combined. However, it has been documented that different RSs exert different physiological effects. In a study using a porcine model, RS3 increased fecal nitrogen excretion compared to RS2 [5]. The composition of the human gut microbiota was affected in different manners, depending on the type of RS consumed (RS2 vs. RS4) [6]. Given these differences, clinical trials on specific resistant starch preparations are necessary to confirm the beneficial physiological effects.

As noted previously, RS4 includes starches that have a variety of chemical modifications to reduce digestibility. VERSAFIBE™ 1490 resistant starch is a distarch phosphate derived from potato that has been modified using phosphorus oxychloride [7]. Distarch phosphate is resistant to digestion due to the presence of diester phosphate crosslinks within and between starch molecules. Phosphated distarch phosphate is a similar type of RS4 with additional monophosphate esters, although the monophosphate esters do not substantially affect digestibility [8,9].

Resistant starch type 4, specifically distarch phosphate and phosphate distarch phosphate, is a relatively new form of resistant starch, with the earliest clinical trials on phosphated distarch phosphate published in 2010. The evidence on phosphated distarch phosphate RS4, albeit limited, supports improvement of metabolic endpoints such as reduced post-prandial glucose response and reduced serum lipids, after the ingredient is consumed [10–13]. To date, only one study examined post-prandial blood glucose response to distarch phosphate (consumed in a beverage) [14]. The aforementioned study demonstrated that distarch phosphate did not contribute to the post-prandial glycemic response, and this effect needed to be confirmed when the ingredient is incorporated into a solid, baked food with mixed nutrients. The present study assessed the acute, post-prandial glycemic and insulinemic response to a cookie containing RS4 in the form of distarch phosphate (VERSAFIBE 1490 resistant starch) in healthy adults. This is the first clinical study to examine these outcomes in a solid food containing distarch phosphate RS4.

2. Materials and Methods

2.1. Study Subjects

This study was conducted in accordance with the ethical principles outlined in the Declaration of Helsinki and approved by the Institutional Review Board (IRB Services, Aurora, ON, Canada). Clinical study visits were held at a clinical research facility (KGK Synergize, London, Ontario, Canada). Healthy subjects were recruited to participate in this study. Subjects that met the inclusion criteria (18 years of age or older, body mass index (BMI) 18.0–29.9 kg/m^2, fasting glucose $\leq$6.0 mmol/L; if female, not of childbearing potential (e.g., taking oral contraceptives, past hysterectomy)) and exclusion criteria (diagnosed metabolic or chronic diseases (e.g., type-2 diabetes); cancer diagnosis or treatment within 5 years; gastrointestinal problems; bowel cleansing during prior week; current medications to control blood glucose; blood cholesterol and/or blood pressure; smoker; use of medical marijuana; alcohol or drug abuse treatment in past 12 months; allergy or sensitivity to study products; blood donation in prior 2 months; if female, currently pregnant, currently breastfeeding, or planning to become pregnant) were qualified to participate in the study. Subjects provided informed consent and were randomly assigned to a treatment order at the time of enrollment: "control cookie-fiber cookie" or "fiber cookie-control cookie". A senior staff member not involved in the study procedures generated two randomization lists—one list for males and one list for females—by www.randomization.com. Fourteen male participants were randomized into seven blocks by utilizing a randomization seed 10,087 and fourteen female participants were randomized into seven blocks by utilizing a randomization seed 11,065. A total of twenty-eight subjects were enrolled in the study. Subject flow through the study is described in Figure 1.

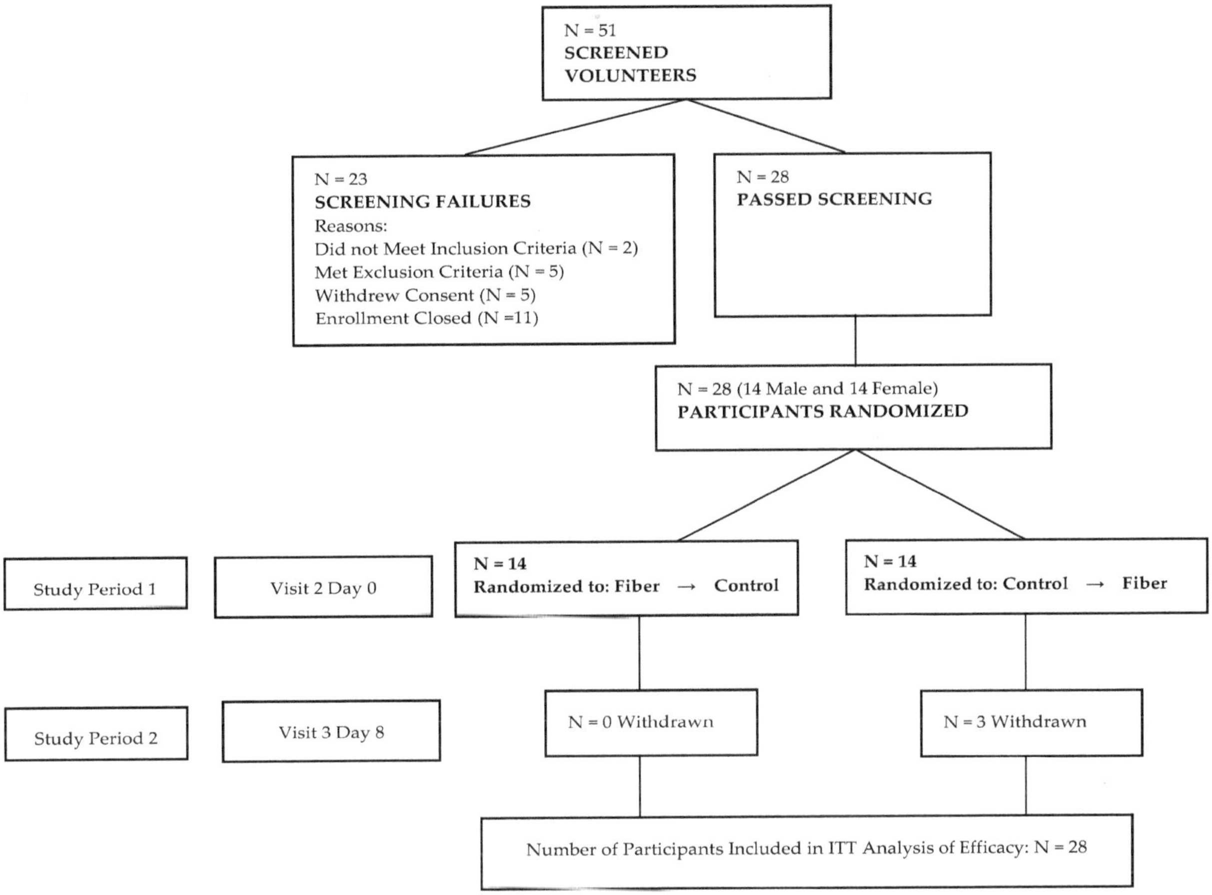

Figure 1. Subject flow through study.

2.2. Study Design

This study was a double-blind, randomized, controlled, cross-over intervention study. Fifty-one subjects were screened, and 28 subjects were enrolled in the study (Figure 1). The subjects participated in two 24-h study periods that began the evening before the clinical study visit. Prior to each clinical study visit, the subjects consumed a standard dinner meal. Subjects arrived at the study center the following morning, after fasting for 12 h. Fasting blood samples (intravenous and capillary) were taken prior to study product consumption. Both intravenous and capillary blood samples were taken because previous reports indicated differences in blood glucose measures, depending on the sampling technique [15]. The study product (cookie) was consumed with 250 mL water. Intravenous and capillary blood samples were taken at 15, 30, 45, 60, 90, and 120 min after cookie consumption. Biochemical analyses were conducted by Life Labs (Hamilton, ON, Canada). Subjects completed a seven-day washout period between study visits.

2.3. Study Foods

The fiber cookie contained 25 g of VERSAFIBE™ 1490 resistant starch (Ingredion Incorporated, Bridgewater, NJ, USA), which was the primary source of fiber in the cookie. VERSAFIBE™ 1490 resistant starch is a resistant starch type 4 with 90% dietary fiber (AOAC 991.43). VERSAFIBE™ 1490 resistant starch is produced from food grade potato starch. The raw food starch is slurried in water and maintained at a temperature not exceeding 100° F. The pH of the slurry is raised not to exceed pH 12 in the presence of salt. To phosphorylate the starch, phosphorus oxychloride is added to the slurry while maintaining the reaction pH. After the phosphorylation step is complete, the pH is neutralized with acid. The starch is washed, dewatered, and dried to a moisture content not to exceed 18%.

The fiber cookie and control cookie were matched for fat, protein, and total carbohydrate (Table 1). Nutrient composition of the cookies was calculated using Genesis R&D Food Labeling Software (ESHA Research, Salem, OR, USA). The cookies were identical in appearance. The cookies were packaged in an opaque enveloped with an alpha-numeric code for identification. Neither the study subjects nor the investigators knew the identity of the cookies. The subjects rated the cookies on appearance, texture, flavor and acceptance using modified visual analog scale with demarcations at whole numbers 1–10. The subjects were not trained sensory panelists.

Table 1. Nutrient composition of cookies.

Per Serving, As-Eaten	Control Cookie	Fiber Cookie
Weight (g)	47.02	48.00
Calories (kcal)	214.7	129.7
Fat (g)	3.99	3.92
Saturated fat (g)	0.56	0.54
Protein (g)	5.36	4.92
Total Carbohydrates (g)	36.84	36.84
Available Carbohydrates (g)	36.28	12.71
Dietary Fiber (g) *	0.55	24.13
Sugars (g)	11.51	11.72

* Fiber cookie contained VERSAFIBE 1490 resistant starch.

2.4. Sample Size Calculation

The sample size of 28 subjects was determined based on the primary outcome of detecting a difference in incremental area under the curve from 0 to 120 minutes ($iAUC_{0\text{-}120min}$) intravenous blood glucose at 80% power, 0.05 alpha, and expected subject dropout rate of 12.5%.

2.5. Statistical Analysis

Incremental area under the curve (iAUC) was calculated using the trapezoidal approximation but only included the positive area components above the baseline value [16]. The maximum concentration (Cmax) was taken to be the highest concentration within the respective time interval. The iAUC calculations as well as the Cmax values were reported and compared for each product group.

Each numeric outcome was assessed for normality using visual representations (histogram, quantile-quantile plot, etc.) and the Shapiro–Wilk normality test. Outcomes that were log-normally or square root normally distributed were analyzed in the logarithmic or square root domain respectively. Non-normal variables were analyzed by appropriate non-parametric tests (see below). All summary statistics were reported non-transformed, arithmetic means.

Numerical efficacy endpoints were formally tested for significance between groups by a linear mixed model with a fixed effect for study product group and a random effect for each participant [17]. The concentrations of the analytes at each time point included a covariate for the baseline value. Numerical endpoints that are intractably non-normal were assessed by the Wilcoxon sign-rank test. All statistical analysis was completed using the R Statistical Software Package Version 3.2.2 (R Core Team, 2015) for Microsoft Windows. Linear mixed models were run using the "nlme" package [18]. Statistical significance was achieved at $p < 0.05$.

3. Results

3.1. Demographics

Subject demographics are shown in Table 2. All of the subjects were healthy. The demographic characteristics are consistent with the typical North American adult population.

Table 2. Subject demographics.

Mean ± SD	All Participants (n = 28)
Age (y)	42.8 ± 18.5
Sex (male/female)	14/14
Race (white/nonwhite)	23/5
Weight (kg)	71.3 ± 12.0
Body Mass Index (kg/m^2)	24.7 ± 3.3
Fasting blood glucose (mmol/L)	5.03 ± 0.34

3.2. Post-Prandial Blood Glucose and Insulin Response

Three subjects who were randomized to the "control cookie-fiber cookie" sequence did not complete the second treatment. Blood samples obtained for up to two subjects in each treatment group could not be analyzed for the metabolite of interest. The sample size for each group and each outcome is noted in the footnote of Table 3.

Table 3. Post-prandial glucose and insulin iAUC and Cmax §.

Mean ± SD	Control Cookie	Fiber Cookie	p-Value §
Intravenous blood glucose *			
$iAUC_{0\text{-}120min}$ (mmol/L *·h)	1.31 ± 0.75	0.73 ± 0.90	0.004
$Cmax_{0\text{-}120min}$ (mmol/L *·h)	6.83 ± 0.90	6.29 ± 0.82	0.001
Capillary blood glucose †			
$iAUC_{0\text{-}120min}$ (mmol/L *·h)	2.35 ± 0.94	1.22 ± 1.18	<0.001
$Cmax_{0\text{-}120min}$ (mmol/L *·h)	7.22 ± 1.00	6.60 ± 1.00	0.005
Intravenous serum insulin ‡			
$iAUC_{0\text{-}120min}$ (pmol/L *·h)	229 ± 124	124 ± 94	<0.001
$Cmax_{0\text{-}120min}$ (pmol/L *·h)	280 ± 129	215 ± 94	0.007

§ iAUC = incremental area under the curve, Cmax = maximum concentration * n = 27 control cookie, n = 25 fiber cookie; † n = 26 control cookie, n = 23 fiber cookie; ‡ n = 27 control cookie, n = 25 fiber cookie; § iAUC intravenous blood glucose and iAUC intravenous serum insulin datasets were square root transformed prior to statistical analysis; Cmax intravenous blood glucose and Cmax intravenous serum insulin datasets were log transformed prior to statistical analysis.

Mean post-prandial intravenous blood glucose, capillary glucose, and intravenous serum insulin concentration over the two-hour study period are shown in the time-course graphs (Figure 2A–C). Intravenous blood glucose was significantly lower at 45 min after the fiber cookie was consumed, compared to the control cookie. Capillary blood glucose concentrations were significantly lower at 15, 30, 45, 60, 90, and 120 min after the fiber cookie was consumed, compared to the control cookie. At 45, 60, 90, and 120 min, intravenous blood insulin concentrations were significantly lower after subjects consumed the fiber cookie compared to the control cookie.

The significant reductions at individual time points for glucose and insulin values reflected significant reductions in iAUC and Cmax. After consuming the fiber cookie, the subjects experienced a 44% reduction in intravenous blood glucose $iAUC_{0\text{-}120min}$ compared to the control cookie (p = 0.004, Table 3). This was largely driven by a significant, 8% reduction in intravenous blood glucose $Cmax_{0\text{-}120min}$ after consuming the fiber cookie compared to the control cookie (p = 0.001). A similar response was noted for capillary blood glucose measures, with a significant, 48% reduction in $iAUC_{0\text{-}120min}$ and a significant 9% reduction in $Cmax_{0\text{-}120min}$. Intravenous blood insulin was significantly lower for $iAUC_{0\text{-}120min}$ (46% lower), and $Cmax_{0\text{-}120min}$ (23% lower), after subjects consumed the fiber cookie, compared to the control. The decrease in insulin concentrations after consuming the fiber cookie reflect the decreased intravenous and capillary blood glucose concentrations.

The subject ratings were favorable and did not differ between groups (Table 4).

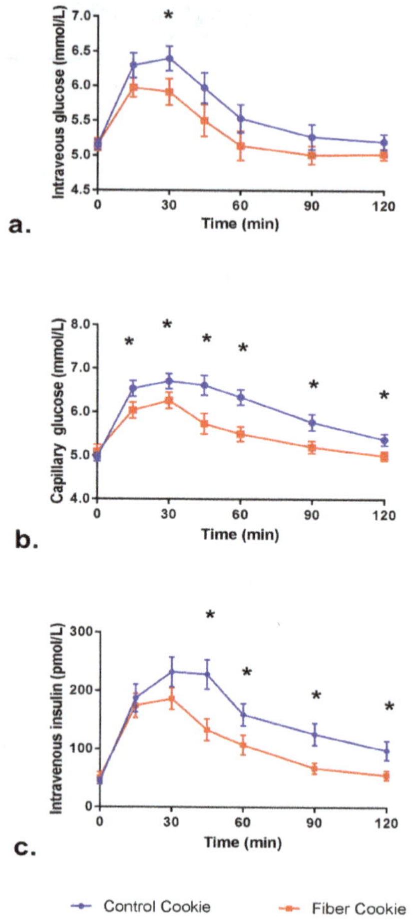

Figure 2. Post-prandial blood measurements over 120 min (**a**) intravenous blood glucose; (**b**) capillary blood glucose; (**c**) intravenous insulin concentrations. Data are presented as means ± SEM. * = Fiber cookie and control cookie were significantly different ($p < 0.05$).

Table 4. Sensory ratings of the fiber cookie and control cookie.

Question	Fiber Cookie	Control Cookie	Between Group p Value [§]
	Mean ± SD (n)	Mean ± SD (n)	
Rate the appearance of the cookie	5.69 ± 2.02 (26)	5.61 ± 1.89 (28)	0.811
Rate the texture of the cookie	6.23 ± 2.07 (26)	5.93 ± 2.07 (28)	0.525
Rate the flavor of the cookie	6.46 ± 2.14 (26)	6.79 ± 1.62 (28)	0.355
What is your overall acceptance of the cookie?	6.54 ± 2.21 (26)	6.50 ± 1.58 (28)	0.970

[§] Between group comparisons were made using RM-ANOVA not adjusted for baseline. Probability values $p \leq 0.05$ are statistically significant.

4. Discussion

Dietary fiber has been long acknowledged for reducing post-prandial blood glucose and insulin concentrations through mechanisms of delayed nutrient absorption or replacement of digestible carbohydrates [19]. The RS4 used in this trial, VERSAFIBE 1490 resistant starch, replaced digestible carbohydrates from refined flour when formulated into processed foods such as bakery items. This fiber maintains sensory attributes of the final food while increasing dietary fiber and decreasing available carbohydrate content. Resistant starch type 4 is a broad class of resistant starches that have been chemically modified to reduce digestibility. The particular ingredient used in this study contains phosphodiester cross-links in the distarch phosphate molecules that reduce swelling and enzyme accessibility [8,9,20]. Previous work demonstrated the low glycemic response to distarch phosphate when mixed with water alone [14]. When the resistant starch type 4 was added to a dextrose beverage, the glycemic response was the same as the dextrose beverage alone. This demonstrates that the RS4 does not affect bioavailability of other carbohydrates, and the changes in post-prandial glycemic response are due to the nondigestible nature of the carbohydrate. The dietary fiber content is consistent when analyzed with both AOAC method 991.43 and AOAC method 2009.01, which indicates that the RS4 is heat-stable and resistant to prolong enzymatic digestion (unpublished data). We expect the RS4 content and dietary fiber content to be similar in the ingredient as well as the final food product (cookie).

Resistant starch type 4 may exert additional mechanisms to reduce post-prandial glycemic response, in addition to strictly replacing available carbohydrate. In a study where the treatments were matched for available carbohydrate, the RS4 treatment, phosphated distarch phosphate, resulted in significantly lower blood glucose $iAUC_{0\text{-}120min}$, peak blood glucose, blood insulin $iAUC_{0\text{-}120min}$ and peak insulin in healthy adults [10]. Additional research is needed to further define the mechanisms by which RS4 lowers post-prandial blood glucose response when treatments are matched for available carbohydrate.

The $iAUC_{0\text{-}120min}$ and $Cmax_{0\text{-}120min}$ for blood glucose were significantly lower after subjects consumed the fiber cookie compared to the control cookie, regardless of the sampling method. As noted by previous researchers, the absolute blood glucose values differ when measured intravenously or through capillary sampling [15]. When individual time points were compared, the capillary sampling method yielded significantly lower values after the fiber cookie was consumed at 45, 60, 90, and 120 min, whereas the intravenous sampling method yielded significantly different blood glucose values at 45 min, only. This can be attributed to the larger variability in blood glucose values when intravenous sampling was used. Previous researchers also noted this phenomenon [15]. Intravenous insulin $iAUC_{0\text{-}120min}$ and Cmax were lower after the subjects consumed the fiber cookie compared to the control cookie, which corresponds to the observed changes in blood glucose.

Resistant starch type 4, such as distarch phosphate, has functional properties that allow it to replace refined grain flour in product formulations. As a result, the available carbohydrates in a food can be reduced while maintaining the same sensory properties [2]. This provides the opportunity to formulate desirable foods with added health benefits such as improved post-prandial blood glucose management.

Reduced post-prandial glycemic response is a beneficial health effect for healthy individuals as well as individuals with compromised carbohydrate metabolism (e.g., pre-diabetes, Type 2 diabetes) The results from this study demonstrate how replacing refined flour with RS4 in a baked good (cookie) reduces post-prandial glucose and insulin response in healthy adults. Further research is warranted in individuals with compromised carbohydrate metabolism.

Acknowledgments: This study was funded by Ingredion Incorporated.

Author Contributions: J.P.Z. conceived and designed the experiments; M.L.S. and J.P.Z. wrote the paper.

References

1. Birt, D.F.; Boylston, T.; Hendrich, S.; Jane, J.L.; Hollis, J.; Li, L.; McClelland, J.; Moore, S.; Phillips, G.J.; Rowling, M.; et al. Resistant starch: Promise for improving human health. *Adv. Nutr.* **2013**, *4*, 587–601. [CrossRef] [PubMed]
2. Maningat, C.C.; Seib, P.A. Rs4-Type Resistant Starch: Chemistry, Functionality and Health Benefits. In *Resistant Starch: Sources, Applications and Health Benefits*; Shi, Y.C., Maningat, C.C., Eds.; John Wiley & Sons: Hoboken, NJ, USA, 2013; pp. 43–77.
3. Shen, D.; Bai, H.; Li, Z.; Yu, Y.; Zhang, H.; Chen, L. Positive effects of resistant starch supplementation on bowel function in healthy adults: A systematic review and meta-analysis of randomized controlled trials. *Int. J. Food Sci. Nutr.* **2017**, *68*, 149–157. [CrossRef] [PubMed]

4. Bindels, L.B.; Walter, J.; Ramer-Tait, A.E. Resistant starches for the management of metabolic diseases. *Curr. Opin. Clin. Nutr. Metab. Care* **2015**, *18*, 559–565. [CrossRef] [PubMed]
5. Heijnen, M.-L.A.; Beynen, A.C. Consumption of retrograded (rs3) but not uncooked (rs2) resistant starch shifts nitrogen excretion from urine to feces in cannulated piglets. *J. Nutr.* **1997**, *127*, 1828–1832. [PubMed]
6. Martínez, I.; Kim, J.H.; Duffy, P.R.; Schlegel, V.L.; Walter, J. Resistant starches types 2 and 4 have differential effects on the composition of the fecal microbiota in human subjects. *PLoS ONE* **2010**, *5*, e15046. [CrossRef] [PubMed]
7. IngredionIncorporated. Technical Specifications: Versafibe 1490 tm Resistant Starch. Available online: http://www.ingredion.us/content/dam/ingredion/technical-documents/na/VERSAFIBE%201490%20%20%2006400400%20%20%20Technical%20Specification.pdf (accessed on 15 December 2016).
8. Woo, K.S.; Seib, P.A. Cross-linked resistant starch: Preparation and properties. *Cereal Chem.* **2002**, *79*, 819–825. [CrossRef]
9. Sang, Y.J.; Seib, P.A.; Herrera, A.I.; Prakash, O.; Shi, Y.-C. Effects of alkaline treatment on the structure of phosphorylated wheat starch and its digestibility. *Food Chem.* **2010**, *118*, 323–327. [CrossRef]
10. Al-Tamimi, E.K.; Seib, P.A.; Snyder, B.S.; Haub, M.D. Consumption of cross-linked resistant starch (rs4(xl)) on glucose and insulin responses in humans. *J. Nutr. Metab.* **2010**. [CrossRef] [PubMed]
11. Haub, M.D.; Hubach, K.L.; Al-Tamimi, E.K.; Ornelas, S.; Seib, P.A. Different types of resistant starch elicit different glucose reponses in humans. *J. Nutr. Metab.* **2010**. [CrossRef] [PubMed]
12. Nichenametla, S.N.; Weidauer, L.A.; Wey, H.E.; Beare, T.M.; Specker, B.L.; Dey, M. Resistant starch type 4-enriched diet lowered blood cholesterols and improved body composition in a double blind controlled cross-over intervention. *Mol. Nutr. Food Res.* **2014**, *58*, 1365–1369. [CrossRef] [PubMed]
13. Upadhyaya, B.; McCormack, L.; Fardin-Kia, A.R.; Juenemann, R.; Nichenametla, S.; Clapper, J.; Specker, B.; Dey, M. Impact of dietary resistant starch type 4 on human gut microbiota and immunometabolic functions. *Sci. Rep.* **2016**, *6*, 28797. [CrossRef] [PubMed]
14. Haub, M.D.; Louk, J.A.; Lopez, T.C. Novel resistant potato starches on glycemia and satiety in humans. *J. Nutr. Metab.* **2012**, *2012*, 478043. [CrossRef] [PubMed]
15. Wolever, T.M.; Vorster, H.H.; Bjorck, I.; Brand-Miller, J.; Brighenti, F.; Mann, J.I.; Ramdath, D.D.; Granfeldt, Y.; Holt, S.; Perry, T.L.; et al. Determination of the glycaemic index of foods: Interlaboratory study. *Eur. J. Clin. Nutr.* **2003**, *57*, 475–482. [CrossRef] [PubMed]
16. Wolever, T.M. Effect of blood sampling schedule and method of calculating the area under the curve on validity and precision of glycaemic index values. *Br. J. Nutr.* **2004**, *91*, 295–301. [CrossRef] [PubMed]
17. Cnaan, A.; Laird, N.M.; Slasor, P. Using the general linear mixed model to analyse unbalanced repeated measures and longitudinal data. *Stat. Med.* **1997**, *16*, 2349–2380. [CrossRef]
18. Pinheiro, J.; Bates, D.; DebRoy, S.; Sarkar, D.; R Core Team. *Nlme: Linear and Nonlinear Mixed Effects Models*; R Foundation: Vienna, Austria, 2015.
19. Medicine, I.O. Dietary, Functional, and Total Fiber. In *Dietary Reference Intakes for Energy, Carbohydrate, Fiber, Fat, Fatty Acids, Cholesterol, Protein, and Amino Acids*; National Academies Press: Washington, DC, USA, 2005; pp. 339–421.
20. Janzen, J.G. Digestibility of starch and phosphate starches by pancreatin. *Starke* **1969**, *21*, 231–235. [CrossRef]

13

Effect of Fibre Supplementation on Body Weight and Composition, Frequency of Eating and Dietary Choice in Overweight Individuals

Vicky A. Solah [1,*], Deborah A. Kerr [1], Wendy J. Hunt [1], Stuart K. Johnson [1], Carol J. Boushey [2], Edward J. Delp [3], Xingqiong Meng [4], Roland J. Gahler [5], Anthony P. James [1,6], Aqif S. Mukhtar [1,7], Haelee K. Fenton [1] and Simon Wood [1,8,9]

1 School of Public Health, Faculty of Health Sciences, Curtin University, Perth WA 6845, Australia; d.kerr@curtin.edu.au (D.A.K.); w.hunt@curtin.edu.au (W.J.H.); s.johnson@curtin.edu.au (S.K.J.); T.P.James@curtin.edu.au (A.P.J.); Aqif.Mukhtar@curtin.edu.au (A.S.M.); h.fenton@curtin.edu.au (H.K.F.); simonwood@shaw.ca (S.W.)

2 Epidemiology Program, University of Hawaii Cancer Center, Honolulu, HI 96813, USA; cjboushey@cc.hawaii.edu

3 Video and Image Processing Laboratory, School of Electrical and Computer Engineering, Purdue University, West Lafayette, IN 47907, USA; ace@ecn.purdue.edu

4 Flinders Centre for Innovation in Cancer, School of Medicine, Flinders University, Adelaide 5001, Australia; rosie.meng@flinders.edu.au

5 Factors Group R & D, Burnaby, BC V3N4S9, Canada; rgahler@naturalfactors.com

6 Curtin Health Innovation Research Institute, Faculty of Health Sciences, Curtin University, Perth WA 6845, Australia

7 Centre for Population Health Research, Faculty of Health Sciences, Curtin University, Perth WA 6845, Australia

8 InovoBiologic Inc., Calgary, AB Y2N4Y7, Canada

9 Food, Nutrition and Health Program, University of British Columbia, Vancouver, BC V6T1Z4, Canada

* Correspondence: v.solah@curtin.edu.au;

Abstract: Fibre supplementation can potentially reduce energy intake and contribute to weight loss. The mechanism may be reduced frequency of eating, resulting in reduced food consumption. The objective of this research was to determine the effectiveness of fibre supplementation with PolyGlycopleX® (PGX®), on body weight and composition, frequency of eating and dietary intake in 118 overweight adults. In a three-arm, parallel, blind, randomised controlled trial participants were randomised to one of three groups; 4.5 g PGX as softgels (PGXS), 5 g PGX granules (PGXG) or 5 g rice flour (RF) control. Prior to supplementation and at 12 weeks, participants captured before and after images of all food and beverages consumed within 4 days using a mobile food record app (mFR). The mFR images were analysed for food group serving sizes and number of eating occasions. In the PGXG group, per-protocol analysis showed there was a significant reduction in waist circumference (2.5 cm; $p = 0.003$). Subgroup analysis showed that PGXG supplementation at the recommended dose resulted in a reduction in body weight (-1.4 ± 0.10 kg, $p < 0.01$), body mass index (BMI) reduction (-0.5 ± 0.10, $p < 0.01$), reduced number of eating occasions (-1.4 ± 1.2, $p < 0.01$) and a reduced intake of grain food (-1.52 ± 1.84 serves, $p = 0.019$). PGXG at the recommended dose resulted in a reduction in weight and BMI which was significantly greater than that for RF ($p = 0.001$). These results demonstrate the potential benefits of PGX fibre in controlling frequency of eating and in weight loss.

Keywords: fibre; weight; waist circumference; frequency; eating; PolyGlycopleX® (PGX)

1. Introduction

The burden of chronic disease in many countries is increasing concomitant with the percentage of the population with a high body mass index (BMI) [1]. Providing tools to improve the healthiness of the food environment and assisting people to make healthy food choices are important in the prevention of excessive weight gain [1].

Dietary pattern evidence has shown that higher dietary quality i.e. consumption of mainly whole grains, vegetables, fruit, nuts, legumes, seafood, plant protein and low-fat dairy leads to marked reductions in all-cause, cardiovascular disease and cancer mortality [2,3]. Similarly, a healthy dietary pattern which includes consumption of fruits, vegetables, grains, combined with a lower intake of sweets, red meat and processed meat, lowers the risk of developing colorectal cancer [4].

Evidence supports the role of dietary fibre in improving metabolic health. A higher intake of fibre is associated with increased satiety and reduced energy intake and therefore may be important in obesity management [5–11].

Total fibre is the sum of both dietary fibre (complete, intrinsic non-digestible plant carbohydrates, lignin) and functional fibres (non-digestible carbohydrates that have been isolated but still have beneficial physiological effects) [12]. What constitutes a 'beneficial physiological effect' and the level of evidence required for this to be substantiated remains unspecified [13]. Solubility or the ability of a fibre to dissolve in water will affect water holding capacity, viscosity and fermentability [11]. The properties of fibre that are associated with appetite, energy intake and body weight include solubility [11]. Solubility remains a common classification technique, although it has been suggested that fibres should be categorised according to functional properties such as viscosity and fermentability [14], since not all fibre is equal in delivering a beneficial physiological effect.

PolyGlycopleX (PGX) is a commercial functional fibre complex, manufactured by a proprietary process (EnviroSimplex®) from three dietary fibres: konjac glucomannan, sodium alginate, and xanthan gum [9]. PGX is a soluble viscous non-starch polysaccharide complex that has been identified as contributing to improved satiety, lipidaemia and glycaemia [8–10,15,16].

In the modern food environment both portion size and frequency of eating have increased in the population [17]. Mattes [17] has suggested that increased frequency of eating is a major factor in weight gain and is linked to the increased energy intake and rising BMI trends. In addition to frequency of eating, the types and amount of food and beverages consumed at an eating occasion may influence energy intake. Aljuraiban et al. [18] suggest that modifying eating behaviour through more frequent meals of low energy density and high nutrient quality may be an important approach to controlling obesity.

A challenge for understanding the contribution of dietary factors is our ability to measure diet. This is even more difficult in overweight and obese participants who are more prone to misreporting or underreporting their energy intake [19,20]. In addition, details such as time of eating is important in examining eating frequency and are difficult to accurately capture with paper-based methods. Advancement in technology has made available new image-based food recording systems such as those using a mobile food record app (mFR) [21–25]. Among the advantages of mFRs is the provision of real-time data capture which allows for the extraction of information from the images on the timing and location of the eating occasion, without relying on individuals to report these details [22,23]. Thus the mFR app allows for more accurate capture of time of eating while reducing the burden to the participant of reporting food consumption [23,24]. A unique aspect of this study was the use of the mFR to capture frequency of eating and dietary intake.

The objective of this research was to determine the effectiveness of diet supplementation with the viscous and gel-forming fibre, PolyGlycopleX (PGX), on body weight and composition and to determine if frequency of eating and diet can explain subsequent changes in 118 overweight adults.

2. Materials and Methods

2.1. Study Design

A three-arm, parallel, blind, randomised control trial was conducted to determine whether PGX supplementation would promote weight loss and reduce waist circumference and BMI, change dietary patterns and reduce the frequency of eating or number of eating occasions. Participants (118 in total) were divided between three groups, 4.5 g PGX as softgels (PGXS), 5 g PGX granules (PGXG) and 5 g rice flour (RF) control, (Figure 1) and were assessed at baseline and 12 weeks. This trial was registered with the Australian New Zealand Clinical Trials Registry (reference ACTRN12614000701628).

The food images sent via the mFR were stored by a participant identification number (ID) only. No personal information was stored with the images. The research was conducted in accordance with the principles proposed by the Australian Association for Research in Education (AARE), the Australian Vice-Chancellor's Committee (AVCC) and the National Health and Medical Research Council (NHMRC). The study was conducted in accordance with the Declaration of Helsinki and ethics approval was granted by the Human Research Ethics Committee, Curtin University (reference HR170/2014).

2.2. Study Participants

Participants, aged 25–70 years and with BMI 25–35 kg/m^2 were recruited through advertisements on Curtin University radio, as well as email communication systems. Individuals that expressed interest were screened for eligibility by completing a screening questionnaire. Participants were excluded if they were: (a) pregnant; (b) unable to complete the 12-week study; (c) undertaking extreme forms of exercise or dieting; (d) unable to attend the study centre; or (e) had an allergy to any food ingredient used in the study; (f) had previous or current renal, liver or respiratory failure; (g) had previous gastric or weight-loss surgery; (h) had any malabsorption conditions or (i) had current or recent dietary fibre supplementation. The participant flow diagram (Figure 1) lists the reasons for exclusion. Once assessed as eligible, further details of the study were provided and informed consent obtained.

2.3. Baseline Assessments

Participants who met the selection criteria had height, weight and waist circumference anthropometric measurements taken at baseline. A portable stadiometer was used to measure height; weight was measured using a pre-calibrated digital scale and waist was measured as described by Norton and Olds [26]. To electronically record food consumption, iPods with mFR application installed were given to the participants, who were asked to keep a 4-day mFR at baseline and during the twelfth week of the study.

Before beginning their baseline image-based 4-day food record, all participants received a 30-minute interactive training session by a single researcher who conducted individual or small group training sessions using PowerPoint slides on how to connect the iPod to the Wi-Fi and how to use the mFR app. Training sessions were held at Curtin University in a room with Wi-Fi access. The inclusion of a fiducial marker (a checkerboard pattern of known shape, size and colour) in all food record images gave a known reference of dimension and markings to assist with food identification and portion size estimation [25]. During training, participants were able to practice taking before and after images using food models. Collected food record images were automatically uploaded from the iPod touch, when in Wi-Fi range. The iPods were coded with the participant ID ensuring each image was tagged with the participant ID, date and time of eating occasion. Participant ID was used to identify the images on the server. The server was accessible by researchers only via password.

Prior to the commencement of supplementation and during the twelfth week of the study, participants took before and after images of all foods and drinks (excluding water) consumed over four consecutive days. Food consumption during the entire study was ad libitum.

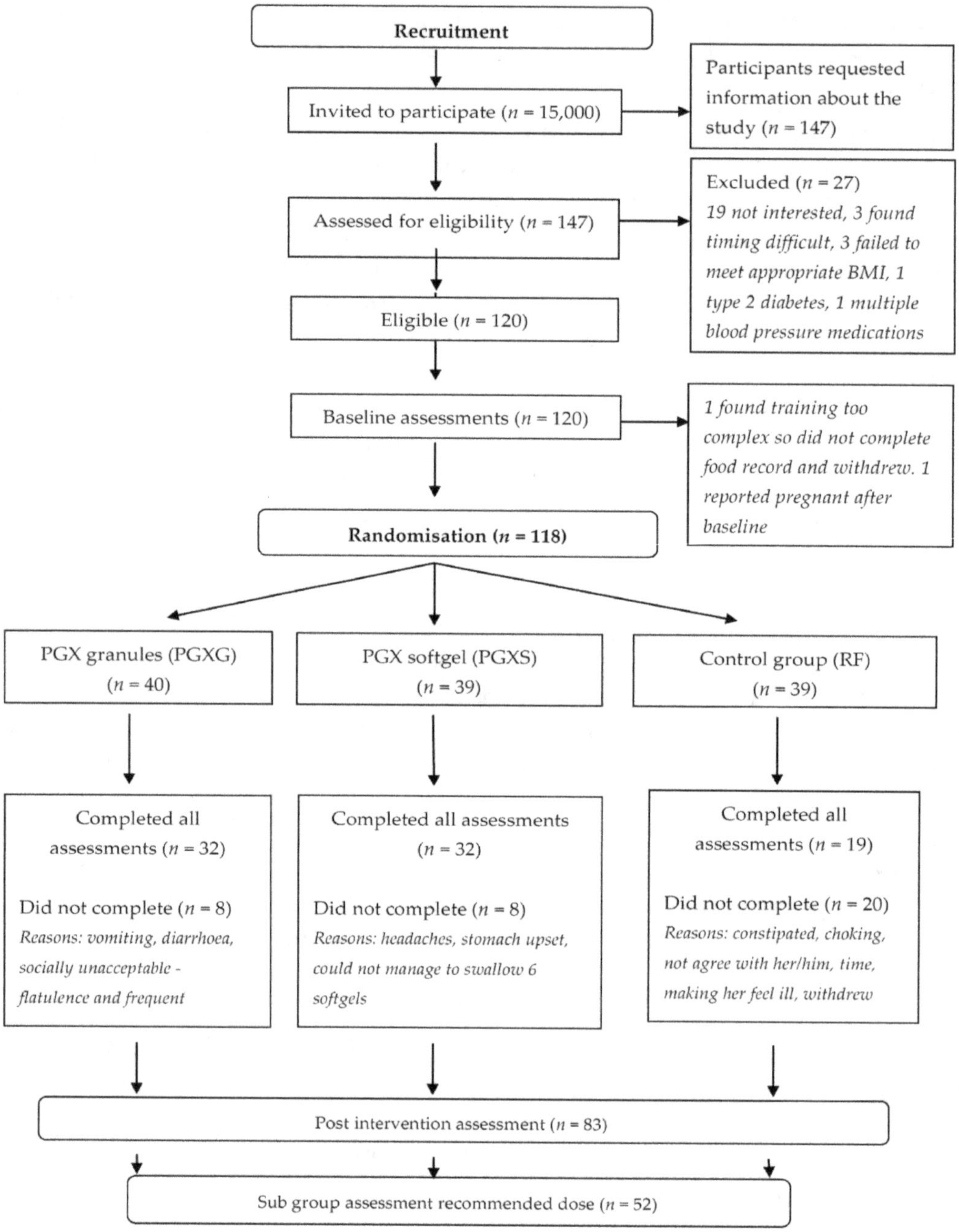

Figure 1. Participant flow diagram. RF: rice flour.

2.4. PGX Supplementation

The PGXS, PGXG and RF control supplements were provided to participants in a carry bag containing a 12-week supply labelled with a three-digit code. PGXG and the control were provided as 5 g individual doses in identical foil sachets and PGXS was provided in plain white jars each containing one month's supply. Research staff were blinded to the treatment allocation until all analyses were completed.

In Arm 1 (PGXS) instructions were provided in writing and verbally to the participants: "Take 1–2 softgels three times a day in week 1, 2–4 softgels three times a day in week 2 and 4–6 softgels, three times a day in week 3 to week 12". The recommended dose was four (4) to six (6) softgels containing 0.64 g fibre each, three times a day. This represented a supplement of dietary of between 7.6–11.4 g/day. Participants were also asked to consume 500 mL water with every softgel dose. Participants in Arm 2 were instructed to consume 5 g of PGXG containing 4.4 g fibre provided in a single dose foil sachet taken three times a day just before or with meals over the 12-week intervention period. This represented a supplement of dietary fibre of 12.2 g/day. Those in Arm 3 were provided with 5 g of RF containing 4 g fibre in the same dose format as the PGXG, representing 12 g fibre/day. RF was selected due to its neutral taste and hypoallergenicity, and it has a similar dietary fibre content, energy, colour and texture to PGX [7]. The recommended dose was 1 sachet, three times per day. Directions were "Stir 1 sachet into your meal or in a drink and consume immediately. You must consume 500mL of water each time you take a sachet." Participants were also advised that "If you have any discomfort, reduce the dose to 1 sachet a day for week 1, 2 sachets for week 2 and 3 sachets week 3 to week 12. Contact the researcher to discuss any issues." Participants were informed of the importance of consuming water with the supplement as well as the possible gastrointestinal effects of fibre such as diarrhoea, bloating and flatulence as described in research by Kacinik et al. [7]. All participants were instructed to record their daily sachet or softgel intake and report in person to the researcher at the end of week 12 of the intervention.

2.5. Post-Intervention Assessments

At the end of the 12-week intervention period, measurement of participants' height, weight and waist circumference were repeated, along with the 4-day mFR being repeated during week 12. At the end of the 12-week intervention, during the final meeting participants reported the number of doses to the interviewer and data were recorded in participant files.

2.6. Dietary Analysis

A researcher reviewed the 4-day food record images and as needed, confirmed the content of images with participants. Eating occasions were defined as all food and beverages (except water) and were taken from the image metadata and any additional notes supplied by the participant. Eating occasions were categorised as beverage only, food only, single item, food and beverage or fibre only. The images of fibre also allowed dose of fibre taken to be determined. Analysis was conducted to measure any change in eating occasions from baseline to study week 12.

Images were analysed and eating occasions, types of foods and serving sizes were entered into a database specifically designed to capture the number of eating occasions and food groups according to the Australian Guide to Healthy Eating food group serves (vegetables, fruit, grain (cereal) foods, mostly wholegrain and/or high cereal fibre varieties, lean meats and poultry, fish, eggs, tofu, nuts and seeds and legumes/beans, milk, yoghurt cheese and/or alternatives, mostly reduced fat) (NHMRC 2013) plus junk food (Table 1).

The primary outcome variables measured at baseline and at the end of the intervention were: changes in weight, waist circumference and BMI; eating occasions and foods consumed each day classified as serves of junk food (energy-dense nutrient poor), grain (cereal), meat, dairy, fruits and vegetables for the three intervention groups. Within each intervention group, participants were further categorised into fibre dose compliance level and number of eating occasions and the primary outcomes for this subgroup were also evaluated.

2.7. Statistical Analysis

Per-protocol analyses were performed and reported. The distribution of all outcome variables, weight, waist and BMI were checked by construction of histograms to check normality. A mixed effect model with clustering of participants' ID and robust variance-covariance estimation were used to assess outcome variables. For per-protocol analysis, only those who completed the study at week 12 were included and missing values were not imputed. Further analysis of subgroups by actual dose consumed was performed and reported. All tests were two tailed and a p value < 0.05 was regarded as statistically significant. All analyses were performed using Stata MP 14.1 (Stata Corp., College Station, TX, USA).

Table 1. Serve size in g or mL National Health and Medical Research Council (NHMRC), 2013 [27]. Fibre is 1 serve (g), with 2.5 serves daily minimum recommended dose.

Grains				Vegetable	Fruit	Meats			Dairy		Junk Food		Fibre *	
Bread	Porridge cooked	Muesli/Oats raw	Rice Pasta cooked			Beef Lamb Pork	Chicken	Fish	Milk	Cheese	Meat pie	Donut or Cake	PGXS	PGXG
40	120	30	75–120 (1/2 cup)	75	150	65	80	100	250 mL	40	60	40	3.8	4.4

* Dose determined by study. PGXS = PGX softgel, PGXG = PGX granules.

3. Results

3.1. Baseline Characteristics

3.1.1. Per-Protocol Analysis

Baseline measurements showing of all recruited participant characteristics according to treatment group are shown in Table 2. There were 92 females and 28 males, evenly distributed across the three treatment groups. In total 83 of the 118 participants (63% retention) completed the 12-week study. Greater attrition was observed in the first two weeks of the supplementation for participants who reported stomach upsets and diarrhoea after PGXG consumption (attrition = 6); who reported diarrhoea, headaches, difficulty swallowing recommended PGXS dose (attrition = 6) and during the first six weeks of supplementation in the RF group (attrition = 15) due to constipation and feeling ill.

Baseline data (Table 2) shows the characteristics of study participants randomised (n = 118) and shows that at baseline there were no significant differences ($p > 0.05$) in age, height, weight, waist circumference, BMI and food group servings across three groups. At baseline PGXS participants had similar baseline frequency of eating (number of eating occasions) to the PGXG and RF participants but those allocated to the PGXG intervention had a significantly greater number of eating occasions per day than those allocated to the RF intervention ($p = 0.04$) (Table 2).

Table 2. Characteristics of all recruited study participants randomised at baseline (n = 120) comparing groups.

All Participants	PGXS (n = 40)	PGXG (n = 40)	RF (n = 40)
Men	9	10	9
Women	31	30	31
Mean ± SD			
Age (years)	42.2 ± 16.0	46.5 ± 14.0	43.3 ± 16.8
Height (cm)	167.4 ± 9.1	167.3 ± 9.0	166.4 ± 7.9
Weight (kg)	82.7 ± 16.8	80.9 ± 16.6	81.3 ± 17.7
Waist (cm)	89.8 ± 12.8	90.7 ± 12.1	88.4 ± 14.3
Body Mass Index (BMI, kg/m^2)	29.4 ± 4.8	28.7 ± 4.4	29.2 ± 4.8
Eating occasions per day	5.4 ± 2.8	6.3 ± 2.0	4.8 ± 2.1
Food group servings (mean daily serves ± SD)			
Fruit (150 g)	0.8 ± 0.8	1.0 ± 1.0	1.1 ± 1.2
Vegetable (75 g)	2.4 ± 1.5	2.6 ± 1.4	2.5 ± 1.1
Grain (cereal) (40 g bread, 75–120 g cooked rice, pasta etc. or 500 kJ)	3.8 ± 1.8	4.3 ± 2.2	4 .0 ± 1.5
Dairy (250 mL milk, 40 g cheese or 500–600 kJ)	1.3 ± 0.9	1.6 ± 0.8	1.3 ± 0.8
Junk food (60 g meat pie or hot chips, 40 g donut or cake)	3.5 ± 1.9	3.1 ± 1.6	3.0 ± 1.7
Meat (65 g meat, 100 g fish or 500–699 kJ)	1.0 ± 0.7	1.6 ± 0.8	1.4 ± 0.7
Alcohol (150 mL)	0.5 ± 0.8	0.4 ± 0.5	0.1 ± 0.2

PGXS = PGX softgel, PGXG = PGX granules, RF = Rice Flour. SD = Standard Deviation.

3.1.2. Subgroup Analysis

Baseline measurements according to treatment group showing participant characteristics of all who consumed the recommended dose of fibre supplements are shown in Table 3. Baseline data (Table 3) shows the characteristics of study participants (n = 54) and shows that at baseline there were no significant differences ($p > 0.05$) in weight, waist circumference and BMI across three groups. PGXG and RF intervention sub-group numbers of eating occasions per day were not significantly different to each other or to the baseline group but the PGXS subgroup number of eating occasions was 7.4 times per day (Table 3).

Table 3. Characteristics of study participants randomised at baseline (n = 54) comparing subgroups who consumed the recommended dose of fibre supplements.

All Participants	PGXS (n = 17)	PGXG (n = 18)	RF (n = 17)	p Value
Body weight (kg)	76.5 ± 15.9	87.7 ± 20.2	78.3 ± 15.0	0.62
BMI (kg/m^2)	27.2 ± 4.5	28.7 ± 5.2	28.3 ± 5.2	0.64
Waist (cm)	84.8 ± 12.2	89.2 ± 20.4	87.1 ± 13.8	0.59
Eating occasions per day	7.4 ± 2.5	6.0 ± 2.0	5.5 ± 2.6	$p > 0.05$

PGXS = PGX softgel, PGXG = PGX granules, RF = Rice Flour.

3.2. *Effect of Intervention on Body Weight and Body Composition*

3.2.1. Per-Protocol Analysis

Per-protocol analysis revealed a significant reduction in waist circumference at week 12 of minus 2.5cm (Confidence Interval = −3.9, −0.8, p = 0.003) for those in the PGXG group (Table 4). No effect was seen on waist circumference for the PGXS and RF groups ($p > 0.05$). There was no effect of the PGXS or PGXG interventions on weight and BMI.

3.2.2. Subgroup Analysis

Analyses of the subgroup who consumed the recommended dose of fibre supplements showed a significant weight loss and reduction in BMI in the PGXG intervention compared to baseline (Table 5). However, the PGXS subgroup did not show a significant weight change during the intervention period. Compared to effect of the intervention on weight seen in the RF subgroup, that of the PGXG subgroup was significantly greater (p = 0.001).

Table 4. Change in participant characteristics from baseline to week 12 of the interventions of all participants who completed the interventions (per-protocol analysis).

All Participants	PGXS (n = 32)	PGXG (n = 32)	RF (n = 19)
Body weight (kg)	0.47 ± 1.85	−0.49 ± 0.34	−0.03 ± 0.58
BMI (kg/m^2)	0.15 ± 0.65	−0.17 ± 0.13	0.01 ± 0.20
Waist (cm)	−0.17 ± 2.92	**−2.50 ± 0.60 p = 0.03**	−1.3 ± 1.0
Eating occasions per day	−0.60 ± 1.5	**−0.82 ± 1.28 p = 0.01**	−0.22 ± 1.72
Food group servings (mean daily serves ± SD)			
Fruit (150 g) [1]	−0.2 ± 0.76	0.08 ± 0.7	−0.18 ± 0.75
Vegetable (75 g) [1]	−0.07 ± 1.11	−0.34 ± 1.22	−0.23 ± 0.64
Grain (cereal)	0.21 ± 1.73	−0.79 ± 1.66	−0.51 ± 1.23
Dairy	0.11 ± 0.63	−0.22 ± 0.64	0.07 ± 0.35
Junk food	−0.14 ± 2.00	−0.57 ± 1.29	0.28 ± 2.12
Meat	0.08 ± 0.59	0.01 ± 0.79	−0.09 ± 0.78
Alcohol	−0.22 ± 0.73	0.17 ± 0.99	−0.02 ± 0.26
Fibre (3.8–4.4 g) [1]	1.89 ± 0.91	2.17 ± 0.71	2.35 ± 0.58

Bold values denote significant within treatment effect. PGXS = PGX softgel, PGXG = PGX granules, RF = Rice Flour.
[1] 1 serve of fruit = 150 g, 1 serve vegetable = 75 g, 1 serve fibre = 3.8 to 4.4 g.

Table 5. Change in participant characteristics from baseline to week 12 of the PGXS, PGXG and RF interventions in the subgroup analysis of those who consumed the recommended dose of fibre supplements.

All Participants	PGXS ($n = 17$)	PGXG ($n = 18$)	RF ($n = 17$)
Body weight (kg)	0.22 ± 1.61	**−1.4 ± 0.10 $p < 0.01$**	−0.03 ± 0.58
BMI (kg/m^2)	0.07 ± 0.59	**−0.5 ± 0.10 $p < 0.01$**	0.01 ± 0.20
Waist (cm)	−1.04 ± 2.28	−1.2 ± 1.00	−1.3 ± 1.0
Eating occasions per day	−1.3 ± 1.9	**−1.4 ± 1.20 $p < 0.01$**	−0.22 ± 1.72
Food group servings (mean daily serves ± SD)			
Fruit (150 g)	−0.43 ± 0.59	**−0.63 ± 0.57 $p = 0.022$**	−0.18 ± 0.75
Vegetable (75 g)	−0.35 ± 0.96	−0.82 ± 1.31	−0.23 ± 0.64
Grain (cereal)	−0.93 ± 1.47	**−1.52 ± 1.84 $p = 0.019$**	−0.51 ± 1.23
Dairy	−0.05 ± 0.56	**−0.59 ± 0.50 $p = 0.012$**	0.07 ± 0.35
Junk food	−0.17 ± 1.48	−0.76 ± 0.85	0.28 ± 2.12
Meat	−0.06 ± 0.62	0.18 ± 0.90	−0.09 ± 0.78
Alcohol	−0.50 ± 0.98	0.11 ± 0.32	−0.02 ± 0.26
Fibre supplement serves (serving size 4.5–5 g)	2.6 ± 0.47	2.82 ± 0.24	2.35 ± 0.58

Bold values denote significant within treatment effect. PGXS = PGX softgel, PGXG= PGX granules, RF = Rice Flour. SD = standard deviation.

3.3. *Number of Eating Occasions and Food Group Servings*

Collection of mFR images required participants to use the iPod provided by the study to record images before and after each eating occasion during the 4-day food record (Figure 2).

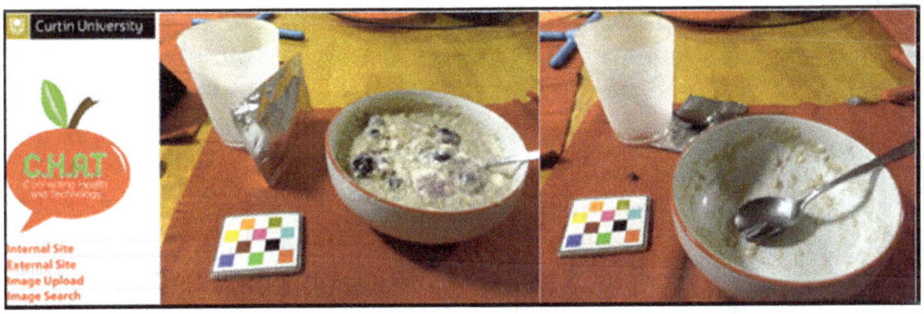

Figure 2. Before and after images of an eating occasion with foil sachet containing PGXG and fiducial marker captured with the mobile food record App on an iPod.

3.3.1. Per-Protocol Analysis

Analysis was conducted to measure change in number of eating occasions from baseline to week 12 of the interventions. The number of eating occasions was significantly reduced in the PGXG group ($p = 0.01$) during the intervention (Table 4). No significant differences in number of eating occasions between baseline and week 12 were observed in the groups PGXS and RF or in food group servings in any of the intervention groups (Table 4) in per-protocol analyses.

3.3.2. Subgroup Analysis

For the subgroup analysis, the participants who consumed PGXG at the recommended dose of 2.5 to 3 times per day, significantly reduced their eating occasions by 1.4 ± 1.2 (CI −2.1, −0.6, $p < 0.01$) during the intervention period (Table 5).

Likewise, the participants who consumed PGXG at the recommended dose significantly reduced their daily intake of fruit (−0.63 ± 0.57 serves, $p = 0.02$), dairy (−0.59 ± 0.50 serves, $p = 0.01$) and grain food (−1.52 ± 1.84 serves, $p = 0.02$) during the intervention (Table 5). Analysis of types of foods in the mFR showed that 1.6 to 2 serves of the grain food consumed at baseline were white bread for these participants. This consumption of white bread for the PGXG group also dropped significantly to 0.74 serves per day at 12 weeks of intervention.

3.4. Adverse Events

Adverse effects reported by the participants were mild and agreed with common reported reactions to increased fibre, for example those reported by Kacinik et al. (2011) [7] where for PGX supplementation, 30.9 % of participants reported diarrhoea, bloating and flatulence whereas for rice flour consumption 7.8% reported constipation.

4. Discussion

This 12 week randomised controlled study showed that when consumed at the recommended dose (subgroup), the PGXG intervention gave a reduction in BMI and body weight, the number of eating occasions per day and consumption of servings of grain food.

The weight loss and BMI reduction observed for the PGXG intervention is most likely a result of compliance to the recommended dose, resulting in 64% of participants who consumed PGXG at the recommended dose losing weight and reducing BMI. The average 1.4-kg weight loss found in our study of overweight adults for the PGX per-protocol intervention is in agreement with previous research by Lyon et al. [28] who found a weight loss in women of 1.6 kg with 12 weeks PGX supplementation. Pal et al. [29] reported obese adults on 12-week supplementation of both artificially sweetened and flavoured PGX and psyllium lost weight (1.6 kg and 1.1 kg respectively).

On an individual basis, the highest weight loss in the PGXS group (per-protocol) was 4.4 kg, with a waist circumference decrease of 5.5 cm. However, in this group a weight gain of 6.3 kg and waist circumference increase was 9.6 cm was also recorded in one participant. This high variance in change in weight and waist circumference resulted in a non-significant weight loss for this group. Data collected by personal communication at the 6-week visit showed five participants in the PGXS group reporting that they expected PGXS to be a "magic bullet" for weight loss, which was an unexpected issue that requires consideration in future research. Protocol in future research may involve education of participants on using PGX to control appetite.

The significant reduction in waist circumference observed in the present study for PGXG per-protocol group of 2.5 cm was similar in magnitude to that reported in a study by Reimer et al. [8] where PGX consumption over 14 weeks resulted in a significant reduction of 1.96 cm in waist circumference. The significant reduction in BMI of 0.5 observed in the present study for PGXG sub-group was in contrast to Reimer [8] who found no significant differences in BMI compared to baseline.

The findings from our study that PGXS and PGXG consumption (per-protocol groups) did not affect weight is similar to research on PGX consumption by Kacinik et al. [7] who reported no significant differences in weight loss between PGX and the placebo groups in a study involving a low-calorie diet of 1000 kcal/day for both treatments. There was also no weight loss recorded in a three-week study by Reimer et al. [30] where PGX was pre-mixed with breakfast cereal and consumed with yogurt. In our study participants were not on an energy restricted diet nor were the PGX and RF doses mixed with other products.

The use of the mFR allowed our research to determine level of compliance to the recommended dose of the PGXG subgroup by reviewing the images collected. The mFR image analysis of the foods eaten, serving sizes and number of eating occasions per day enabled important information about the dietary pattern of the overweight participants to be collected. The reduced number of eating occasions found with the PGXG subgroup, translated into reduced consumption of grain food of 1.52 serves ($p = 0.019$), mainly being a reduction in consumption of white bread.

Research by Kerr et al. [23] reported a reduction in consumption of energy-dense nutrient-poor (EDNP) foods as a result of tailored dietary feedback using the mFR. In the present study there was a non-significant reduction in junk food consumption of 0.57 in the PGXG per-protocol group and 0.76 serves in the PGXG subgroup. Pollard et al. [31] also found overweight people were more likely than those who were a healthy weight to decrease their intake grain food when trying to lose weight, supporting the reduced grain food trend found in this research. Small reductions in conscious or mindful energy intake can improve weight gain [32] and the choice to reduce grain food intake found in this research may have been the contributor to weight loss. Although we observed a reduction in daily intake of fruit and dairy, which is not desirable based on dietary guidelines [27], the magnitude of this change was minor.

Data from the mFR showed participants in all groups, other than the PGXG subgroup, appeared to make no changes to their eating pattern, as after 12 weeks of intervention, food group servings were not significantly different to baseline. This finding is supported by previous studies [32–34] where it was reported that humans tend to consume a consistent weight or volume of food from day to day. While participants reported feeling full in previous PGXS and PGXG research [9,10,35,36], most participants in this study did not appear to use appetite to change their eating patterns, except in the PGXG subgroup who consumed the recommended dose, most likely resulting reduced appetite and reduced food intake.

Dietary feedback using the mFR indicated a reduction of 1 serve white bread, each day, which may have been a contributor to the reduction of 40 g in weight daily in the PGXG per-protocol group [27]. In a previous study, a reduction of 31.5 g carbohydrate per day was recorded at 12 weeks after PGX supplementation using a 3-day food and drink diary [29]. The 3-day food and drink diary does not provided details on type carbohydrates foods, whereas the mFR reports provided detail of types of foods and serving sizes. Dietary intake records collected using the mFR can reduce the bias found in auto-assessment [24].

In the present study, PGXG was taken with 500 mL water immediately before or with a meal. The PGXG was mixed in the water, in juice or mixed into the meal. The mechanism for weight loss in the PGXG sub-group in the present study may have been as a result of reducing dietary energy density of the meals with which it was consumed by increasing the fibre and water content of meals while maintaining the volume of food eaten [37,38]. Decreasing dietary energy density has been shown to be useful in long-term weight loss [39].

The detailed dietary feedback from the mFR enabled this research to determine weight loss was possible when PGXG at the recommended dose was consumed and the reduction in the number of eating occasions may be part of the mechanism for this effect. Previous research indicates that a possible mechanism behind the appetite and body weight reduction effects of PGX may be related to circulating gut hormones [30]. Reimer et al. [30] reported increased peptide YY, which can slow gastric emptying and decreased ghrelin (an appetite stimulant) on consumption of PGX. More work is required to confirm the physiological mechanisms controlling these effects of PGX.

The detailed dietary feedback from the mFR enabled this research to more accurately determine food group changes after 12 weeks. The reason the PGXS, and PGXG per-protocol groups did not reduce their weight may be because they did not reduce the number of eating occasions or change their daily intake of the foods and continued to consume the amount and type of food usually eaten. In addition, research by Polidori et al. [40] reports that weight loss leads to increased appetite, and appetite increases by approximately 100 kcal/day per kg of lost weight. The reason fibre such as PGXG helps some individuals in the control of appetite and not others requires more research.

Limitation

Meals and consumption of test products were self-administered; the possibility of non-compliance could not be avoided. In the current study misreporting of intake may have occurred due to participants not taking images of all food and beverages consumed. In addition, the assessment of food group serves by a trained analyst may not be sensitive enough to detect changes in dietary intake.

5. Conclusions

Supplementation with PGX at the recommended dose resulted in a reduction in body weight (kg), BMI (kg/m^2), reduced frequency of eating and reduced intake of white bread. The weight loss and BMI reduction from baseline to 12 weeks was significantly greater for PGXG at the recommended dose than for the RF treatment. Dietary assessment using the mFR provided detailed information enabling accurate analysis of the number of eating occasions and changes to food group servings per day. Further research on reducing the frequency eating of specific foods, such as junk food is warranted. These results demonstrate the potential benefits of PGX fibre in controlling frequency of eating and in weight loss.

Acknowledgments: PGX® and PolyGlycopleX® are registered trademarks of InovoBiologic Inc., Calgary, AB, Canada. Financial support for the submitted work was provided by Factors Group, Australia Pty Ltd. RJG owns the Factors Group of Companies, which retains an interest in PGX. SW receives consulting fees from InovoBiologic Inc.

Author Contributions: V.A.S., D.A.K., W.J.H., X.M., S.K.J. and S.W. designed and conducted the research; C.J.B., D.A.K. and E.J.D. developed the mFR part of this research; R.J.G. critically reviewed the study design; X.M., V.A.S., A.S.M. and D.A.K. analysed the data; V.A.S., D.A.K., W.J.K., S.K.J., C.J.B., E.J.D., X.M., A.P.J., A.S.M., H.K.F. and S.W. wrote the paper; all authors read and approved the final manuscript.

References

1. Swinburn, B.; Kraak, V.; Rutter, H.; Vandevijvere, S.; Lobstein, T.; Sacks, G.; Gomes, F.; Marsh, T.; Magnusson, R. Strengthening of accountability systems to create healthy food environments and reduce global obesity. *Lancet* **2015**, *385*, 2534–2545. [CrossRef]
2. Liese, A.D.; Krebs-Smith, S.M.; Subar, A.F.; George, S.M.; Harmon, B.E.; Neuhouser, M.L.; Boushey, C.J.; Schap, T.E.; Reedy, J. The Dietary Patterns Methods Project: Synthesis of findings across cohorts and relevance to dietary guidance. *J. Nutr.* **2015**, *145*, 393–402. [CrossRef] [PubMed]
3. Reedy, J.; Krebs-Smith, S.M.; Miller, P.E.; Liese, A.D.; Kahle, L.L.; Park, Y.; Subar, A.F. Higher diet quality is associated with decreased risk of all-cause, cardiovascular disease, and cancer mortality among older adults. *J. Nutr.* **2014**, *144*, 881–889. [CrossRef] [PubMed]
4. Tayyem, R.F.; Bawadi, H.A.; Shehadah, I.; Agraib, L.M.; AbuMweis, S.S.; Al-Jaberi, T.; Al-Nusairr, M.; Bani-Hani, K.E.; Heath, D.D. Dietary patterns and colorectal cancer. *Clin. Nutr.* **2016**, in press. [CrossRef] [PubMed]
5. Delzenne, N.M.; Cani, P.D. A place for dietary fiber in the management of the metabolic syndrome. *Curr. Opin. Clin. Nutr. Metab. Care* **2005**, *8*, 636–640. [CrossRef] [PubMed]
6. Kristensen, M.; Jensen, M.G. Dietary fibres in the regulation of appetite and food intake. Importance of viscosity. *Appetite* **2011**, *56*, 65–70. [CrossRef] [PubMed]
7. Kacinik, V.; Lyon, M.; Purnama, M.; Reimer, R.A.; Gahler, R.; Green, T.J.; Wood, S. Effect of PGX, a novel functional fibre supplement, on subjective ratings of appetite in overweight and obese women consuming a 3-day structured, low-calorie diet. *Nutr. Diabetes* **2011**, *1*, 1–8. [CrossRef] [PubMed]
8. Reimer, R.A.; Yamaguchi, H.; Eller, L.K.; Lyon, M.R.; Gahler, R.J.; Kacinik, V.; Juneja, P.; Wood, S. Changes in visceral adiposity and serum cholesterol with a novel viscous polysaccharide in Japanese adults with abdominal obesity. *Obesity* **2013**, *21*, E379–E387. [PubMed]
9. Solah, V.; Brand-Miller, J.; Atkinson, F.; Gahler, R.; Kacinik, V.; Lyon, M.; Wood, S. Dose-response effect of a novel functional fibre, PolyGlycopleX, PGX, on satiety. *Appetite* **2014**, *77*, 72–76. [CrossRef] [PubMed]
10. Solah, V.A.; O'Mara-Wallace, B.; Meng, X.; Gahler, R.J.; Kerr, D.A.; James, A.P.; Fenton, H.K.; Johnson, S.K.; Wood, S. Consumption of the Soluble Dietary Fibre Complex PolyGlycopleX® Reduces Glycaemia and Increases Satiety of a Standard Meal Postprandially. *Nutrients* **2016**, *8*, 268. [CrossRef] [PubMed]
11. Wanders, A.J.; Van Den Borne, J.J.G.C.; De Graaf, C.; Hulshof, T.; Jonathan, M.C.; Kristensen, M.; Mars, M.; Schols, H.A.; Feskens, E.J.M. Effects of dietary fibre on subjective appetite, energy intake and body weight: A systematic review of randomized controlled trials. *Obes. Rev.* **2011**, *12*, 724–739. [CrossRef] [PubMed]
12. Slavin, J.; Green, H. Dietary fibre and satiety. *Nutr. Bull.* **2007**, *32*, 32–42. [CrossRef]

13. Mann, J.I.; Cummings, J.H. Possible implications for health of the different definitions of dietary fibre. *Nutr. Metab. Cardiovasc. Dis.* **2009**, *19*, 226–229. [CrossRef] [PubMed]
14. Slavin, J.L. Dietary fibre and body weight. *Nutrition* **2005**, *21*, 411–418. [CrossRef] [PubMed]
15. Brand-Miller, J.C.; Atkinson, F.S.; Gahler, R.J.; Kacinik, V.; Lyon, M.R; Wood, S. Effects of PGX, a novel functional fibre, on acute and delayed postprandial glycaemia. *Eur. J. Clin. Nutr.* **2010**, *64*, 1488–1493. [CrossRef] [PubMed]
16. Brand-Miller, J.C.; Atkinson, F.S.; Gahler, R.J.; Kacinik, V.; Lyon, M.R.; Wood, S. Effects of added PGX®, a novel functional fibre, on the glycaemic index of starchy foods. *Br. J. Nutr.* **2012**, *108*, 245–248. [CrossRef] [PubMed]
17. Mattes, R. Energy intake and obesity: Ingestive frequency outweighs portion size. *Physiol. Behav.* **2015**, *134*, 110–118. [CrossRef] [PubMed]
18. Aljuraiban, G.S.; Chan, Q.; Griep, L.M.O.; Brown, I.J.; Daviglus, M.L.; Stamler, J.; Van Horn, L.; Elliott, P.; Frost, G.S.; INTERMAP Research Group. The impact of eating frequency and time of intake on nutrient quality and Body Mass Index: The INTERMAP Study, a Population-Based Study. *J. Acad. Nutr. Diet.* **2015**, *115*, 528–536. [CrossRef] [PubMed]
19. Thompson, F.E.; Subar, A.F. Dietary Assessment Methodology. In *Nutrition in the Prevention and Treatment of Disease*, 3rd ed.; Coulston, A.M., Boushey, C.J., Ferruzzi, M.G., Eds.; Elsevier Academic Press: San Diego, CA, USA, 2013.
20. Meng, X.; Kerr, D.A.; Zhu, K.; Devine, A.; Solah, V.A.; Wright, J.; Binns, C.W.; Prince, R.L. Under-reporting of energy intake in elderly Australian women is associated with a higher body mass index. *J. Nutr. Health Aging* **2013**, *17*, 112–118. [CrossRef] [PubMed]
21. Bosch, M.; Zhu, F.; Khanna, N.; Boushey, C.J.; Delp, E.J. Combining global and local features for food identification in dietary assessment. *IEEE Trans. Image Process.* **2011**, *2011*, 1789–1792. [PubMed]
22. Harray, A.J.; Boushey, C.J.; Pollard, C.M.; Delp, E.J.; Ahmad, Z.; Dhaliwal, S.S.; Mukhtar, S.A.; Kerr, D.A. A novel dietary assessment method to measure a healthy and sustainable diet using the Mobile Food Record: Protocol and methodology. *Nutrients* **2015**, *7*, 5375–5395. [CrossRef] [PubMed]
23. Kerr, D.A.; Pollard, C.M.; Howat, P.; Delp, E.J.; Pickering, M.; Kerr, K.R.; Dhaliwal, S.S.; Pratt, I.S.; Wright, J.; Boushey, C.J. Connecting Health and Technology (CHAT): Protocol of a randomized controlled trial to improve nutrition behaviours using mobile devices and tailored text messaging in young adults. *BMC Public Health* **2012**, *12*, 477. [CrossRef] [PubMed]
24. Kerr, D.A.; Harray, A.J.; Pollard, C.M.; Dhaliwal, S.S.; Delp, E.J.; Howat, P.A.; Pickering, M.R.; Ahmad, Z.; Meng, X.; Pratt, I.S.; et al. The connecting health and technology study: A 6-month randomized controlled trial to improve nutrition behaviours using a mobile food record and text messaging support in young adults. *Int. J. Behav. Nutr. Phys. Act.* **2016**, *13*, 52. [CrossRef] [PubMed]
25. Zhu, F.; Bosch, M.; Khanna, N.; Boushey, C.J.; Delp, E.J. Multiple hypotheses image segmentation and classification with application to dietary assessment. *IEEE J. Biomed. Health Inform.* **2015**, *19*, 377–388. [CrossRef] [PubMed]
26. Norton, K.; Olds, T. *Anthropometrica*; University of New South Wales Press: Sydney, Australia, 2000.
27. National Health and Medical Research Council. Eat for Health. Australian Dietary Guidelines Summary. Canberra: Australian Government, Department of Health and Ageing. 2013. Available online: http://www.nhmrc.gov.au/_files_nhmrc/publications/attachments/n55a_australian_dietary_guidelines_susumma_131014.pdf (accessed on 2 February 2015).
28. Lyon, M.; Wood, S.; Pelletier, X.; Donazzolo, Y.; Gahler, R.; Bellisle, F. Effects of a 3-month supplementation with a novel soluble highly viscous polysaccharide on anthropometry and blood lipids in nondieting overweight or obese adults. *J. Hum. Nutr. Diet.* **2011**, *24*, 351–359. [CrossRef] [PubMed]
29. Pal, S.; Ho, S.; Gahler, R.J.; Wood, S. Effect on body weight and composition in overweight/obese Australian adults over 12 months consumption of two different types of fibre supplementation in a randomized trial. *Nutr. Metab.* **2016**, *13*, 82. [CrossRef] [PubMed]
30. Reimer, R.A.; Pelletier, X.; Carabin, I.G.; Lyon, M.; Gahler, R.; Parnell, J.A.; Woods, S. Increased plasma PYY levels following supplementation with functional fiber PolyGlycopleX in healthy adults. *Eur. J. Clin. Nutr.* **2010**, *64*, 1186–1191. [CrossRef] [PubMed]

31. Pollard, C.M.; Pulker, C.; Meng, X.; Denham, F.; Solah, V.; Scott, J.A.; Kerr, D.A. Cereal foods consumption trends and factors associated with changing intake, among Western Australian adults, 1995 to 2012. *FASEB J.* **2016**, *30*, 409.
32. Hill, J.O. Can a small-changes approach help address the obesity epidemic? A report of the Joint Task Force of the American Society for Nutrition, Institute of Food Technologists, and International Food Information Council. *Am. J. Clin. Nutr.* **2009**, *89*, 477–484. [CrossRef] [PubMed]
33. Bell, E.A.; Castellanos, V.H.; Pelkman, C.L.; Thorwart, M.L.; Rolls, B.J. Energy density of foods affects energy intake in normal-weight women. *Am. J. Clin. Nutr.* **1998**, *67*, 412–420.
34. Bell, E.A.; Rolls, B.J. Energy density of foods affects energy intake across multiple levels of fat content in lean and obese women. *Am. J. Clin. Nutr.* **2001**, *73*, 1010–1018. [PubMed]
35. Solah, V.A.; Meng, X.; Wood, S.; Gahler, R.J.; Kerr, D.A.; James, A.P.; Pal, S.; Fenton, H.K.; Johnson, S.K. Effect of training on the reliability of satiety evaluation and use of trained panellists to determine the satiety effect of dietary fibre: A randomised controlled trial. *PLoS ONE* **2015**, *10*, e012. [CrossRef] [PubMed]
36. Yong, M.K.; Solah, V.A.; Johnson, S.K.; Meng, X.; Kerr, D.A.; James, A.P.; Fenton, H.K.; Gahler, R.J.; Wood, S. Effects of a viscous-fibre supplemented evening meal and the following un-supplemented breakfast on post-prandial satiety responses in healthy women. *Physiol. Behav.* **2016**, *154*, 34–39. [CrossRef] [PubMed]
37. Rolls, B.J.; Castellanos, V.H.; Halford, J.C.; Kilara, A.; Panyam, D.; Pelkman, C.L.; Smith, G.P.; Thorwart, M.L. Volume of food consumed affects satiety in men. *Am. J. Clin. Nutr.* **1998**, *67*, 1170–1177. [PubMed]
38. Rolls, B.J. The relationship between dietary energy density and energy intake. *Physiol. Behav.* **2009**, *97*, 609–615. [CrossRef] [PubMed]
39. Ello-Martin, J.A.; Roe, L.S.; Ledikwe, J.H.; Beach, A.M.; Rolls, B.J. Dietary energy density in the treatment of obesity: A year-long trial comparing 2 weight-loss diets. *Am. J. Clin. Nutr.* **2007**, *85*, 1465–1477. [PubMed]
40. Polidori, D.; Sanghvi, A.; Seeley, R.J.; Hall, K.D. How strongly does appetite counter weight loss? Quantification of the feedback control of human energy intake. *Obesity* **2016**, *24*, 2289–2295. [CrossRef] [PubMed]

14

Effects of Commercial Apple Varieties on Human Gut Microbiota Composition and Metabolic Output Using an In Vitro Colonic Model

Athanasios Koutsos [1,2,*], Maria Lima [2], Lorenza Conterno [2], Mattia Gasperotti [3], Martina Bianchi [2], Francesca Fava [2], Urska Vrhovsek [3], Julie A. Lovegrove [1] and Kieran M. Tuohy [2]

1 Hugh Sinclair Unit of Human Nutrition and the Institute for Cardiovascular and Metabolic Research (ICMR), Department of Food and Nutritional Sciences, University of Reading, Whiteknights, P.O. Box 226, Reading RG6 6AP, UK; j.a.lovegrove@reading.ac.uk

2 Nutrition & Nutrigenomics Unit, Department of Food Quality and Nutrition, Research and Innovation Centre, Fondazione Edmund Mach (FEM), Via Mach 1, 38010 San Michele all'Adige, TN, Italy; Lima80in@yahoo.co.in (M.L.); lorenza.conterno@oliocru.it (L.C.); martina.bianchi.1@gmail.com (M.B.); francesca.fava@fmach.it (F.F.); kieran.tuohy@fmach.it (K.M.T.)

3 Metabolomics Unit, Department of Food Quality and Nutrition, Research and Innovation Centre, Fondazione Edmund Mach (FEM), Via Mach 1, 38010 San Michele all'Adige, TN, Italy; mattiagasperotti84@gmail.com (M.G.); urska.vrhovsek@fmach.it (U.V.)

* Correspondence: athanasios.koutsos@reading.ac.uk;

Abstract: Apples are a rich source of polyphenols and fiber. A major proportion of apple polyphenols escape absorption in the small intestine and together with non-digestible polysaccharides reach the colon, where they can serve as substrates for bacterial fermentation. Animal studies suggest a synergistic interaction between apple polyphenols and the soluble fiber pectin; however, the effects of whole apples on human gut microbiota are less extensively studied. Three commercial apple varieties—Renetta Canada, Golden Delicious and Pink Lady—were digested and fermented in vitro using a batch culture colonic model (pH 5.5–6.0, 37 °C) inoculated with feces from three healthy donors. Inulin and cellulose were used as a readily and a poorly fermentable plant fiber, respectively. Fecal microbiota composition was measured by 16S rRNA gene Illumina MiSeq sequencing (V3-V4 region) and Fluorescence in Situ Hybridization. Short chain fatty acids (SCFAs) and polyphenol microbial metabolites were determined. The three apple varieties significantly changed bacterial diversity, increased Actinobacteria relative abundance, acetate, propionate and total SCFAs ($p < 0.05$). Renetta Canada and Golden Delicious significantly decreased Bacteroidetes abundance and increased Proteobacteria proportion and bifidobacteria population ($p < 0.05$). Renetta Canada also increased *Faecalibacterium prausnitzii*, butyrate levels and polyphenol microbial metabolites ($p < 0.05$). Together, these data suggest that apples, particularly Renetta Canada, can induce substantial changes in microbiota composition and metabolic activity in vitro, which could be associated with potential benefits to human health. Human intervention studies are necessary to confirm these data and potential beneficial effects.

Keywords: apples; polyphenols; proanthocyanidins; fiber; pectin; gut microbiota; in vitro batch culture fermentation; microbial metabolites; Illumina 16S rRNA gene sequencing; Fluorescence in situ hybridization (FISH)

---

1. Introduction

Evidence suggests that plant-derived dietary polyphenols and fiber possess health-promoting properties [1]. Apples are among the most popular and frequently consumed fruits in the world and a rich source of both polyphenols and fiber [2]. Epidemiological and dietary intervention studies suggest that frequent apple consumption is associated with a reduced risk of chronic pathologies such as cardiovascular disease, obesity and cancer [2,3]. However, up to 90–95% of dietary polyphenols are not absorbed in the small intestine [4] and together with non-digestible polysaccharides from apples reach the colon almost intact, where they can interact with the gut microbiota [2]. This interaction is reciprocal. Firstly, polyphenols and fiber undergo an extensive microbial bioconversion producing phenolic acids and short chain fatty acids (SCFAs), respectively, well-known to have positive health effects [5]. Secondly, polyphenols, fiber and/or their metabolic products modulate the gut microbiota composition by inhibiting pathogenic bacteria and stimulating beneficial bacteria, therefore acting as potential prebiotics [5].

Dietary fiber constituents in apples include insoluble fiber, mainly cellulose and hemicellulose and soluble fiber, mainly pectin. In vitro studies, using human fecal inoculum, have shown that pectin is fermented to SCFAs (acetate, propionate and butyrate) by several intestinal bacteria genera including *Bacteroides*, eubacteria, clostridia and bifidobacteria [6,7]. However, a recent study suggested a high selectivity at the species level [8]. Apples also contain a variety of polyphenols including dihydrochalcones, flavonols, hydroxycinnamates and flavanols (catechin and proanthocyanidins (PAs)) [9]. PAs, the major polyphenolic class in apples, also known as condensed tannins, are oligomers and polymers of flavanols and the most likely to reach the colon [2]. In an in vitro study, apple PAs have been shown to be converted to polyphenol microbial metabolites, mainly phenylpropionic, phenylacetic and benzoic acid derivatives. [10]. The study also reported reduced saccharolytic fermentation, suggesting potential antimicrobial properties of PAs. However, the specific bacteria composition was not explored [10].

In vivo, extraction juices from apple pomace, rich in polyphenols and fiber, have been shown to increase *Lactobacillus*, *Bifidobacterium*, *Bacteroidaceae* species, *Eubacterium rectale* cluster as well as SCFAs in rats [11,12]. Licht et al. (2010) [13] considered pectin, among apple components, responsible for a decrease in *Bacteroides* spp. and an increase in *Clostridium coccoides* and butyrate in rats [13]. Likewise, apple pectin restored the Firmicutes/Bacteroidetes ratio to normal in obesity-induced rats [14]. Decreased Firmicutes/Bacteroidetes ratio was similarly seen in mice with the administration of apple PAs, which also increased the proportion of *Akkermansia* [15]. However, a rat cecum fermentation showed that apple polyphenols and pectin are more effective in combination implying a synergistic effect [16]. Data available from human studies are still limited [2]. In a small scale trial of eight people, two apples per day for two weeks significantly increased bifidobacteria while reducing *Enterobacteriaceae* and lecithinace-positive clostridia, including *C. perfringens* [17]. In a more recent four-week study of 23 healthy subjects, whole apple and pomace intake lowered fecal pH but there were no changes in gut microbiota composition [18].

Thus, to date, the effects of apple components on gut microbiota have been explored mainly in animals and using extracted juices [11,12], PAs [15] or pectin [14] alone. There are no in vitro studies investigating the effects of whole apples using human fecal inoculum and only recently studies with apple components have focused on the entire gut community instead of targeted taxa [13,15]. The aim of the current work was to assess the effect of three commercial apple varieties—Renetta Canada, Golden Delicious and Pink Lady—on human gut microbiota composition and metabolic activity in vitro, compared to inulin (a prebiotic) and cellulose (poorly fermented). Illumina 16S rRNA sequencing was used to provide a broad picture of the microbial community architecture. Bacteria of specific interest (i.e., bifidobacteria and *Faecalibacterium prausnitzii*) were enumerated using the quantitative 16S rRNA probe based method, FISH. The production of SCFAs (acetate, propionate and butyrate) was also measured. Finally, disappearance of apple polyphenols and formation of microbial-derived metabolites were monitored throughout the fermentation using a targeted LC-MS based metabolomics approach.

2. Materials and Methods

2.1. Fecal Donors

Fecal donors, two males and one female, were in good health and aged between 30 and 50. They had not received antibiotic treatment for at least 3 months prior to stool collection, had not knowingly consumed pre- or probiotic supplements prior to experiment, and had no history of bowel disorders. The three healthy donors were informed of the study aims and procedures and provided their verbal consent for their fecal matter to be used for the experiments, in compliance with the ethics procedures required at the University of Reading and Fondazione Edmund Mach.

2.2. Materials

Enzymes for the apples digestion and chemicals for the batch culture basal nutrient medium were purchased from Sigma-Aldrich (St. Louis, MO, USA) and Applichem (Darmstadt, Germany), unless otherwise stated. For the chemical standards of polyphenols and microbial metabolites as well as the LC-MS reagents more information can be found in Vrhovsek et al. (2012) [19] and Gasperotti et al. (2014) [20].

2.3. Apples and Controls

The three commercial apple varieties, Renetta Canada, Golden Delicious and Pink Lady were purchased from a local shop in the Trentino region in north Italy. The apples' macronutrient composition was analyzed by Campden BRI laboratories, UK, whereas the detailed polyphenol content was measured in our laboratory in Fondazione Edmund Mach based on Vrhovsek et al. (2012) [19]. Inulin (from dahlia tubers) and cellulose were used as a readily and a poorly fermentable plant fiber, respectively.

2.4. Preparation of Phospholipid Vesicles

A protocol was followed according to Mandalari et al. (2008) [21], with some modifications, for the preparation of the phospholipid vesicles and the simulation of the in vitro gastric and duodenal digestion as described below. Egg L-α-phosphatidylcholine (PC, lecithin grade 1, 99% purity, Lipid Products, Surrey, UK), 6.5 mL of a stock solution (127 mmol/L in chloroform/methanol), was placed into a round-bottom flask, and dried under rotary evaporation to make a thin phospholipid film. The lipid film was further dried overnight under vacuum to remove any remaining solvent. Then, it was hydrated with the addition of 170 mL of warm saline (150 mmol/L NaCl, pH 2.5, at 37 °C). The flask was flushed with argon to prevent oxidation and was placed in an orbital shaker (170 rpm, 37 °C) for 30 min together with five 2 mm diameter glass beads. A PC nanoemulsion was then produced using a Branson Ultrasonics sonifier S-450 (Branson Ultrasonics, Danbury, CT, USA) equipped with a 13 mm titanium horn (30% of amplitude). The temperature of the liquid kept below 60 °C with ice.

2.5. In Vitro Gastric and Duodenal Digestion

A ratio of 4 g of apples for 12.4 mL gastric phase volume (acidic saline) considered appropriate after preliminary experiments and according to Mandalari et al. (2008) [21]. Initially, 96 g of each apple variety were grated with their skin and added to 146 mL of the sonicated and filtrated PC vesicle suspension. The pH was adjusted to 2.5 using HCl and acidic saline (150 mmol/L NaCl, pH 2.5) was added to a total volume of 298 mL. Then, the PC vesicle suspension together with gastric pepsin and lipase were added so that the final concentrations were 2.4 mmol/L, 146 units/mL and 60 units/mL, respectively. The digestion was performed in an orbital shaker (170 rpm, 37 °C) for 2 h. The in vitro gastric digestion was followed by duodenal digestion. The pH was raised to 6.5 using NaOH and the following were added: 4 mmol/L sodium taurocholate, 4 mmol/L sodium glycodeoxycholate,

11.7 mmol/L $CaCl_2$, 0.73 mmol/L Bis-Tris buffer (pH 6.5), 5.9 units/mL α-chymotrypsin, 104 units/mL trypsin, 3.2 μg/mL colipase, 54 units/mL pancreatic lipase and 25 units/mL alpha-amylase. The total volume of 340 mL was reached by the addition of saline (150 mmol/L NaCl, pH 6.5) and the final PC concentration was 2.1 mmol/L. The duodenal digestion was performed for 1 h in the shaking incubator (170 rpm, 37 °C). Then, samples were transferred to 1 kDa MWCO (molecular weight cut off) cellulose dialysis tubing (Spectra/Por® 6, Spectrum Europe, Breda, Netherlands) and dialyzed overnight against NaCl (10 mmol/L) at 4 °C to remove low molecular mass digestion products. The dialysis fluid was changed and dialysis continued for an additional 2 h. Finally, apples were frozen at −20 °C and then freeze-dried until use. Inulin and cellulose (19.2 g each, equivalent with the dry content of 96 g of apples) were also digested and dialyzed using the same protocol.

2.6. Fecal Batch-Culture Fermentation and Samples Collection

The fermentation profile of the three commercial apples, the prebiotic inulin and the poorly fermented cellulose was determined using anaerobic, stirred, pH and temperature controlled fecal batch cultures. Glass water-jacketed vessels (300 mL) were sterilized and filled aseptically with 180 mL of pre-sterilized basal nutrient medium according to Sanchez-Patan et al. 2012 [22]. The pH was adjusted to 5.5–6.0 and kept between this range throughout the experiment with the automatic addition of NaOH or HCI (0.5 M), to mimic the conditions located in the proximal region of the human large intestine. The medium was then gassed overnight with oxygen free nitrogen to maintain anaerobic conditions. The following day and before the inoculation, each of the 5 vessels was dosed with 2 g of the appropriate substrate/treatment (inulin, cellulose, Renetta Canada, Golden Delicious or Pink Lady) for a final concentration of 1% (*w*/*v*). Fresh human fecal samples were collected in an anaerobic jar and were processed within 1 h. Fecal slurry was prepared by homogenizing the feces in pre-reduced phosphate buffered saline (PBS). The temperature was set to 37 °C using a circulating water-bath and the vessels were inoculated with 20 mL fecal slurry (10% *w*/*v* of fresh human feces) to a final concentration of 1% (*w*/*v*). Batch cultures were run under these controlled conditions for a period of 24 h, during which samples were collected at 4 time points (0, 5, 10 and 24 h) for FISH, SCFA, precursors polyphenols and polyphenol microbial metabolites. Pellets were stored at −80 °C for DNA extraction. Fermentations were conducted in triplicate using three healthy fecal donors.

2.7. DNA Extraction, Amplification and Sequencing

DNA was extracted from each sample (available for 0, 10 and 24 h time points) using the FastDNA Spin Kit for Feces (MP Biomedicals, UK). Nucleic acid purity was tested on NanoDropTM 8000 Spectrophotometer (Thermo Fisher Scientific). Total genomic DNA was then subjected to PCR amplification by targeting a ~460-bp fragment of the 16S rRNA variable region V3-V4 using the specific bacterial primer set 341F (5′ CCTACGGGNGGCWGCAG 3′) and 806R (5′ GACTACNVGGGTWTCTAATCC 3′) with overhang Illumina adapters. PCR amplification of each sample was carried out using 25 μL reactions with 1 μM of each primer, following the Illumina Metagenomic Sequencing Library Preparation Protocol for 16S Ribosomal RNA Gene Amplicons. The PCR products were checked on 1.5% agarose gel and cleaned from free primers and primer dimer using the Agencourt AMPure XP system (Beckman Coulter, Brea, CA, USA) following the manufacturer's instructions. Subsequently dual indices and Illumina sequencing adapters Nextera XT Index Primer (Illumina) were attached by 7 cycles PCR (16S Metagenomic Sequencing Library Preparation, Illumina). The final libraries, after purification by the Agencourt AMPure XP system (Beckman), were analyzed on a Typestation 2200 platform (Agilent Technologies, Santa Clara, CA, USA) and quantified using the Quant-IT PicoGreen dsDNA assay kit (Thermo Fisher Scientific) by the Synergy2 microplate reader (Biotek). Finally, all the libraries were pooled in an equimolar way in a final amplicon library and analyzed on a Typestation 2200 platform (Agilent Technologies, Santa Clara, CA, USA). Barcoded library was sequenced on an Illumina® MiSeq (PE300) platform

(MiSeq Control Software 2.0.5 (Illumina, San Diego, CA, USA) and Real-Time Analysis software 1.16.18 (Illumina, San Diego, CA, USA)).

2.8. Sequence Data Analysis

Demultiplexed sequences were further processed using the Quantitative Insight Into Microbial Ecology (QIIME) open-source software package [23] using the following workflow: Forward and reverse Illumina reads (300 bp each) were joined using the fastq-join method [24], quality filtering was performed using 19 as the minimum Phred quality score and chimeric sequences were identified and removed using usearch 6.1. Then, sequences were assigned to operational taxonomic units (OTUs) using the QIIME implementation of UCLUST algorithm at 97% similarity threshold [25]. Representative sequences for each OTU were assigned to different bacterial taxonomic levels -phylum (p.), class (c.), order (o.), family (f.) and genus (g.)—by using Greengenes database release (May 2013).

The number of sequences collected that fulfilled quality control requirements (Phred quality score $\geq$20) yielded 1,647,935 (Sequence length mean $\pm$ SD, 450 $\pm$ 12). After removing chimeric sequences, a total of 1,621,799 reads remained, meaning that the used usearch61 algorithm reduced the dataset by approximately 1.6%. Using 97% as a homology cutoff value 4530 species-level OTUs were identified. For alpha and beta diversity tests all samples were subsampled to an equal number of reads (11,708 reads per sample which constitutes to 90% of the most indigent sample in the dataset). For further downstream analysis, the dataset was filtered to consider only those OTUs that were present in all samples at a relative abundance >0.005% (486 OTUs).

2.9. Enumeration of Bacterial Groups with Fluorescence In Situ Hybridization (FISH)

Changes in bacterial populations were determined using genus- and group-specific 16S rRNA gene-targeted oligonucleotide probes, labeled with Cy3 fluorescent dye, applying the FISH method [22]. The used oligonucleotide probes were: Bif164 specific for the *Bifidobacterium* spp. [26] and Fpra655 specific for the *Faecalibacterium prausnitzii* genus [27]. For total bacterial cell stain, the fixing of the samples onto the Teflon slides was performed as normal and the slides were incubated for 10 minutes in 50 mL of PBS with the addition of 50 μL of SYBR Green to a final concentration of 1:1000 [28].

2.10. Analysis of Short Chain Fatty Acids (SCFAs)

Analysis of SCFAs was performed using the method by Zhao et al. (2006) [29] with slight modifications. Briefly, 1 mL aliquots of 10% (*w*/*v*) fecal suspension in sterile 1 M PBS (pH 7.2) were dispensed into 1.5 mL tubes and centrifuged at 13,000× *g* for 5 min to pellet bacteria and other solids. Supernatants were then transferred into clean 1.5 mL tubes and frozen at 20 °C until required. On the day of the analysis samples were defrosted on ice and acidified to pH 2–3 by the addition of one volume of 6 M HCl to three volumes of sample. After 10 min incubation at room temperature, samples were centrifuged at 13,000× *g* for 5 min and filtered using a 0.2 μm polycarbonate syringe. One volume of 10 mM 2-ethylbutyirc acid was added to four volumes of sample as the internal standard. Calibration was done using standard solutions of acetic acid, propionic acid, i-butyric acid and n-butyric acid (Sigma-Aldrich, Schnelldorf, Germany) in acidified water (pH 2). SCFAs were determined by gas-liquid chromatography coupled with mass spectrometry on a Thermo Trace GC Ultra (Thermo Fisher Scientific, Austin, TX, USA) fitted with a FFAP column (Restek Stabilwax-DA; 30 m × 0.25 mm; 0.25 μm fth) and a flame-ionization detector. Peaks were integrated using Thermo Scientific Xcalibur data system (Thermo Fisher Scientific, Austin, TX, USA). All SCFAs showed a linear range between at least 0.5–20 mM with a coefficient of linearity R^2 > 0.999. LOD and LOQ were below 0.5 mM.

2.11. Analysis of Precursor Polyphenols and Polyphenol Microbial Metabolites

The determination of precursor polyphenols was performed according to Vrhovsek et al. (2012) [19] whereas the polyphenol microbial metabolites according to Gasperotti et al. (2014) [20].

Briefly, a previously developed targeted metabolomic method was performed with an ultra-performance liquid chromatographic system coupled to tandem mass spectrometry system with electrospray ionization (UHPLC-ESI-MS/MS). Before injection, batch culture supernatants were defrosted, centrifuged (13,000 rpm, 5 min), filtered (0.22 μm) and trans-cinnamic acid-d5 (5 μg/mL) was added as the first internal standard. Then, samples were dried under nitrogen and reconstituted in methanol:water (1:1, *v*/*v*) containing rosmarinic acid (1 μg/mL) as the second internal standard. Samples were finally shaken for 10 min in an orbital shaker, centrifuged for 5 min at 16,000 rpm and injected (2 μL) into the UHPLC–MS/MS system. Data processing was performed using Waters MassLynx 4.1 (Waters, Milford, CT, USA) and TargetLynx software (Waters, Milford, CT, USA). Details of the liquid chromatography and mass spectrometry are described in Vrhovsek et al. (2012) [19] and Gasperotti et al. (2014) [20].

2.12. Statistical Analysis

For the sequencing data analysis, the QIIME pipeline version 1.9.1 [23] was used. Within community diversity (alpha diversity) was calculated using observed OTUs, Chao1 and Shannon indexes with 10 sampling repetitions at each sampling depth. Analysis of similarity (ANOSIM) and the ADONIS test were used to determine statistical differences between samples (beta diversity) following the QIIME compare_categories.py script and using weighted and unweighted phylogenetic UniFrac distance matrices. Principal Coordinate Analysis (PCoA) plots were generated using the QIIME beta diversity plots workflow. The biplot function was used to visualize samples and taxa in the PCoA space. For the rest of the data analysis the SPSS IBM version 21 (SPSS Inc., Chicago, IL, USA) was used. One-way ANOVA was used to determine differences between fermentation treatments (inulin, cellulose, Renetta Canada, Golden Delicious and Pink Lady) at the same time point (0, 5, 10 or 24 h), followed by the least significant difference (LSD) *post hoc* test. A repeated measures ANOVA was used to explore the differences within the same treatment/vessel (inulin, cellulose, Renetta Canada, Golden Delicious or Pink Lady) with all the time points (0, 5, 10 and 24 h) as within factor and with LSD as the *post hoc* test. In addition to these analyses, the p values were corrected using false discovery rate (FDR) to account for multiple testing at the lower bacterial taxonomical level (67 taxa). $p \leq 0.05$ was considered statistically significant.

3. Results

3.1. Composition of Apples

The fiber and polyphenol content of the three fresh apples is shown in Table 1 (detailed nutrient composition analysis is presented in the Supplementary File, Table S1). Renetta Canada had the highest total polyphenol content (276 mg/100 g) followed by Golden Delicious (132 mg/100 g) and Pink Lady (94 mg/100 g). The total fiber content was similar among the apple varieties (Table 1).

Table 1. Composition analysis of Renetta Canada, Golden Delicious and Pink Lady *.

Components	Renetta Canada	Golden Delicious	Pink Lady
Total dietary fiber (AOAC) (g/100 g)	2.6	2.4	2.4
Soluble fiber (AOAC) (g/100 g)	1.6	1.3	0.9
Insoluble fiber (AOAC) (g/100 g)	1.0	1.1	1.5
Polyphenols (mg/100 g)			
Flavanols			
(+)—Catechin	1.07	0.16	0.17
(−)—Epicatechin	10.9	2.8	2.8
Procyanidin B1	6.6	0.95	0.78
Procyanidin B2 + B4 (as B2)	18.3	6.1	4.8
Proanthocyanidin (as cyanidin)	169.2	91.5	62.1

Table 1. *Cont.*

Components	Renetta Canada	Golden Delicious	Pink Lady
Hydroxycinnamates			
Chlorogenic acid	61	18.7	17.5
Neochlorogenic acid	0.04	0.04	0.01
Cryptochlorogenic acid	0.98	0.67	0.15
Flavonols			
Quercetin-3-glucoside	0.99	6.9	3.1
Quercetin-3-rhamnoside	0.65	2.7	1.7
Rutin	0.09	0.44	0.19
Kaempferol-3-rutinoside	0.002	0.011	0.002
Isorhamnetin-3-glucoside	0.001	0.002	0.001
Dihydrochalcones			
Phlorizin	5.9	1.5	0.8
Anthocyanins			
Cyanidin 3-galactoside	0.006	0.017	0.027
Benzoic Acid Derivatives			
Vanillin	0.008	0.006	0.003
Vanillic acid	0.001	0.003	0.002

* For each apple variety a mixture of three fresh whole apples was analyzed.

3.2. Changes in Fecal Bacterial Alpha and Beta Diversity

The diversity of gut microbiota within a community was measured with alpha diversity indices (within-sample richness), in particular the number of observed OTUs, the Chao1 estimator of species richness and the Shannon entropy and these are shown in Figure 1. At 0 h there were no differences between the treatments. At 10 h the observed OTUs, species richness (Chao1) as well as Shannon entropy were significantly lower with all the apple treatments compared to inulin or cellulose. At 24 h the same statistical differences as the 10 h time point were shown for the observed OTUs and species richness, with the exception of Shannon entropy, where Renetta Canada and inulin had lower values compared to the other apples or cellulose ($p < 0.05$). All alpha diversity indices decreased over time within every treatment throughout the fermentation ($p < 0.05$).

When the bacterial diversity between samples (for all the data set) was examined (beta diversity) a clustering was shown according to fecal donor (ANOSIM and ADONIS test, $p = 0.01$ and $p = 0.001$ ($R^2 = 34\%$), respectively) (Figure 2) and time point (ANOSIM and ADONIS test, $p = 0.01$ and $p = 0.001$ ($R^2 = 11\%$), respectively) (Figure S1), as demonstrated with principal coordinate analysis (PCoA) based on an unweighted (qualitative) phylogenetic UniFrac distance matrix. The clustering was less distinct but still significant according to donor (ANOSIM and ADONIS test, $p = 0.01$ and $p = 0.001$ ($R^2 = 29\%$), respectively) and time (ANOSIM and ADONIS test, $p = 0.01$ and $p = 0.001$ ($R^2 = 30\%$), respectively) when based on a weighted (quantitative) phylogenetic UniFrac distance matrix (Figure 2 and Figure S1, respectively). There was no significant effect of treatment on beta diversity for all the data set together (all time points and donors), ANOSIM test, $p = 0.81$ and $p = 0.59$ and ADONIS test, $p = 0.95$, $R^2 = 7\%$ and $p = 0.55$, $R^2 = 8.5\%$, according to an unweighted and a weighted UniFrac distance matrix, respectively (Figure S2). The 6 core genera which influenced overall variance the most in the samples were *Bacteroides, Bifidobacterium, Megamonas, Ruminococcaceae* unassigned genus, *Lachnospiraceae* unassigned *genus and Faecalibacterium* (Figure 2, Figures S1 and S2).

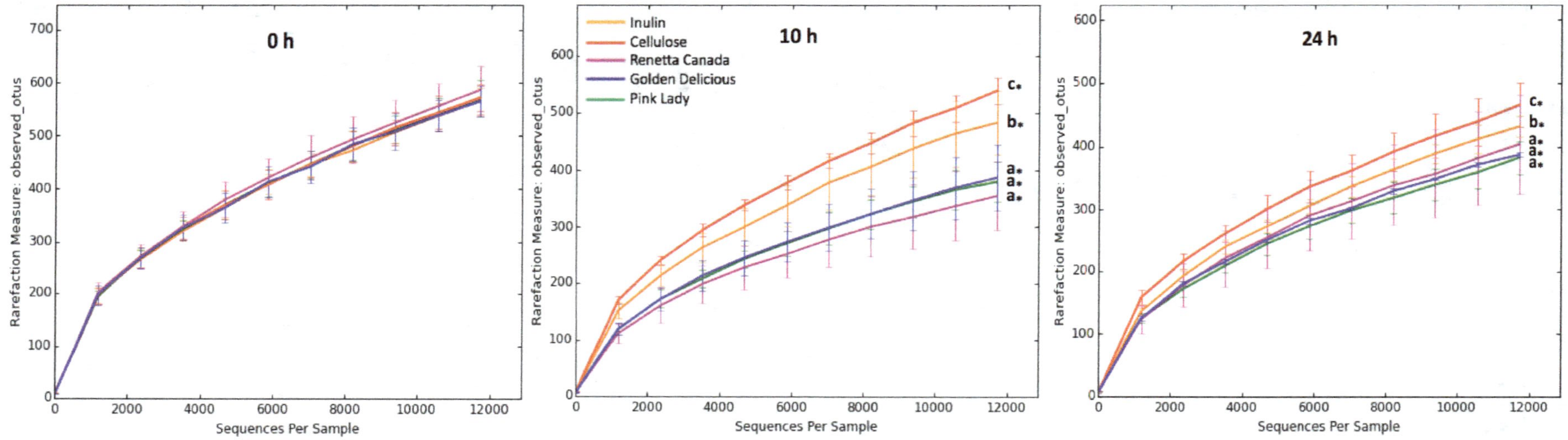

Treatment	Chao1 (0 h)	Shannon (0 h)	Chao1 (10 h)	Shannon (10 h)	Chao1 (24 h)	Shannon (24 h)
Inulin	1076 ± 43	6.36 ± 0.36	931 ± 91 ^{b,*}	5.32 ± 0.53 ^{b,*}	811 ± 37 ^{b,*}	4.88 ± 0.32 ^{a*}
Cellulose	1091 ± 26	6.39 ± 0.43	1030 ± 66 ^{c,*}	5.99 ± 0.27 ^{c,*}	849 ± 89 ^{c,*}	5.72 ± 0.29 ^{c,*}
Renetta Canada	1124 ± 84	6.49 ± 0.28	673 ± 113 ^{a,*}	4.28 ± 0.71 ^{a,*}	774 ± 135 ^{a,*}	4.78 ± 0.63 ^{a,*}
Golden Delicious	1064 ± 46	6.35 ± 0.41	724 ± 125 ^{a,*}	4.57 ± 0.64 ^{a,*}	737 ± 31 ^{a,*}	5.20 ± 0.07 ^{b,*}
Pink Lady	1115 ± 67	6.47 ± 0.27	748 ± 69 ^{a,*}	4.63 ± 0.66 ^{a,*}	769 ± 48 ^{a,*}	5.14 ± 0.47 ^{b,*}

Figure 1. Alpha diversity (within-sample richness) rarefaction curves based on the observed number of Operational Taxonomic Units, OTUs (image), average Chao1 and Shannon indexes (±SEM) in 24-h in vitro batch culture fermentations inoculated with human feces (n = 3 healthy donors) and administrated with inulin, cellulose, Renetta Canada, Golden Delicious and Pink Lady as the substrates (treatments). Samples were analyzed at 0, 10 and 24 h. Ten sampling repetitions were calculated at an even sampling depth of 11708 sequences. Significant differences ($p < 0.05$) between treatments at the same time point are indicated with different letters. * Significant differences ($p < 0.05$) from the 0 h time point within the same treatment.

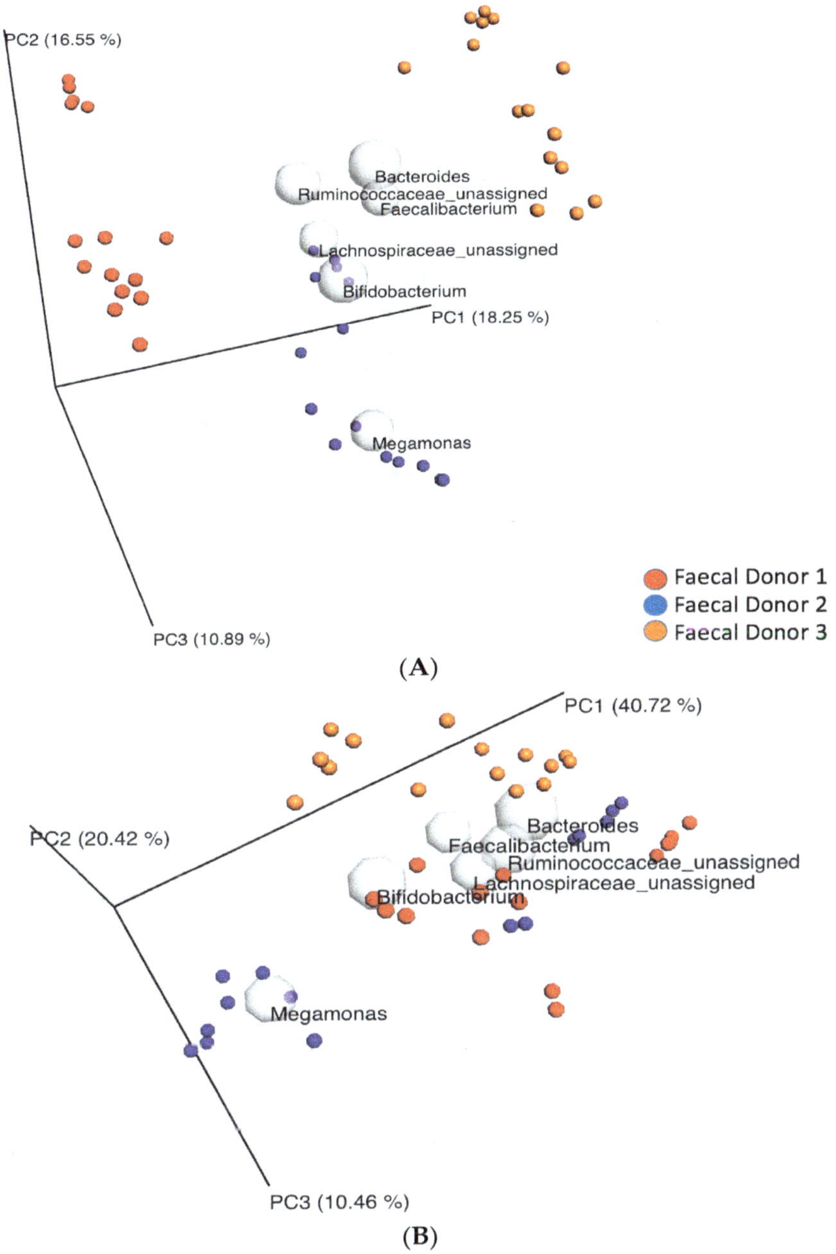

Figure 2. Principal coordinate analysis (PCoA) plots of 16S rRNA gene profiles based on (**A**) unweighted (qualitative) and (**B**) weighted (quantitative) phylogenetic UniFrac distance matrices calculated from a rarefied OTU table (11708 reads per sample) showing a clustering between donors (ANOSIM and ADONIS test, p = 0.01 and p = 0.001, respectively) for the whole data set (24-h in vitro batch culture fermentations inoculated with human feces (n = 3 healthy donors) and administrated with inulin, cellulose, Renetta Canada, Golden Delicious and Pink Lady as the substrates/treatments). Samples were analyzed at 0, 10 and 24 h. Each color represents a different donor. The gray spherical coordinates indicate taxonomic vectors of the 6 most prevalent taxa at the genus level. The size of each sphere is proportional to the mean relative abundance and approximates the causing variance throughout the plotted samples.

3.3. Fecal Bacterial Relative Abundance at the Phylum Level

The total sequence reads used in this study were classified into 7 phyla and one phylum was noted as unassigned. In particular, the bacterial communities, at time 0 h in all cultures, were dominated by bacteria belonging to Firmicutes (58–64%), Bacteroidetes (27–34%), Actinobacteria (5–7%) and Proteobacteria (1.5–2.0%) phylum, whereas a small percentage (0.1–0.3%) belonged to Cyanobacteria,

Lentisphaerae, Tenericutes and an unassigned phylum (Figure 3). Treatment did not have any significant effect on the relative abundance of phylum level at time 0 h and 10 h. However, at time 24 h Actinobacteria relative abundance differed significantly among all five treatments ($p = 0.017$), where supplementation with all the apple varieties led to a higher abundance compared to cellulose ($p < 0.05$). Focusing on changes over time for each treatment separately (Figure 3), Firmicutes abundance remained unaffected, whereas Bacteroidetes significantly decreased over time with inulin ($p = 0.012$), Renetta Canada ($p = 0.002$) and Golden Delicious ($p = 0.019$). Actinobacteria proportion was significantly increased over time with all the apple varieties (Renetta Canada, $p = 0.05$, Golden Delicious, $p = 0.011$ and Pink Lady, $p = 0.018$). Finally, Proteobacteria abundance was also significantly increased with cellulose ($p = 0.021$), Renetta Canada ($p = 0.012$) and Golden Delicious ($p = 0.02$) (Figure 3).

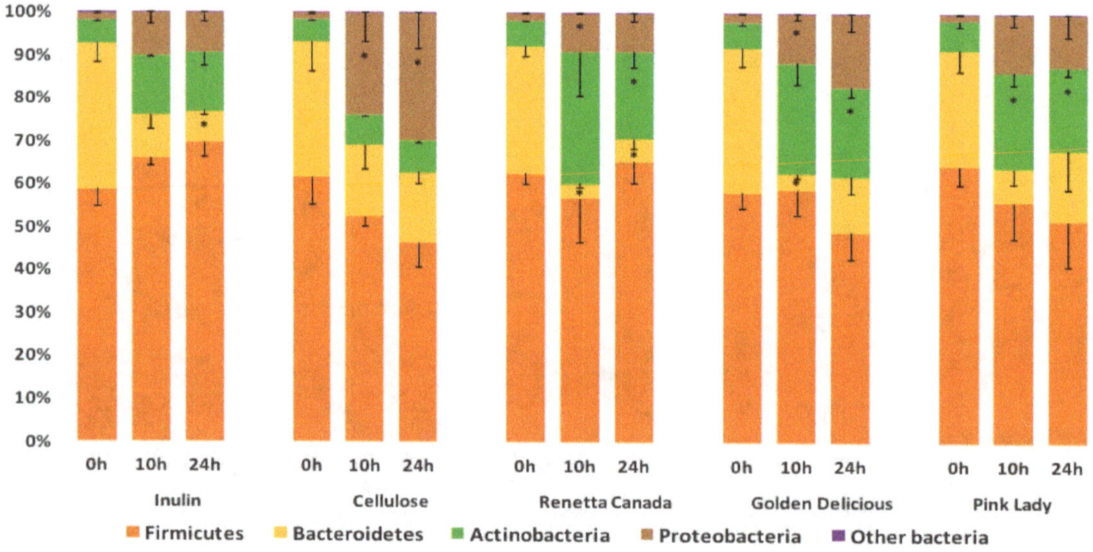

Figure 3. Changes in bacterial phyla (relative abundances (%)) throughout 24-h in vitro batch culture fermentations inoculated with human feces ($n = 3$ healthy donors) and administrated with inulin, cellulose, Renetta Canada, Golden Delicious and Pink Lady as the substrates (treatments). Samples were analyzed at 0, 10 and 24 h. Values are mean (%) with SEM (the negative error value is shown). Other bacteria represent Cyanobacteria, Lentisphaerae, Tenericutes and an unassigned phylum. * Significant differences from the 0 h time point within the same treatment ($p < 0.05$, FDR corrected).

3.4. Fecal Bacterial Relative Abundance at the Genus Level

At the lowest taxonomic level, 67 distinct bacterial taxa were detected. Of these, 46 were identified at the genus level, 15 at the family level, 5 at the order level and one was unassigned. At 0 h there were no differences between the treatments in bacterial taxa relative abundance. At 10 h, treatment had an effect on the abundance of g. *Oscillospira*, g. *Ruminococcus*, g. *Parabacteroides*, g. *Bilophila*, unassigned f. *Lachnospiraceae*, unassigned f. *Mogibacteriaceae* and unassigned and unclassified o. Clostridiales, which remained significant after the FDR correction for multiple testing for o. unassigned Clostridiales and f. *Mogibacteriaceae*, with cellulose administration showing higher proportions of these taxa compared to the other treatments (Table 2). Notably, *Bifidobacterium* g. abundance differed among all treatments at 10 h, with the highest proportion after Renetta Canada and Golden Delicious administration, however, this lost significance with FDR correction (Table 2). Significant differences, before correction, between treatments were also observed at 24 h on the relative abundance of g. *Faecalibacterium*, g. *Butyricimonas*, g. *Bifidobacterium* and unassigned o. Clostridiales. Additional details on the relative abundance of bacterial taxa at 10 and 24 h for the different treatments are shown in Table 2. Focusing on changes over time for each treatment separately, there were significant changes in the relative abundance of specific taxa however, these were not always significant after correction and presented as supplementary information (Table S2).

Table 2. Changes in bacterial taxa relative abundance (%) at 10 h and 24 h of in vitro batch culture fermentations inoculated with human feces (n = 3 healthy donors) and administrated with inulin, cellulose, Renetta Canada, Golden Delicious and Pink Lady as the substrates (treatments).

Phylum	Class	Order	Family	Genus	Time Point	Inulin (%)	Cellulose (%)	Renetta Canada (%)	Golden Delicious (%)	Pink Lady (%)	p *	p # (FDR-Corrected)
Firmicutes	Clostridia	Clostridiales	*Lachnospiraceae*	unassigned	10 h	4.3 ± 1.3^{a}	9 ± 0.9^{b}	2.6 ± 0.7^{a}	$5 \pm 2^{a,b}$	2.9 ± 1.2^{a}	0.040	0.336
Firmicutes	Clostridia	Clostridiales	*[Mogibacteriaceae]*	unassigned	10 h	0.15 ± 0.01^{b}	0.14 ± 0.01^{b}	0.08 ± 0.02^{a}	0.05 ± 0.01^{a}	0.06 ± 0.01^{a}	0.001	0.040
Firmicutes	Clostridia	Clostridiales	*Ruminococcaceae*	*Oscillospira*	10 h	0.66 ± 0.1^{b}	1 ± 0.1^{c}	0.32 ± 0.03^{a}	0.3 ± 0.1^{a}	0.23 ± 0.07^{a}	0.001	0.052
Firmicutes	Clostridia	Clostridiales	*Ruminococcaceae*	*Ruminococcus*	10 h	$1.4 \pm 0.3^{a,b}$	1.8 ± 0.5^{b}	0.63 ± 0.43^{a}	0.41 ± 0.18^{a}	0.45 ± 0.17^{a}	0.050	0.369
Firmicutes	Clostridia	Clostridiales	unassigned	unassigned	10 h	1.8 ± 0.1^{b}	2.8 ± 0.3^{c}	0.82 ± 0.24^{a}	0.76 ± 0.16^{a}	0.81 ± 0.12^{a}	0.000	0.009
Firmicutes	Clostridia	Clostridiales	unclassified	unclassified	10 h	0.68 ± 0.12^{b}	1.4 ± 0.23^{c}	$0.47 \pm 0.1^{a,b}$	$0.33 \pm 0.03^{a,b}$	$0.59 \pm 0.27^{a,b}$	0.013	0.215
Bacteroidetes	Bacteroidia	Bacteroidales	*Porphyromonadaceae*	*Parabacteroides*	10 h	0.72 ± 0.2^{b}	1.9 ± 0.6^{c}	$0.4 \pm 0.1^{a,b}$	$0.37 \pm 0.04^{a,b}$	$0.56 \pm 0.1^{a,b}$	0.022	0.264
Actinobacteria	Actinobacteria	Bifidobacteriales	*Bifidobacteriaceae*	*Bifidobacterium*	10 h	4.7 ± 2.4^{a}	2.8 ± 0.2^{a}	24.3 ± 8.7^{b}	19.4 ± 4.2^{b}	$16.2 \pm 2.1^{a,b}$	0.028	0.273
Proteobacteria	Deltaproteobacteria	Desulfovibrionales	*Desulfovibrionaceae*	*Bilophila*	10 h	0.33 ± 0.03^{a}	1.7 ± 0.6^{b}	0.17 ± 0.01^{a}	0.24 ± 0.08^{a}	0.26 ± 0.05^{a}	0.024	0.264
Firmicutes	Clostridia	Clostridiales	*Ruminococcaceae*	*Faecalibacterium*	24 h	17 ± 3.7^{c}	4.6 ± 2.2^{a}	$16 \pm 5.5^{b,c}$	$5.9 \pm 1.9^{a,b}$	5.4 ± 1.4^{a}	0.049	0.950
Firmicutes	Clostridia	Clostridiales	unassigned	unassigned	24 h	1.2 ± 0.3^{a}	2.5 ± 0.6^{b}	0.36 ± 0.05^{a}	0.75 ± 0.19^{a}	0.86 ± 0.19^{a}	0.007	0.482
Bacteroidetes	Bacteroidia	Bacteroidales	*[Odoribacteraceae]*	*Butyricimonas*	24 h	$0.04 \pm 0.01^{a,b}$	0.09 ± 0.03^{b}	0.03 ± 0.01^{a}	0.02 ± 0.01^{a}	0.02 ± 0.01^{a}	0.044	0.950
Actinobacteria	Actinobacteria	Bifidobacteriales	*Bifidobacteriaceae*	*Bifidobacterium*	24 h	$6.3 \pm 4.6^{a,b}$	2.6 ± 0.2^{a}	14.9 ± 2.5^{b}	15.2 ± 2.6^{b}	$10.4 \pm 3^{a,b}$	0.050	0.950

* ANOVA analysis to verify whether the relative abundance of a given taxa is different between the treatments within the same time point. # The p value after correction for multiple tests (67 taxa) with the false discovery rate (FDR) method. Different letters (a, b, c) indicate significant differences ($p < 0.05$) between treatments at the same time point. Brackets indicate suggested but not verified names. Values are mean ± SEM.

3.5. Changes in Selected Fecal Bacterial Populations Measured with FISH

Changes in *Bifidobacterium* spp., *Faecalibacterium prausnitzii* and total bacteria were also assessed by FISH (Figure 4). At 0 h there were no significant changes between the treatments. At 5 h bifidobacteria numbers increased significantly with Renetta Canada compared to cellulose ($p = 0.004$) and inulin ($p = 0.047$); bifidobacteria also increased with Golden Delicious as the treatment compared to cellulose ($p = 0.007$). At 10 h bifidobacteria and total bacteria increased significantly with all the apple varieties compared to cellulose ($p < 0.05$); with total bacteria also increasing with inulin compared to cellulose ($p = 0.009$). Bifidobacteria also increased at 10 h with Renetta Canada compared to inulin ($p = 0.036$). At 24 h *Faecalibacterium prausnitzii* increased significantly with Renetta Canada compared to the other apples ($p < 0.05$). All apple varieties and inulin increased *Faecalibacterium prausnitziii* compared to cellulose ($p < 0.05$). Inulin and Golden Delicious also had higher *Faecalibacterium prausnitziii* numbers at 24 h compared to Pink Lady ($p = 0.004$ and $p = 0.032$ respectively) (Figure 4). Finally, at 24 h total bacteria increased significantly with all the apple varieties and inulin compared to cellulose ($p < 0.05$).

Following changes over time for the same treatment, a significant increase in bifidobacteria population, from 0 h, was observed for Renetta Canada (compared to 5, 10 and 24 h ($p < 0.05$)) and Golden Delicious (compared to 10 and 24 h ($p < 0.05$)). Furthermore, inulin also increased *Bifidobacterium* spp. at 5 h ($p = 0.044$) compared to the 0 h value, but to a lesser extent compared to Renetta Canada and Golden Delicious. *Faecalibacterium prausnitzii* population was significantly higher after 24 h only for Renetta Canada compared to 0 h ($p = 0.049$), while it decreased significantly after the administration of cellulose (at 24 h compared to 0 h, $p = 0.02$). Apart from the cellulose treatment (significant decrease at 10 h, $p = 0.028$) there were no significant changes over time in total bacteria population with any of the other treatments (Figure 4).

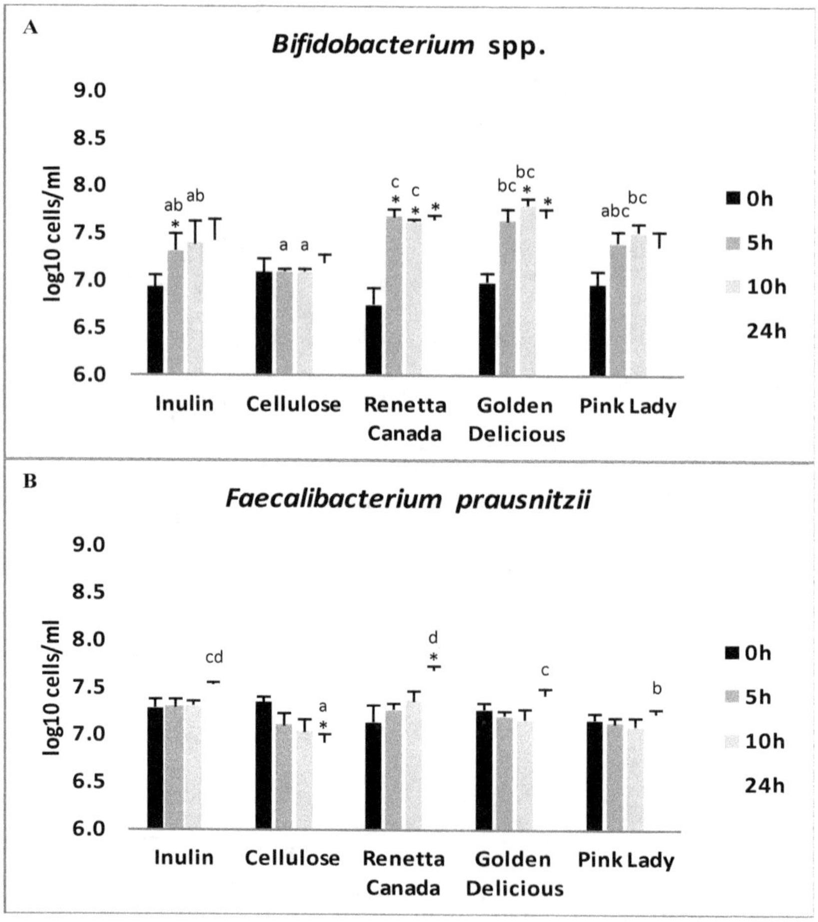

Figure 4. *Cont.*

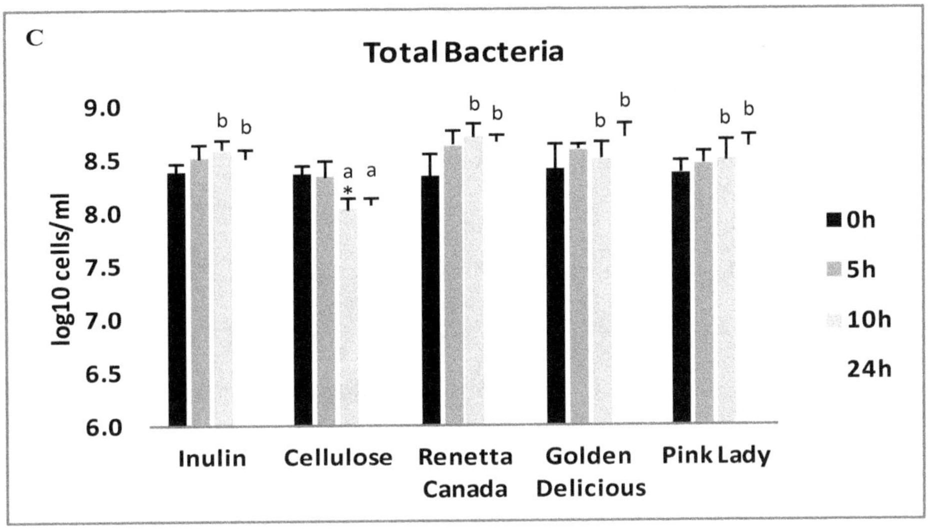

Figure 4. Changes in bacterial populations ((**A**) *Bifidobacterium* spp.; (**B**) *Faecalibacterium prausnitzii* and (**C**) Total Bacteria) throughout 24-h in vitro batch culture fermentations inoculated with human feces ($n = 3$ healthy donors) and administrated with inulin, cellulose, Renetta Canada, Golden Delicious and Pink Lady as the substrates (treatments). Samples were collected at 0, 5, 10 and 24 h. Results are expressed as $\log_{10}$ cells/mL of batch culture medium and values are mean ± SEM of the three fermentations. Significant differences ($p < 0.05$) between treatments at the same time point are indicated with different letters. * Significant differences ($p < 0.05$) from the 0 h time point within the same treatment.

3.6. SCFAs Production

Changes in SCFAs concentrations over time with the different treatments are shown in Table 3. All apples varieties significantly increased the concentration of acetic, propionic and total SCFAs ($p < 0.05$), but only Renetta Canada increased butyric acid among the apples ($p < 0.05$). Inulin significantly increased the concentrations of acetic, butyric and total SCFAs ($p < 0.05$) but these remained lower compared to the apple varieties. Cellulose increased butyric acid and total SCFAs but to a much lesser extent compared to inulin and the apple varieties ($p < 0.05$). There were no significant changes between the treatments at the same time point (0, 5, 10 or 24 h).

3.7. Changes in Precursor Polyphenols

A list of the precursor polyphenols and polyphenol microbial metabolites together with their multiple reaction monitoring (MRM) conditions are presented in Table S3. Changes in the concentration of precursor polyphenols, during the fecal fermentation, are shown in Table S4. Proanthocyanidin, kaempferol-3-rutinoside, rutin, isorhamentin-3-glucoside and cyanidin 3-galactoside were measured only in fresh apples whereas procyanidin A2, quercetin, kaempferol, isorhamnetin, laricitrin, phloretin, luteolin and ellagic acid were measured only in batch cultures.

Changes between the three apple varieties were observed at 0 h. In particular, Renetta Canada treatment resulted in significant higher concentrations of (+)-catechin, (−)-epicatechin, procyanidin A2, procyanidin B1, phloretin, phlorizin and vanillin compared to Golden Delicious and Pink Lady (Table S4). On the other hand, treatment with Golden Delicious resulted in higher ($p < 0.05$) levels of quercetin-3-glc compared to Pink Lady and Renetta Canada and higher quercetin-3-rha compared to Renetta Canada (Table S4). There were no significant changes in the concentration of precursor polyphenols at 5, 10 or 24 h.

Changes in the concentration of precursor polyphenols were observed over time throughout the fecal fermentation of the three apple varieties. In particular, significant reductions throughout the fermentation were detected for (+)-catechin (Renetta Canada), (−)-epicatechin (Renetta Canada and Golden Delicious), procyanidin A2 (Renetta Canada, Golden Delicious and Pink Lady), neochlorogenic acid (Golden Delicious), cryptochlorogenic acid (Golden Delicious), quercetin-3-glc (Renetta Canada, Golden Delicious and Pink Lady), quercetin-3-rha (Renetta Canada, Golden Delicious and Pink Lady), kaempferol (Renetta Canada), isorhamnetin (Renetta Canada), phlorizin (Renetta Canada and Golden Delicious) and vanillin (Renetta Canada and Golden Delicious) (Table S4).

Table 3. SCFA concentrations (mmol/L) throughout 24-h in vitro batch culture fermentations inoculated with human feces (n = 3 healthy donors) and administrated with inulin, cellulose, Renetta Canada, Golden Delicious and Pink Lady as the substrates (treatments).

Substrate	Time (h)	Acetic Acid (mmol/L)	p [a]	Propionic Acid (mmol/L)	p [a]	Butyric Acid (mmol/L)	p [a]	Total SCFAs (mmol/L)	p [a]
Inulin	0	2.2 ± 0.1	0.050	0.8 ± 0.1	0.185	1 ± 0.3	0.013	4.1 ± 0.6	0.049
	5	9.5 ± 5.4		2.8 ± 1.4		4.4 ± 2.8		16.8 ± 9.6	
	10	11 ± 2.1		2.9 ± 0.8		5.5 ± 1 *		19.3 ± 3.3 *	
	24	17.3 ± 2.1 *		6.9 ± 2.6		11 ± 0.5 *		35.4 ± 4.6 *	
Cellulose	0	4.8 ± 2.9	0.062	1.4 ± 0.8	0.062	1.2 ± 0.6	0.041	7.5 ± 4.2	0.022
	5	5 ± 1.3		1.9 ± 0.5		2.3 ± 0.2 *		9.2 ± 2.3	
	10	13.5 ± 5.2		3.3 ± 1		2.8 ± 0.6		19.5 ± 5.6 *	
	24	13.1 ± 1.1		3.4 ± 0.1		3.5 ± 1		20 ± 1.5	
Renetta Canada	0	1 ± 0.1	0.034	0.5 ± 0.1	0.020	0.5 ± 0.1	0.025	3 ± 0.3	0.044
	5	11.5 ± 2.7		4.6 ± 2.6		2 ± 0.5		18.1 ± 3.9	
	10	19 ± 2.2 *		5.6 ± 2.1		3.7 ± 0.6 *,#		28.4 ± 1.8 *	
	24	28.1 ± 6 *,#		8.8 ± 2.6 #,^		16.9 ± 6.1		53.7 ± 11.4 *	
Golden Delicious	0	2 ± 0.4	0.034	0.6 ± 0.1	0.016	0.5 ± 0.2	0.057	3.1 ± 0.7	0.008
	5	13.9 ± 5.8		4.2 ± 1.6		1.9 ± 0.7		20 ± 6.7	
	10	15.3 ± 3 *		4.7 ± 1.9		4.9 ± 1.6		25 ± 3.1 *	
	24	23.7 ± 2.8 *		7.8 ± 1.9 #,^		13.3 ± 5.1		44.8 ± 7.2 *,#	
Pink Lady	0	1.8 ± 0.3	0.049	0.5 ± 0.1	0.020	0.4 ± 0.1	0.044	2.7 ± 0.5	0.040
	5	8.3 ± 2.3		3.2 ± 1.5		1.1 ± 0.2		12.6 ± 2.9	
	10	22.8 ± 8		6 ± 2.2		4 ± 1.2		32.8 ± 9.7	
	24	26.2 ± 3.8 *,#		8.8 ± 2 #,^		13 ± 2.8		48 ± 7.9 *,#,^	

Results are expressed as mmol/L of batch culture medium and values are mean ± SEM of the three fermentations. [a] Difference over time within the same treatment (ANOVA). * Significant different from 0 h time point $p < 0.05$, # Significant different from 5 h time point, $p < 0.05$, ^ Significant different from 10 h time point, $p < 0.05$.

3.8. Formation of Polyphenol Microbial Metabolites

The formation of polyphenol microbial metabolites throughout the fecal fermentation of the three apple varieties is shown in Figures 5 and 6. Significant increases were observed over time for 3-hydroxyphenylacetic acid (Renetta Canada and Pink Lady, p = 0.034 and p = 0.043, respectively), 3,4-dihydroxyphenylacetic acid (Renetta Canada, p = 0.05), 3-(4-hydroxyphenyl)propionic acid (Pink Lady, p = 0.009), hydroferulic acid (Renetta Canada, p = 0.046), 4-hydroxybenzoic acid (Pink Lady, p = 0.017) and pyrocatechol (Pink Lady, p = 0.049). In contrast, significant decreases throughout the fermentation were shown for caffeic acid (Renetta Canada and Golden Delicious, p = 0.000 and p = 0.001, respectively), p-coumaric acid (Renetta Canada and Golden Delicious, p = 0.001 and p = 0.001, respectively), trans-ferulic (Renetta Canada and Golden Delicious, p = 0.002 and p = 0.003, respectively) and trans-isoferulic (Renetta Canada, $p = 0.001$), as these metabolites can also appear as precursor polyphenols in apples (Figure S3). There were no significant changes in the concentration of the polyphenol microbial metabolites between the three apple varieties when each time point (0, 5, 10 or 24 h) was explored separately, with the exception of caffeic acid and p-coumaric acid (significantly higher concentration with Renetta Canada fermentation compared to Golden Delicious and Pink Lady at 0 h) and t-ferulic acid (significantly higher concentration with Renetta Canada compared to Pink Lady at 0 h).

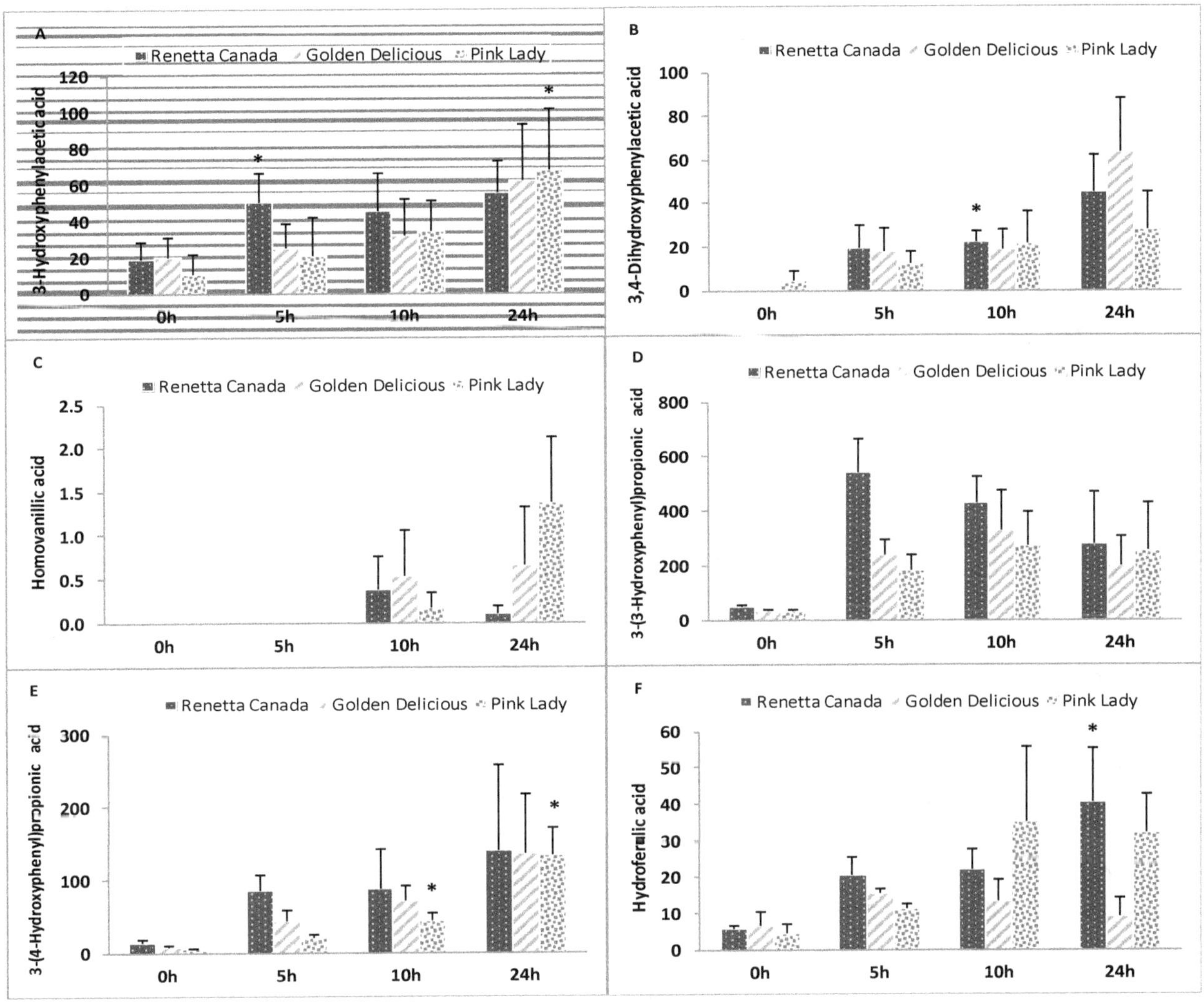

Figure 5. Changes in phenylacetic ((**A**) 3-Hydroxyphenylacetic acid; (**B**) 3,4-Dihydroxyphenylacetic acid and (**C**) Homovanillic acid) and phenylpropionic acid ((**D**) 3-(3-Hydroxyphenyl)propionic acid; (**E**) 3-(4-Hydroxyphenyl)propionic acid and (**F**) Hydroferulic acid) derivatives throughout 24-h in vitro batch culture fermentations inoculated with human feces ($n = 3$ healthy donors) and administrated with Renetta Canada, Golden Delicious and Pink Lady as the substrates (treatments). Samples were collected at 0, 5, 10 and 24 h. Results are expressed as ng/mL of batch culture medium and values are mean $\pm$ SEM of the three fermentations. * Significant differences ($p < 0.05$) from the 0 h time point within the same treatment.

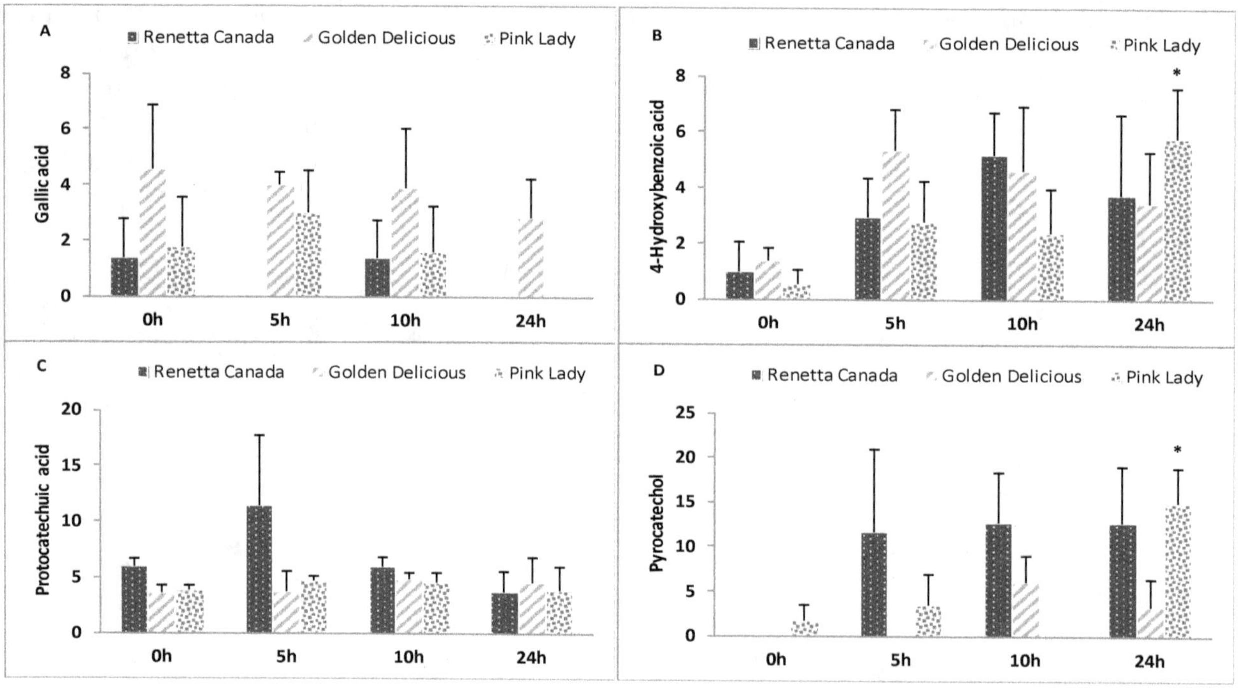

Figure 6. Changes in benzoic acid derivatives ((**A**) Gallic acid; (**B**) 4-Hydroxybenzoic acid; (**C**) Protocatechuic acid and (**D**) Pyrocatechol) throughout 24-h in vitro batch culture fermentations inoculated with human feces ($n = 3$ healthy donors) and administrated with Renetta Canada, Golden Delicious and Pink Lady as the substrates (treatments). Samples were collected at 0, 5, 10 and 24 h. Results are expressed as ng/mL of batch culture medium and values are mean ± SEM of the three fermentations. * Significant differences ($p < 0.05$) from the 0 h time point within the same treatment.

4. Discussion

The present in vitro study showed that whole apples can effectively modify both the human fecal microbiota composition and metabolic output. Effects on the bacterial community were observed at phylum and genus/species level. Actinobacteria relative abundance increased with all the tested apple varieties (Renetta Canada, Golden Delicious and Pink Lady). Increases in Actinobacteria have been observed in humans after intake of pectin [30], resistant starch [31] and pomegranate extract [32] and in rats fed with wild blueberries [33]. This increase can be explained by *Bifidobacterium* spp. growth, an important member of the Actinobacteria phylum. Although this did not remain significant with Illumina sequencing after multiple testing correction in the current study, the FISH results showed that *Bifidobacterium* spp. population increased significantly after the administration with Renetta Canada and Golden Delicious varieties. Notably, *Bifidobacterium* is considered a beneficial member of the gut microbiota by inhibiting the growth of pathogens, synthesizing certain vitamins (e.g., folate) and reducing serum cholesterol [2]. This observation is consistent with previous studies showing a bifidogenic effect with extraction juices from apple pomace in rats [12] and with the administration of two apples daily for two weeks in eight human subjects [17]. In contrast, Masumoto et al. (2016) [15], using a high throughput metagenomics technique, have reported decreased relative abundance of *Bifidobacterium* in diet-induced obese mice after the administration of apple PAs [15]. In our study, inulin, a known prebiotic, increased bifidobacteria to a lesser extent than apples. Inulin structure can affect its utilization by gut bacteria and many isolated bifidobacteria cannot utilize long-chain inulin [8] but they can grow on short-chain length structures (i.e., fructo-oligosaccharides) [34]. The inulin in the current study was a commercial isolate from dahlia tubers and details of its structure were not available.

Within the Firmicutes phylum, *Faecalibacterium prausnitzii* population (measured with the quantitative FISH) increased with Renetta Canada administration. *F. prausnitzii* is a key butyrate-producer, with anti-inflammatory properties, that may offer potential health benefits, especially in patients with inflammatory bowel disease (IBD) [35,36]. Renetta Canada increased butyrate, a major energy source for the colonocytes, which is particularly beneficial to the gut mucosa [37]. In support of our results *F. prausnitzii* strains have been shown to utilize apple pectin for growth [8,38] and increase butyrate concentration [13,39]. *F. prausnitzii* levels were unaffected by Golden Delicious and Pink Lady, and although the concentration of pectin was not determined, Renetta Canada had 19% and 44% higher soluble fiber content compared with Golden Delicious and Pink Lady, respectively. These data suggest that at least for *F. prausnitzii*, pectin may have played a major role.

Bacteroidetes relative abundance decreased with inulin, Renetta Canada and Golden Delicious. *Bacteroides* is considered a dominant bacterial group in the large intestine and the main Bacteroidetes member, along with the *Prevotella*. Licht et al. (2010) reported that both whole apples and isolated pectin decreased *Bacteroides* spp. in rats compared to a control diet [13]. Moreover, *Bacteroides* has been shown to decrease after the administration of other polyphenol sources, such as red wine [40] and cocoa [41] in rats, as well as with grape [42] and date extracts [43] in in vitro gut models inoculated with human feces. By contrast, *Bacteroides* species have been shown to increase with apple pomace juice extracts [11] and PAs from *Acacia angustissima* [44] in rats, as well as with red wine in humans [45].

The proportion of Proteobacteria increased after the administration of Renetta Canada and Golden Delicious but to a lesser extent compared to cellulose. However, an increase in *Enterobacteriaceae* family, a major member of Proteobacteria, was not observed. *Enterobacteriaceae*, includes numerous pathogenic bacteria genera, such as *Escherichia*, *Salmonella* and *Yersinia* and has been shown to increase in IBD patients. Increased Proteobacteria with inulin [8], resistant starch [46] and de-alcoholized wine [45] has also been reported elsewhere.

Interestingly, the alpha diversity of gut microbiota, at the OTU level, was lower with the apple treatments compared to inulin or cellulose. This may indicate the selective nature of the apple fermentations towards particular species. The beta diversify analysis showed a partitioning by donor and time, but not with treatment, which indicates that each individual possesses a specific starting population of gut bacteria, a finding consistent with the previously described inter-individual variation in the intestinal microbiota [47,48]. However, despite the variability between donors, there were still treatment-associated changes in gut microbiota composition at phylum and at genus/species level.

In the present study, the conditions of the proximal colon were simulated by creating an environment moderately acidic (pH 5.5–6.0) compared to a more neutral pH in the transverse and distal colon. The majority of the unabsorbed dietary carbohydrates are fermented in the proximal section producing SCFAs, leading to this reduced colonic pH, whereas in the distal section carbohydrate fermentation is generally assumed to be low. The pH affects bacterial growth and SCFA production, especially among bacteria that utilize the same polysaccharides [8,49]. For example, suppression in *Bacteroides* spp. growth was observed at pH values below six [8]. On the other hand, *F. prausnitzii* is more low-pH tolerant [8]. Moreover, a lower pH tends to favor butyrate production [49]. However, in our study, a significant increase in butyrate levels and *F. prausnitzii* population was only shown by Renetta Canada, indicating a treatment effect rather than a pH effect.

Pectin, the main soluble fiber found in apples, is extensively fermented by the gut microbiota to SCFAs, which are an important energy source for colonic health as well as for other tissues and organs [2]. Apart from the aforementioned butyrate increase by Renetta Canada, all apples significantly increased propionate and mainly acetate. Increased SCFAs have been shown with apple pomace juices [11,12]. Acetate serves as an energy source for the liver and peripheral tissues, but is also involved in the metabolic pathways of lipogenesis [50]. Pectin is known to produce relatively large amounts of acetate [51], which can also be utilized by butyrate producers such as *F. prausnitzii* as part of the cross feeding between bacteria [52]. A cross-feeding between *Bifidobacterium* strains and *F. prausnitzii* has been suggested, enhancing butyrate production [53]. Propionate on the other hand, may help to reduce hepatic cholesterol synthesis [54].

The effects of polyphenols on health depend on their bioavailability. Flavanol monomers (i.e., catechin and epicatechin) are readily absorbed in the small intestine, while high molecular weight polyphenols, such as the polymeric PAs, reach the colon almost intact, where they are transformed by the gut bacteria into a complex mixture of simple phenolic acids [55]. In the present study, the degradation of precursor apple polyphenols started as early as 5 h of fermentation and was complete throughout the 24 h for most of the polyphenolic compounds. Renetta Canada fermentation resulted in higher degradation of precursor polyphenols due to their initial high concentration.

The formation of polyphenol microbial products represent potential beneficial bioactive metabolites, not only locally in the gut but also systematically after their absorption in the colon and their appearance in the blood circulation. Renetta Canada was associated with the production of 3,4-dihydroxyphenylacetic acid and hydroferulic acid, which both have shown to possess anti-inflammatory properties [56]. It has been proposed that 3,4-dihydroxyphenylacetic acid can arise from the microbial catabolism of dimeric PAs [57]. Moreover, microbial metabolites of chlorogenic acids such as dihydroferulic acid showed a high antioxidant activity in vitro [58]. These results are in line with the higher concentration of PAs and chlorogenic acid in Renetta Canada apples. Pink Lady was associated with the formation of 3-(4-hydroxyphenyl)propionic acid and benzoic acid derivatives, in particular 4-hydroxybenzoic acid and pyrocatechol. Benzoic acids such as 4-hydroxybenzoic acid are considered to arise from beta oxidation of phenylpropionic acid derivatives and higher levels have been found after the in vitro fermentation of grape seed flavanols [59]. Pyrocatechol may arise from the dehydroxylation of gallic acid [60], which has been identified as a microbial metabolite and a native compound [61]. In our study, gallic acid concentration remained unaffected throughout the fermentation. Finally, both Renetta Canada and Pink Lady apples increased 3-hydroxyphenylacetic acid concentration. In vitro studies with human fecal inoculum are in line with the identified phenolic acids. In particular, PA catabolism has been associated with the production of 3-hydroxyphenylpropionic acid, 3-phenylpropionic acid, 4-hydroxyphenylpropionic acid and 4-hydroxyphenylacetic acid [62] as the main metabolites, whereas apples and apple components including isolated PAs formed 3-(3,4-dihydroxyphenyl)propionic acid, 3-(3-hydroxyphenyl)propionic acid, 3-phenylpropionic acid, benzoic acid, 2-(3,4-dihydroxyphenyl)acetic acid and 2-(3-hydroxyphenyl)acetic acid [10]. Furthermore, in human subjects, chocolate intake, a rich source of flavanols increased the urinary excretion of 3-hydroxyphenylpropionic acid, ferulic acid, 3,4-dihydroxyphenylacetic acid, 3-hydroxyphenylacetic acid, vanillic acid and 3-hydroxybenzoic acid [63].

In this study, we demonstrated that whole apples could modify the gut microbiota composition and affect the extent of degradation of soluble fiber and polyphenols through the production of SCFAs and phenolic acids, with Renetta Canada variety showing the most beneficial effects. In vitro batch culture models are a quick, simple and cost effective method of mimicking changes in gut microbiota numbers and metabolism [64], although they lack key metabolic functions, such as host immunological interactions, intestinal absorption and physiological components, such as epithelial mucosa, that exist in the human colon. The sample size (n = 3) is consistent with similar studies investigating polyphenols extracts [22,59], prebiotics [65,66] and fruits [43,67], with observed changes consistent with outcomes of human intervention studies [68]. Batch culture vessels contain a basal medium with limited carbohydrate and protein sources, therefore changes in microbiota composition and fermentation metabolites is known to be due to the added substrate, the apple varieties added to the vessels, even with different starting bacterial populations. Finally, although, donors were of similar age, with no gastrointestinal disorders, other characteristics that may affect gut microbiota composition such as diet, exercise and stress levels were not recorded and may have influenced the observed results, and it is recommended that these are provided in future studies.

5. Conclusions

In conclusion, whole apples beneficially modulate the gut microbiota composition and metabolic output in vitro. Renetta Canada variety in particular may have positive consequences for human health by increasing bifidobacteria, *Faecalibacterium prausnitzii* population and producing SCFAs and polyphenol microbial metabolites. It is recommended that the findings of this in vitro study should be confirmed in human intervention trials.

Supplementary Materials:
Figure S1: Principal coordinate analysis (PCoA) plots of 16S rRNA gene profiles based on (A) unweighted (qualitative) and (B) weighted (quantitative) phylogenetic UniFrac distance matrices, colored by time, Figure S2: Principal coordinate analysis (PCoA) plots of 16SrRNA gene profiles based on (A) unweighted (qualitative) and (B) weighted (quantitative) phylogenetic UniFrac distance matrices, colored by treatment, Figure S3: Changes in cinnamic acid derivatives, Table S1: Composition analysis of Renetta Canada, Golden Delicious and Pink Lady, Table S2: Changes in bacterial taxa throughout 24-h in vitro batch culture fermentations inoculated with human feces (n = 3 healthy donors) and administrated with inulin, cellulose, Renetta Canada, Golden Delicious and Pink Lady as the substrates, Table S3: Multiple Reaction Monitoring (MRM) conditions of precursor polyphenols and polyphenol microbial metabolites, Table S4: Changes in precursor polyphenols throughout 24-h in vitro batch culture fermentations inoculated with human feces (n = 3 healthy donors) and administrated with inulin, cellulose, Renetta Canada, Golden Delicious and Pink Lady as the substrates.

Acknowledgments: This study was jointly funded by the University of Reading Research Endowment Trust Fund, Reading, United Kingdom and Fondazione Edmund Mach, San Michele all' Adige, Italy. We kindly thank Domenico Masuero and Evelyn Soini for measuring polyphenols in the three test apples and Silvia Carlin for helping with the SCFA analysis.

Author Contributions: K.M.T., J.A.L., A.K. and M.L. conceived the research and designed the study. A.K. wrote the manuscript. A.K. and M.L. performed the apple digestion and the in vitro batch cultures with the training of L.C. and F.F. A.K. performed the FISH analysis, the MiSeq Illumina sequencing data analysis and statistical analysis. A.K. performed the metabolites annotation, with the advice of L.C. and M.B. M.L. performed the SCFA analysis. M.G., M.L. and U.V. performed the metabolomics polyphenol analysis in fermentation samples. K.M.T. and J.A.L. coordinated the overall project and provided funding. J.A.L. and K.M.T. reviewed and edited the manuscript and all authors approved the final version.

References

1. Wang, X.; Ouyang, Y.Y.; Liu, J.; Zhu, M.M.; Zhao, G.; Bao, W.; Hu, F.B. Fruit and vegetable consumption and mortality from all causes, cardiovascular disease, and cancer: Systematic review and dose-response meta-analysis of prospective cohort studies. *BMJ* **2014**, *349*, 14. [CrossRef] [PubMed]
2. Koutsos, A.; Tuohy, K.M.; Lovegrove, J.A. Apples and cardiovascular health-is the gut microbiota a core consideration? *Nutrients* **2015**, *7*, 3959–3998. [CrossRef] [PubMed]
3. Gerhauser, C. Cancer chemopreventive potential of apples, apple juice, and apple components. *Planta Med.* **2008**, *74*, 1608–1624. [CrossRef] [PubMed]
4. Monagas, M.; Urpi-Sarda, M.; Sanchez-Patan, F.; Llorach, R.; Garrido, I.; Gomez-Cordoves, C.; Andres-Lacueva, C.; Bartolome, B. Insights into the metabolism and microbial biotransformation of dietary flavan-3-ols and the bioactivity of their metabolites. *Food Funct.* **2010**, *1*, 233–253. [CrossRef] [PubMed]
5. Ozdal, T.; Sela, D.A.; Xiao, J.B.; Boyacioglu, D.; Chen, F.; Capanoglu, E. The reciprocal interactions between polyphenols and gut microbiota and effects on bioaccessibility. *Nutrients* **2016**, *8*, 36. [CrossRef] [PubMed]
6. Olano-Martin, E.; Gibson, G.R.; Rastall, R.A. Comparison of the in vitro bifidogenic properties of pectins and pectic-oligosaccharides. *J. Appl. Microbiol.* **2002**, *93*, 505–511. [CrossRef] [PubMed]
7. Chen, J.; Liang, R.-H.; Liu, W.; Li, T.; Liu, C.-M.; Wu, S.-S.; Wang, Z.-J. Pectic-oligosaccharides prepared by dynamic high-pressure nnicrofluidization and their in vitro fermentation properties. *Carbohydr. Polym.* **2013**, *91*, 175–182. [CrossRef] [PubMed]
8. Chung, W.S.F.; Walker, A.W.; Louis, P.; Parkhill, J.; Vermeiren, J.; Bosscher, D.; Duncan, S.H.; Flint, H.J. Modulation of the human gut microbiota by dietary fibres occurs at the species level. *BMC Biol.* **2016**, *14*, 13. [CrossRef] [PubMed]
9. Vrhovsek, U.; Rigo, A.; Tonon, D.; Mattivi, F. Quantitation of polyphenols in different apple varieties. *J. Agric. Food Chem.* **2004**, *52*, 6532–6538. [CrossRef] [PubMed]
10. Bazzocco, S.; Mattila, I.; Guyot, S.; Renard, C.M.G.C.; Aura, A.-M. Factors affecting the conversion of apple polyphenols to phenolic acids and fruit matrix to short-chain fatty acids by human faecal microbiota in vitro. *Eur. J. Nutr.* **2008**, *47*, 442–452. [CrossRef] [PubMed]

11. Sembries, S.; Dongowski, G.; Jacobasch, G.; Mehrlander, K.; Will, F.; Dietrich, H. Effects of dietary fibre-rich juice colloids from apple pomace extraction juices on intestinal fermentation products and microbiota in rats. *Br. J. Nutr.* **2003**, *90*, 607–615. [CrossRef] [PubMed]
12. Sembries, S.; Dongowski, G.; Mehrlaender, K.; Will, F.; Dietrich, H. Physiological effects of extraction juices from apple, grape, and red beet pomaces in rats. *J. Agric. Food Chem.* **2006**, *54*, 10269–10280. [CrossRef] [PubMed]
13. Licht, T.R.; Hansen, M.; Bergstrom, A.; Poulsen, M.; Krath, B.N.; Markowski, J.; Dragsted, L.O.; Wilcks, A. Effects of apples and specific apple components on the cecal environment of conventional rats: Role of apple pectin. *BMC Microbiol.* **2010**, *10*. [CrossRef] [PubMed]
14. Jiang, T.; Gao, X.; Wu, C.; Tian, F.; Lei, Q.; Bi, J.; Xie, B.; Wang, H.Y.; Chen, S.; Wang, X. Apple-derived pectin modulates gut microbiota, improves gut barrier function, and attenuates metabolic endotoxemia in rats with diet-induced obesity. *Nutrients* **2016**, *8*, 126. [CrossRef] [PubMed]
15. Masumoto, S.; Terao, A.; Yamamoto, Y.; Mukai, T.; Miura, T.; Shoji, T. Non-absorbable apple procyanidins prevent obesity associated with gut microbial and metabolomic changes. *Sci. Rep.* **2016**, *6*, 31208. [CrossRef] [PubMed]
16. Aprikian, O.; Duclos, V.; Guyot, S.; Besson, C.; Manach, C.; Bernalier, A.; Morand, C.; Remesy, C.; Demigne, C. Apple pectin and a polyphenol-rich apple concentrate are more effective together than separately on cecal fermentations and plasma lipids in rats. *J. Nutr.* **2003**, *133*, 1860–1865. [PubMed]
17. Shinohara, K.; Ohashi, Y.; Kawasumi, K.; Terada, A.; Fujisawa, T. Effect of apple intake on fecal microbiota and metabolites in humans. *Anaerobe* **2010**, *16*, 510–515. [CrossRef] [PubMed]
18. Ravn-Haren, G.; Dragsted, L.O.; Buch-Andersen, T.; Jensen, E.N.; Jensen, R.I.; Nemeth-Balogh, M.; Paulovicsova, B.; Bergstrom, A.; Wilcks, A.; Licht, T.R.; et al. Intake of whole apples or clear apple juice has contrasting effects on plasma lipids in healthy volunteers. *Eur. J. Nutr.* **2012**. [CrossRef] [PubMed]
19. Vrhovsek, U.; Masuero, D.; Gasperotti, M.; Franceschi, P.; Caputi, L.; Viola, R.; Mattivi, F. A versatile targeted metabolomics method for the rapid quantification of multiple classes of phenolics in fruits and beverages. *J. Agric. Food Chem.* **2012**, *60*, 8831–8840. [CrossRef] [PubMed]
20. Gasperotti, M.; Masuero, D.; Guella, G.; Mattivi, F.; Vrhovsek, U. Development of a targeted method for twenty-three metabolites related to polyphenol gut microbial metabolism in biological samples, using spe and uhplc-esi-ms/ms. *Talanta* **2014**, *128*, 221–230. [CrossRef] [PubMed]
21. Mandalari, G.; Faulks, R.M.; Rich, G.T.; Lo Turco, V.; Picout, D.R.; Lo Curto, R.B.; Bisignano, G.; Dugo, P.; Dugo, G.; Waldron, K.W.; et al. Release of protein, lipid, and vitamin e from almond seeds during digestion. *J. Agric. Food Chem.* **2008**, *56*, 3409–3416. [CrossRef] [PubMed]
22. Sanchez-Patan, F.; Cueva, C.; Monagas, M.; Walton, G.E.; Gibson, G.R.; Quintanilla-Lopez, J.E.; Lebron-Aguilar, R.; Martin-Alvarez, P.J.; Moreno-Arribas, M.V.; Bartolome, B. In vitro fermentation of a red wine extract by human gut microbiota: Changes in microbial groups and formation of phenolic metabolites. *J. Agric. Food Chem.* **2012**, *60*, 2136–2147. [CrossRef] [PubMed]
23. Caporaso, J.G.; Kuczynski, J.; Stombaugh, J.; Bittinger, K.; Bushman, F.D.; Costello, E.K.; Fierer, N.; Pena, A.G.; Goodrich, J.K.; Gordon, J.I.; et al. Qiime allows analysis of high-throughput community sequencing data. *Nat. Methods* **2010**, *7*, 335–336. [CrossRef] [PubMed]
24. Aronesty, E. Comparison of sequencing utilitiy programs. *Open Bioinform. J.* **2013**, *7*, 1–8. [CrossRef]
25. Edgar, R.C. Search and clustering orders of magnitude faster than blast. *Bioinformatics* **2010**, *26*, 2460–2461. [CrossRef] [PubMed]
26. Langendijk, P.S.; Schut, F.; Jansen, G.J.; Raangs, G.C.; Kamphuis, G.R.; Wilkinson, M.H.F.; Welling, G.W. Quantitative fluorescence in-situ hybridization of *Bifidobacterium* spp. with genus-specific 16s ribosomal-rna-targeted probes and its application in fecal samples. *Appl. Environ. Microbiol.* **1995**, *61*, 3069–3075. [PubMed]
27. Hold, G.L.; Schwiertz, A.; Aminov, R.I.; Blaut, M.; Flint, H.J. Oligonucleotide probes that detect quantitatively significant groups of butyrate-producing bacteria in human feces. *Appl. Environ. Microbiol.* **2003**, *69*, 4320–4324. [CrossRef] [PubMed]
28. Daims, H.; Stoecker, K.; Wagner, M. Fluorescence In Situ Hybridization for the detection of prokaryotes. In *Molecular Microbial Ecology*; Osborn, A.M., Smith, C.J., Eds.; Taylor & Francis: New York, NY, USA, 2005.

29. Zhao, G.H.; Nyman, M.; Jonsson, J.A. Rapid determination of short-chain fatty acids in colonic contents and faeces of humans and rats by acidified water-extraction and direct-injection gas chromatography. *Biomed. Chromatogr.* **2006**, *20*, 674–682. [CrossRef] [PubMed]
30. Yang, J.; Martinez, I.; Walter, J.; Keshavarzian, A.; Rose, D.J. In vitro characterization of the impact of selected dietary fibers on fecal microbiota composition and short chain fatty acid production. *Anaerobe* **2013**, *23*, 74–81. [CrossRef] [PubMed]
31. Martinez, I.; Kim, J.; Duffy, P.R.; Schlegel, V.L.; Walter, J. Resistant starches types 2 and 4 have differential effects on the composition of the fecal microbiota in human subjects. *PLoS ONE* **2010**, *5*, 11. [CrossRef] [PubMed]
32. Li, Z.P.; Henning, S.M.; Lee, R.P.; Lu, Q.Y.; Summanen, P.H.; Thames, G.; Corbett, K.; Downes, J.; Tseng, C.H.; Finegold, S.M.; et al. Pomegranate extract induces ellagitannin metabolite formation and changes stool microbiota in healthy volunteers. *Food Funct.* **2015**, *6*, 2487–2495. [CrossRef] [PubMed]
33. Lacombe, A.; Li, R.W.; Klimis-Zacas, D.; Kristo, A.S.; Tadepalli, S.; Krauss, E.; Young, R.; Wu, V.C.H. Lowbush wild blueberries have the potential to modify gut microbiota and xenobiotic metabolism in the rat colon. *PLoS ONE* **2013**, *8*, 8. [CrossRef] [PubMed]
34. Rossi, M.; Corradini, C.; Amaretti, A.; Nicolini, M.; Pompei, A.; Zanoni, S.; Matteuzzi, D. Fermentation of fructooligosaccharides and inulin by bifidobacteria: A comparative study of pure and fecal cultures. *Appl. Environ. Microbiol.* **2005**, *71*, 6150–6158. [CrossRef] [PubMed]
35. Sokol, H.; Pigneur, B.; Watterlot, L.; Lakhdari, O.; Bermudez-Humaran, L.G.; Gratadoux, J.-J.; Blugeon, S.; Bridonneau, C.; Furet, J.-P.; Corthier, G.; et al. Faecalibacterium prausnitzii is an anti-inflammatory commensal bacterium identified by gut microbiota analysis of crohn disease patients. *Proc. Natl. Acad. Sci. USA* **2008**, *105*, 16731–16736. [CrossRef] [PubMed]
36. Machiels, K.; Joossens, M.; Sabino, J.; De Preter, V.; Arijs, I.; Eeckhaut, V.; Ballet, V.; Claes, K.; Van Immerseel, F.; Verbeke, K.; et al. A decrease of the butyrate-producing species roseburia hominis and faecalibacterium prausnitzii defines dysbiosis in patients with ulcerative colitis. *Gut* **2014**, *63*, 1275–1283. [CrossRef] [PubMed]
37. Pryde, S.E.; Duncan, S.H.; Hold, G.L.; Stewart, C.S.; Flint, H.J. The microbiology of butyrate formation in the human colon. *FEMS Microbiol. Lett.* **2002**, *217*, 133–139. [CrossRef] [PubMed]
38. Lopez-Siles, M.; Khan, T.M.; Duncan, S.H.; Harmsen, H.J.M.; Garcia-Gil, L.J.; Flint, H.J. Cultured representatives of two major phylogroups of human colonic faecalibacterium prausnitzii can utilize pectin, uronic acids, and host-derived substrates for growth. *Appl. Environ. Microbiol.* **2012**, *78*, 420–428. [CrossRef] [PubMed]
39. Waldecker, M.; Kautenburger, T.; Daumann, H.; Busch, C.; Schrenk, D. Inhibition of histone-deacetylase activity by short-chain fatty acids and some polyphenol metabolites formed in the colon. *J. Nutr. Biochem.* **2008**, *19*, 587–593. [CrossRef] [PubMed]
40. Dolara, P.; Luceri, C.; de Filippo, C.; Femia, A.P.; Giovannelli, L.; Caderni, G.; Cecchini, C.; Silvi, S.; Orpianesi, C.; Cresci, A. Red wine polyphenols influence carcinogenesis, intestinal microflora, oxidative damage and gene expression profiles of colonic mucosa in f344 rats. *Mutat. Res.-Fundam. Mol. Mech. Mutag.* **2005**, *591*, 237–246. [CrossRef] [PubMed]
41. Massot-Cladera, M.; Perez-Berezo, T.; Franch, A.; Castell, M.; Perez-Cano, F.J. Cocoa modulatory effect on rat faecal microbiota and colonic crosstalk. *Arch. Biochem. Biophys.* **2012**, *527*, 105–112. [CrossRef] [PubMed]
42. Kemperman, R.A.; Gross, G.; Mondot, S.; Possemiers, S.; Marzorati, M.; van de Wiele, T.; Dore, J.; Vaughan, E.E. Impact of polyphenols from black tea and red wine/grape juice on a gut model microbiome. *Food Res. Int.* **2013**, *53*, 659–669. [CrossRef]
43. Eid, N.; Enani, S.; Walton, G.; Corona, G.; Costabile, A.; Gibson, G.; Rowland, I.; Spencer, J.P. The impact of date palm fruits and their component polyphenols, on gut microbial ecology, bacterial metabolites and colon cancer cell proliferation. *J. Nutr. Sci.* **2014**, *3*, e46. [CrossRef] [PubMed]
44. Smith, A.H.; Mackie, R.I. Effect of condensed tannins on bacterial diversity and metabolic activity in the rat gastrointestinal tract. *Appl. Environ. Microbiol.* **2004**, *70*, 1104–1115. [CrossRef] [PubMed]
45. Isabel Queipo-Ortuno, M.; Boto-Ordonez, M.; Murri, M.; Miguel Gomez-Zumaquero, J.; Clemente-Postigo, M.; Estruch, R.; Cardona Diaz, F.; Andres-Lacueva, C.; Tinahones, F.J. Influence of red wine polyphenols and ethanol on the gut microbiota ecology and biochemical biomarkers. *Am. J. Clin. Nutr.* **2012**, *95*, 1323–1334. [CrossRef] [PubMed]

46. Lyte, M.; Chapel, A.; Lyte, J.M.; Ai, Y.F.; Proctor, A.; Jane, J.L.; Phillips, G.J. Resistant starch alters the microbiota-gut brain axis: Implications for dietary modulation of behavior. *PLoS ONE* **2016**, *11*, 22. [CrossRef] [PubMed]
47. Walker, A.W.; Ince, J.; Duncan, S.H.; Webster, L.M.; Holtrop, G.; Ze, X.L.; Brown, D.; Stares, M.D.; Scott, P.; Bergerat, A.; et al. Dominant and diet-responsive groups of bacteria within the human colonic microbiota. *ISME J.* **2011**, *5*, 220–230. [CrossRef] [PubMed]
48. Salonen, A.; Lahti, L.; Salojarvi, J.; Holtrop, G.; Korpela, K.; Duncan, S.H.; Date, P.; Farquharson, F.; Johnstone, A.M.; Lobley, G.E.; et al. Impact of diet and individual variation on intestinal microbiota composition and fermentation products in obese men. *ISME J.* **2014**, *8*, 2218–2230. [CrossRef] [PubMed]
49. Walker, A.W.; Duncan, S.H.; McWilliam Leitch, E.C.; Child, M.W.; Flint, H.J. Ph and peptide supply can radically alter bacterial populations and short-chain fatty acid ratios within microbial communities from the human colon. *Appl. Environ. Microbiol.* **2005**, *71*, 3692–3700. [CrossRef] [PubMed]
50. Zambell, K.L.; Fitch, M.D.; Fleming, S.E. Acetate and butyrate are the major substrates for de novo lipogenesis in rat colonic epithelial cells. *J. Nutr.* **2003**, *133*, 3509–3515. [PubMed]
51. Onumpai, C.; Kolida, S.; Bonnin, E.; Rastall, R.A. Microbial utilization and selectivity of pectin fractions with various structures. *Appl. Environ. Microbiol.* **2011**, *77*, 5747–5754. [CrossRef] [PubMed]
52. Duncan, S.H.; Barcenilla, A.; Stewart, C.S.; Pryde, S.E.; Flint, H.J. Acetate utilization and butyryl coenzyme a (coa): Acetate-coa transferase in butyrate-producing bacteria from the human large intestine. *Appl. Environ. Microbiol.* **2002**, *68*, 5186–5190. [CrossRef] [PubMed]
53. Rios-Covian, D.; Gueimonde, M.; Duncan, S.H.; Flint, H.J.; de los Reyes-Gavilan, C.G. Enhanced butyrate formation by cross-feeding between faecalibacterium prausnitzii and bifidobacterium adolescentis. *FEMS Microbiol. Lett.* **2015**, *362*. [CrossRef] [PubMed]
54. Cheng, H.H.; Lai, M.H. Fermentation of resistant rice starch produces propionate reducing serum and hepatic cholesterol in rats. *J. Nutr.* **2000**, *130*, 1991–1995. [PubMed]
55. Velderrain-Rodriguez, G.R.; Palafox-Carlos, H.; Wall-Medrano, A.; Ayala-Zavala, J.F.; Chen, C.Y.O.; Robles-Sanchez, M.; Astiazaran-Garcia, H.; Alvarez-Parrilla, E.; Gonzalez-Aguilar, G.A. Phenolic compounds: Their journey after intake. *Food Funct.* **2014**, *5*, 189–197. [CrossRef] [PubMed]
56. Larrosa, M.; Luceri, C.; Vivoli, E.; Pagliuca, C.; Lodovici, M.; Moneti, G.; Dolara, P. Polyphenol metabolites from colonic microbiota exert anti-inflammatory activity on different inflammation models. *Mol. Nutr. Food Res.* **2009**, *53*, 1044–1054. [CrossRef] [PubMed]
57. Appeldoorn, M.M.; Vincken, J.P.; Aura, A.M.; Hollman, P.C.H.; Gruppen, H. Procyanidin dimers are metabolized by human microbiota with 2-(3,4-dihydroxyphenyl)acetic acid and 5-(3,4-dihydroxyphenyl)-gamma-valerolactone as the major metabolites. *J. Agric. Food Chem.* **2009**, *57*, 1084–1092. [CrossRef] [PubMed]
58. Gomez-Ruiz, J.A.; Leake, D.S.; Ames, J.M. In vitro antioxidant activity of coffee compounds and their metabolites. *J. Agric. Food Chem.* **2007**, *55*, 6962–6969. [CrossRef] [PubMed]
59. Cueva, C.; Sanchez-Patan, F.; Monagas, M.; Walton, G.E.; Gibson, G.R.; Martin-Alvarez, P.J.; Bartolome, B.; Moreno-Arribas, M.V. In vitro fermentation of grape seed flavan-3-ol fractions by human faecal microbiota: Changes in microbial groups and phenolic metabolites. *FEMS Microbiol. Ecol.* **2013**, *83*, 792–805. [CrossRef] [PubMed]
60. Selma, M.V.; Espin, J.C.; Tomas-Barberan, F.A. Interaction between phenolics and gut microbiota: Role in human health. *J. Agric. Food Chem.* **2009**, *57*, 6485–6501. [CrossRef] [PubMed]
61. Dall'Asta, M.; Calani, L.; Tedeschi, M.; Jechiu, L.; Brighenti, F.; Del Rio, D. Identification of microbial metabolites derived from in vitro fecal fermentation of different polyphenolic food sources. *Nutrition* **2012**, *28*, 197–203. [CrossRef] [PubMed]
62. Deprez, S.; Brezillon, C.; Rabot, S.; Philippe, C.; Mila, I.; Lapierre, C.; Scalbert, A. Polymeric proanthocyanidins are catabolized by human colonic microflora into low-molecular-weight phenolic acids. *J. Nutr.* **2000**, *130*, 2733–2738. [PubMed]
63. Rios, L.Y.; Gonthier, M.P.; Remesy, C.; Mila, L.; Lapierre, C.; Lazarus, S.A.; Williamson, G.; Scalbert, A. Chocolate intake increases urinary excretion of polyphenol-derived phenolic acids in healthy human subjects. *Am. J. Clin. Nutr.* **2003**, *77*, 912–918. [PubMed]
64. Williams, C.F.; Walton, G.E.; Jiang, L.; Plummer, S.; Garaiova, I.; Gibson, G.R. Comparative analysis of intestinal tract models. In *Annual Review of Food Science and Technology*; Doyle, M.P., Klaenhammer, T.R., Eds.; Annual Reviews: Palo Alto, CA, USA, 2015; Volume 6, pp. 329–350.

65. Johnson, L.P.; Walton, G.E.; Psichas, A.; Frost, G.S.; Gibson, G.R.; Barraclough, T.G. Prebiotics modulate the effects of antibiotics on gut microbial diversity and functioning in vitro. *Nutrients* **2015**, *7*, 4480–4497. [CrossRef] [PubMed]
66. Rodrigues, D.; Walton, G.; Sousa, S.; Rocha-Santos, T.A.P.; Duarte, A.C.; Freitas, A.C.; Gomes, A.M.P. In vitro fermentation and prebiotic potential of selected extracts from seaweeds and mushrooms. *LWT -Food Sci. Technol.* **2016**, *73*, 131–139. [CrossRef]
67. Blatchford, P.; Stoklosinski, H.; Walton, G.; Swann, J.; Gibson, G.; Gearry, R.; Ansell, J. Kiwifruit fermentation drives positive gut microbial and metabolic changes irrespective of initial microbiota composition. *Bioact. Carbohydr. Diet. Fibre* **2015**, *6*, 37–45. [CrossRef]
68. Walton, G.E.; van den Heuvel, E.; Kosters, M.H.W.; Rastall, R.A.; Tuohy, K.M.; Gibson, G.R. A randomised crossover study investigating the effects of galacto-oligosaccharides on the faecal microbiota in men and women over 50 years of age. *Br. J. Nutr.* **2012**, *107*, 1466–1475. [CrossRef] [PubMed]

15

A Prospective Study of Different Types of Dietary Fiber and Risk of Cardiovascular Disease: Tehran Lipid and Glucose Study

Parvin Mirmiran [1], Zahra Bahadoran [1,*], Sajad Khalili Moghadam [1], Azita Zadeh Vakili [2] and Fereidoun Azizi [3,*]

1 Nutrition and Endocrine Research Center, Student Research Committee, Research Institute for Endocrine Sciences, Shahid Beheshti University of Medical Sciences, No. 24, Shahid-Erabi St., Yeman St., Velenjak, Tehran 19395-4763, Iran; mirmiran@endocrine.ac.ir (P.M.); sajadkhalili69@gmail.com (S.K.M.)

2 Cellular and Molecular Endocrine Research Center, Obesity Research Center, Research Institute for Endocrine Sciences, Shahid Beheshti University of Medical Sciences, No. 24, Shahid-Erabi St., Yeman St., Velenjak, Tehran 19395-4763, Iran; azitavakili@endocrine.ac.ir

3 Endocrine Research Center, Research Institute for Endocrine Sciences, Shahid Beheshti University of Medical Sciences, No. 24, Shahid-Erabi St., Yeman St., Velenjak, Tehran 19395-4763, Iran

* Correspondence: z.bahadoran@endocrine.ac.ir (Z.B.); azizi@endocrine.ac.ir (F.A.);

Abstract: Background and aim: This study was designed to examine the hypothesis that dietary of intake different types of fiber could modify the risk of cardiovascular disease (CVD) in a large prospective cohort among Iranian adults. Methods: In 2006–2008, we used a validated food frequency questionnaire to assess dietary fiber intake among 2295 health professionals with no previous history of heart disease. Subjects were subsequently followed until 2012 for incidence of CVD events. Multivariate Cox proportional hazard regression models, adjusted for potential confounders were used to estimate the risk of CVD across tertiles of total dietary fiber and different types of fiber. Linear regression models were also used to indicate the association of dietary fiber intakes with changes of cardiovascular risk factors during the follow-up. Results: Mean age of participants (42.8% men) was 38.2 ± 13.4, at baseline. Mean (SD) dietary intake of total fiber was 23.4 (8.9) g/day. After adjustment for cardiovascular risk score and dietary confounders, a significant inverse association was observed between intakes of total, soluble and insoluble dietary fiber and CVD risk, in the highest compared to the lowest tertiles (HR = 0.39, 95% CI = 0.18–0.83, HR = 0.19, 95% CI = 0.09–0.41, and HR = 0.31, 95% CI = 0.14–0.69, respectively). Inverse relations were observed between risk of CVD and dietary fiber from legumes, fruits and vegetables; however, dietary fiber intake from grain and nut sources was not related to risk of CVD. Conclusion: Our findings confirmed that higher intakes of dietary fiber from different sources is associated with CVD events and modify its major risk-related factors.

Keywords: coronary heart disease; dietary fiber; soluble fiber; insoluble fiber

---

1. Introduction

Dietary fiber, by its impact on the glycemic response and other aspects of metabolism, may also have important effects on cardiometabolic pathways [1]. An increasing number of studies have reported a reduced risk of cardiovascular disease (CVD) following regular diets high in fiber. Based on findings from epidemiologic studies regarding the protective effects of fiber intakes, the Dietary Reference Intakes (DRI) recommended consumption of dietary fiber is 14 g/1000 kcal, or 25 and 38 g/day for adult women and men, respectively [2]. Consuming a diet rich in high-fiber foods is also a critical component of the American Heart Association's strategy and other dietary recommendations for cardiovascular disease risk reduction in the general population [3,4].

It has been proposed that dietary fiber could modify underlying CVD risk factors including lipid and lipoprotein metabolism, insulin homeostasis, inflammatory markers and coagulation, and also improve insulin sensitivity, thereby reducing the risk of CVD mortality [5–7]. Although studies showed beneficial effects of soluble, gel-forming fiber on cardiometabolic risk factors, food sources of mainly insoluble fibers, primarily contributed by cereal products, have been the fiber most consistently associated with lower risk of CVD [5]. Findings of some investigations also suggest that the role of dietary fiber is more dependent on its types and sources, rather than the amount of intake [8,9]. Different types or sources of dietary fiber may induce different physiological effects; soluble fiber is responsible for the cholesterol-lowering effect of dietary fiber whereas insoluble fiber interacts with intestinal absorption of foods and contributes to reduction in clotting factors [10,11].

To examine the hypothesis that a greater intake of dietary fiber reduces risk of CVD, and different dietary fiber may lead to different CVD outcomes, we used prospective data from the Tehran Lipid and Glucose Study over a 6-year period to assess the relationship between total dietary fiber, soluble and insoluble fiber, and different fiber sources on the risk of CVD among Iranian adults.

2. Methods

2.1. Study Population

This study was conducted within the framework of the Tehran Lipid and Glucose Study (TLGS), an ongoing community-based prospective study being conducted to investigate and prevent non-communicable diseases in a representative sample in the district 13 of Tehran, the capital city of Iran [12]. During the third phase of the TLGS (2006–2008), of a total of 12,523 subjects who completed the examinations, 4920 were randomly selected for completing the dietary assessment based on their age and sex. The randomization was performed because of cost and complexity of dietary data collection in large populations and also the fact that this process is time-consuming. Finally, the dietary data for 3462 subjects who agreed to participate and completed the food frequency questionnaire (FFQ) were available. The characteristics of participants who completed the validated FFQ were similar to those of the total population in the third phase of TLGS [13]. For the purpose of the current study, among subjects aged ≥19 years, we recruited 2927 adult men and women, with complete data (demographics, anthropometrics, biochemicals). Participants were excluded from the final analysis if they had under- or over-reported energy intakes (<800 kcal/day or >4200 kcal/day, respectively), or were on specific diets (n = 563). Participants were also excluded if they had history of CVD at baseline examination (n = 88). The remaining participants (n = 2276) were followed until March 2012, for a mean duration of 4.7 years from the baseline examination. Participants who had left the study (n = 17) were also excluded and final analyses was conducted on data of 2259 adults (Figure 1).

Written informed consents were obtained from all participants. The study protocol, based on the ethical guidelines of the 1975 Declaration of Helsinki, was approved (ethics committee number: 57ECRIES94/02/15) by the Ethics Research Council of the Research Institute for Endocrine Sciences, Shahid Beheshti University of Medical Sciences.

2.2. Demographic and Anthropometric Measures

Demographics, anthropometrics and biochemical measures were assessed both at baseline (2006–2008) and again at the follow-up examination (2010–2012). Trained interviewers collected information including demographic data, medical history, medication use and smoking habits, using pretested questionnaires. Weight was measured to the nearest 100 g using digital scales, while the subjects were minimally clothed, without shoes. Height was measured to the nearest 0.5 cm, in a standing position without shoes, using a tape meter. Body mass index was calculated as weight (kg) divided by square of the height (m^2). Waist circumference was measured to the nearest 0.1 cm, midway between the lower border of the ribs and the iliac crest at the widest portion, over light clothing, using a soft measuring tape, without any pressure to the body. For blood pressure (BP) measurements, after a 15-min rest in the sitting position, two measurements of BP were taken on the right arm, during a standardized mercury sphygmomanometer; the mean of the two measurements was considered as the participant's BP.

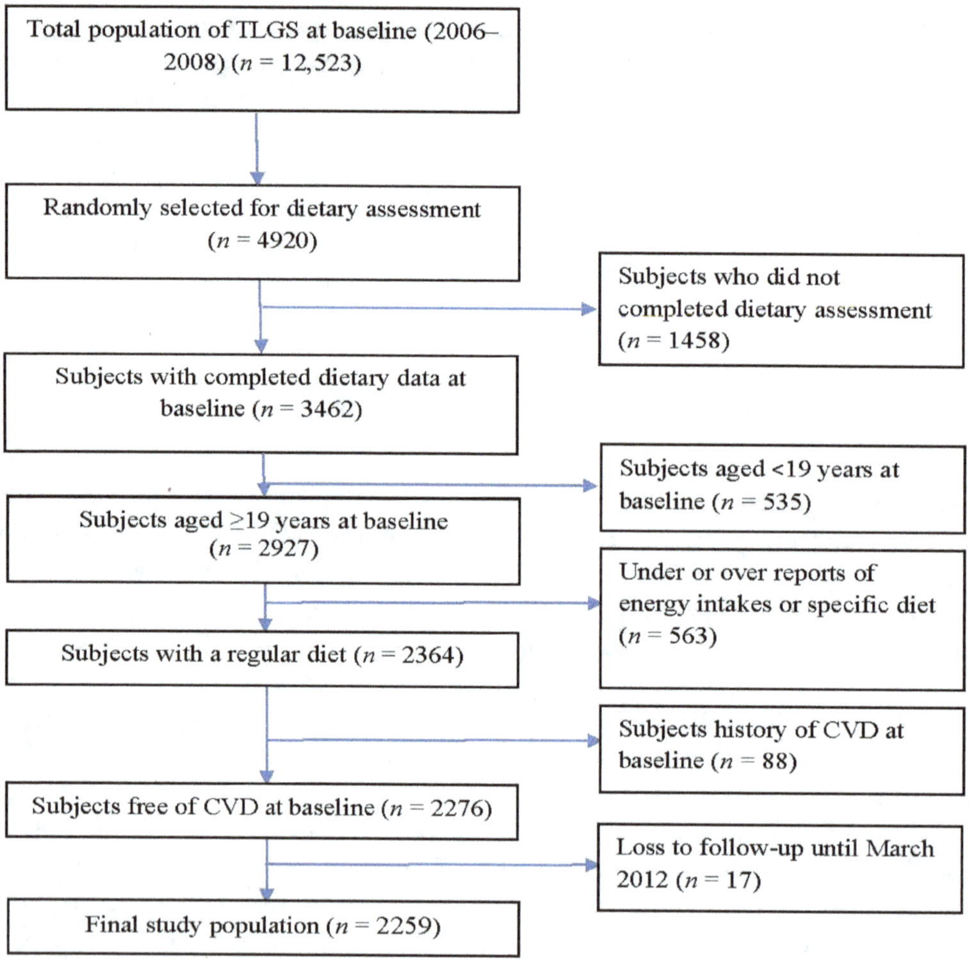

Figure 1. The flowchart of the study population.

2.3. Biochemical Measures

Fasting blood samples were taken after 12–14 h from all study participants, both at baseline and follow-up phase. Serum creatinine levels were assayed using kinetic colorimetric Jaffe method. Fasting serum glucose (FSG) was determined by the enzymatic colorimetric method using glucose oxidase. The standard 2 h serum glucose 2-h SG test was performed for all individuals who were not on anti-diabetic drugs. In a subsample of the population (n = 904), fasting serum insulin (FSI) was measured, by the electrochemiluminescence immunoasaay (ECLIA), using Roche Diagnostics kits and the Roche/Hitachi Cobas e-411 analyzer (GmbH, Mannheim, Germany). Intra- and inter-assay coefficients of variation for insulin were 1.2% and 3.5%, respectively.

Triglyceride (TG) levels were assessed by enzymatic colorimetric analysis with glycerol phosphate oxidase. High-density lipoprotein cholesterol (HDL-C) was measured after precipitation of the apolipoprotein B containing lipoproteins with phosphotungstic acid. Analyses were performed using Pars Azmoon kits (Pars Azmoon Inc., Tehran, Iran) and a Selectra 2 auto-analyzer (Vital Scientific, Spankeren, The Netherlands). Both inter- and intra-assay coefficients of variation of all assays were <5%.

2.4. Dietary Assessment

A 168-item food frequency questionnaire (FFQ) was used at the first examination to assess typical food intakes over the previous year. The validity and reliability of the FFQ had previously been assessed in a random sample, by comparing the data from two FFQs, completed 1 year apart and comparing the data from the FFQs and 12 dietary recalls, respectively; the validity and reliability of the FFQ for total dietary fat were acceptable; correlation coefficients between the FFQ and multiple 24 recalls were 0.59 and 0.38 and those between the two FFQs were 0.43 and 0.42 in male and female subjects, respectively [14]. Study of the reliability, comparative validity and stability of dietary patterns derived from the FFQ also showed that there was a reasonable reliability and validity of the dietary patterns among the population over time [15]. Trained dietitians asked participants to designate their intake frequency for each food item consumed during the past year on a daily, weekly, or monthly basis. Portion sizes of consumed foods reported in household measures were then converted to grams. Energy and nutrient content of foods and beverages were analyzed using the US Department of Agriculture Food Composition Table (FCT) because the Iranian FCT is incomplete, and has limited data on nutrient content of raw foods and beverages [13]. Finally, dietary intakes of participants, including dietary energy and energy density, macronutrients, and micronutrients were determined. In addition to calculating total dietary fiber from all foods, soluble and insoluble dietary fiber intakes were separately calculated. Additionally, we computed dietary fiber from different sources including cereal (traditional breads including barbari, taftoon, sangak, lavash, baguette breads, white rice, and barley), legumes (soya, cowpea, chickpea, broad bean, red bean, white bean, lentil, and split pea), nuts (almond, pistachio, walnut, hazelnut, and peanut), vegetables (green leafy vegetables, roots, starchy vegetables, and other vegetables including cucumber, tomato, scallion, zucchini, eggplant, cauliflower, onion, and garlic) and fruits (cantaloupe, melon watermelon, pear, apricot, cherries, apple, peach, nectarines, figs, grapes, kiwi, grapefruit, tangerine, pomegranate, strawberry, banana, lemons) as well.

2.5. Definition of Terms

History of cardiovascular disease was defined as previous ischemic heart disease and/or cerebrovascular accidents. Family history of premature cardiovascular disease reflected any prior diagnosis of cardiovascular disease in first-degree female relatives, aged <65 years, or first-degree male relatives, aged <55 years. Diabetes was defined as fasting serum glucose ≥126, 2 h serum glucose ≥200 or anti-diabetic medications [16]. Hypertension (HTN) was considered as systolic BP ≥140 mmHg or systolic BP ≥90 mmHg or current use of antihypertensive medications [17]. Homeostatic model assessment of insulin resistance was defined as follows: HOMA-IR = fasting insulin (μU/mL) × fasting glucose (mmol/L)/22.5; this index has been developed as a simple, inexpensive, and validated alternative tool for assessment of insulin resistance in epidemiological studies [18,19]. Insulin resistance was defined as HOMA-IR ≥3.2 [20].

2.6. Definition of Outcome in Our Study

Details of the collection of cardiovascular outcome data have been described elsewhere [21]. Briefly, each participant was followed up for any medical event annually by phone calls. Information of any medical condition or event was collected by a trained nurse, a trained physician and by utilization of data from medical files. The collected data were evaluated and confirmed by an outcome committee consisting of an internist, an endocrinologist, a cardiologist, an epidemiologist and other experts. CHD were included cases of definite myocardial infarction (MI) (diagnostic ECG and biomarkers), probable MI (positive ECG findings plus cardiac symptoms or signs plus missing biomarkers or positive ECG findings plus equivocal biomarkers), and angiographic proven CHD. Cardiovascular disease was defined as any CHD events, stroke (a new neurological deficit that lasted ≥24 h), or CVD death (definite fatal MI, definite fatal CHD, and definite fatal stroke) [22]. The CVD risk score was calculated according to the sex-specific "general CVD" algorithms were derived that incorporated age, total cholesterol, HDL-C, SBP, treatment for HTN, smoking, and diabetes status [23].

2.7. Statistical Methods

Dietary intakes of fiber and other nutrients were adjusted for total energy intake, according to residuals methods [24]. Mean (SD) values and the frequencies (%) of baseline characteristics of the participants, with and without CVD event were compared using independent t test or chi square test, respectively.

Linear associations of baseline intakes of total and different types of dietary fiber with changes of serum lipids, blood pressure and insulin levels during the follow-up period were estimated using linear regression models with adjustment of age, sex, and BMI.

A univariate analysis was performed for potential confounding variables including CVD risk score, dietary intake of total fats (% of energy), sodium (mg/1000 kcal), and vitamin C (mg/1000 kcal); variables with $P_E < 0.2$ in the univariate analyses were selected for the final multivariable models. Adjustment of CVD risk score, as a continuous potential risk factor of CVD, improve the stability of our models in the case of a limited number of events during the study follow-up.

To determine whether the associations of soluble and insoluble fiber intake are independent of each other, we adjusted the models in the presence of each type of the fiber. Similarly, the analyses of fiber from each different source were adjusted for fiber from all of the other sources.

Cox proportional hazard regression was used to assess the hazard ratios (HRs) of dietary fiber intakes for CVD. Time to event was defined by time of censoring or having event, whichever came first. The proportional hazards assumption was tested. We censored participants at the time of other causes of death, leaving the district or being in the study until March 2012 without event. The energy-adjusted amount of dietary fiber and its different types was categorized into tertiles, and the first tertile was given as a reference. Two Cox proportional hazard regression models were defined; model 1 was adjusted for CVD risk score and model 2 was further adjusted for dietary intakes of total fats, sodium and vitamin C. To assess the overall trends of HRs across tertiles of dietary fiber intakes, the median of each tertile was used as a continuous variable in Cox proportional hazard regression models.

All analyses were performed using IBM SPSS for Windows version 19 and STATA version 12 SE (StataCorp LP, College Station, TX, USA), with a two-tailed p value < 0.05 being considered significant.

3. Results

Mean age of participants (42.8% men) was 38.2 $\pm$ 13.4, at baseline. Mean (SD) dietary intake of total fiber was 23.4 (8.9) g/day. Legumes (35.8%), fruits (30.4%), vegetables (27.8%), and grains (24.0%) had greater contributions to total intakes of dietary fiber, respectively. During the average 4.7 $\pm$ 1.4 year of follow-up, 57 participants experienced CVD events; of which the more common events were angiographic proven CVD (40.4%), definite MI (24.6%), unstable angina (12.2%) and stroke (8.8%).

The distributions of the major known CVD risk factors and some biochemical values for the participants who had a CVD event and for those who did not are shown in Table 1. Higher prevalence of diabetes (14.3 vs. 3.9, $p = 0.002$) and HTN (43.9 vs. 8.3, $p = 0.001$), as well as higher rate of medications, including lipid-lowering drugs, anti-hypertensive drugs and aspirin, was observed in subjects with CVD events, compared to the rest of the cohort. Compared with non-CVD subjects, CVD patients were more likely to be older, and had higher BMI, waist circumference, blood pressure, serum creatinine, FPG, TG, TG/HDL-C ratio and CVD risk score at baseline (p for all < 0.05). Compared to non-CVD subjects, CVD patients had also higher intakes of dietary carbohydrate and lower intake of mono-unsaturated fatty acids and fiber (p for all < 0.05).

Results of linear regression showed a significant association between grain fiber intake and baseline CVD risk score ($\beta = 0.05$, 95% CI = 0.02–0.08) as well as changes of HOMA-IR ($\beta = 0.04$, 95% CI = 0.01–0.08) during the study follow-up. Legume fiber was associated with baseline CVD risk score ($\beta = -0.14$, 95% CI = -0.23, -0.04) and changes of HDL-C ($\beta = 0.64$, 95% CI = 0.19–1.08). Furthermore, dietary fiber from vegetables ($\beta = -0.24$, 95% CI = -0.34, -0.15), nuts ($\beta = -0.23$, 95% CI = -0.33, -0.13), fruits ($\beta = -0.18$, 95% CI = -0.28, -0.08) was inversely related to CVD risk score at baseline. Higher intake of dietary fiber from vegetables was related to lower levels of TG ($\beta = -7.4$, 95% CI = -12.7, -2.1) and TG/HDL-C ratio ($\beta = -0.18$, 95% CI = -0.29, -0.03), whereas dietary fiber intake from fruits was inversely related to changes of insulin levels ($\beta = -7.80$, 95% CI = -12.8, -2.7) and DBP ($\beta = -0.50$, 95% CI = -1.08, -0.03); compared to baseline values, higher intake of fruit-based fiber was also related to higher HDL-C levels ($\beta = 0.54$, 95% CI = 0.09–0.98).

Table 1. Baseline characteristics of the participants.

	Participants with CVD Outcome ($n = 57$)	Participants without CVD Outcome ($n = 2202$)	p Value
Age (years)	58.6 ± 9.7	37.3 ± 13.0	0.001
Male (%)	59.6	42.5	0.001
Smoking (%)	26.3	22.7	0.31
Body mass index (m^2/kg)	28.4 ± 4.4	26.5 ± 4.8	0.005
Lipid-lowering drugs (%)	10.5	1.5	0.001
Anti-hypertensive drugs (%)	14.3	1.5	0.001
Aspirin (%)	8.9	2.3	0.001
Waist circumference (cm)	97.2 ± 10.1	88.0 ± 13.2	0.001
Serum creatinine (μmol/L)	1.13 ± 0.18	1.03 ± 0.15	0.001
Systolic blood pressure (mmHg)	130 ± 17.4	109 ± 14.9	0.001
Diastolic blood pressure (mmHg)	80.2 ± 10.6	72.5 ± 10.3	0.001
Fasting blood glucose (mg/dL)	106 ± 39.9	88.5 ± 16.7	0.001
Serum triglycerides (mg/dL)	190 ± 107	132 ± 78.0	0.001
HDL-C (mg/dL)	40.2 ± 8.0	43.3 ± 10.4	0.03
TG/HDL-ratio	5.0 ± 3.2	3.4 ± 2.7	0.001
Serum insulin	7.4 ± 3.4	8.8 ± 4.9	0.13
HOMA-IR	1.5 ± 0.8	1.9 ± 0.8	0.28
Hyperinsulinemia (%)	12.5	17.6	0.57
Diabetes (%)	14.3	3.9	0.002
Hypertension (%)	43.9	8.3	0.001
Cardiovascular disease risk score	22.1	21.2	0.001
Dietary intakes			
Total fats (g/day)	74.1 ± 2.5	79.5 ± 0.4	0.03
Saturated fats (g/day)	24.8 ± 1.8	27.1 ± 0.3	0.22
Mono-unsaturated fat (g/day)	21.9 ± 1.0	27.6 ± 0.2	0.01
Sodium (mg/day)	4883 ± 410	4421 ± 66	0.26
Total carbohydrate (g/day)	337 ± 5.8	323 ± 0.9	0.02
Total fiber (g/day)	25.3 ± 1.1	29.0 ± 0.2	0.003

Data are mean ± SD unless stated otherwise (independent t-test for continuous variables and chi-square test for dichotomous variables was used.

There was also a significant negative association between fiber from nuts with body weight changes during the study period ($\beta = -2.01$, $p < 0.05$); no significant association was observed between other sources of dietary fiber or total fiber with changes of body weight.

The hazard ratios (95% CIs) of CVD across tertiles of dietary fiber and its categories are shown in Table 2. After adjustment of all potential confounding variables, a lower risk of CVD was observed in the highest compared to the lowest tertile of total dietary fiber intakes (HR = 0.39, 95% CI = 0.18–0.83, p for trend = 0.05). Soluble and insoluble dietary fiber was also negatively related to risk of CVD (HR = 0.19, 95% CI = 0.09–0.41, and HR = 0.31, 95% CI = 0.14–0.69) with a significant decreasing trend across increasing intakes (p for trend < 0.01).

Table 3 shows HRs (95% CIs) across tertile categories of different dietary sources of fiber. Dietary intake of grain and nut fiber had no significant association with the risk of CVD, whereas legume fiber intake was inversely related to risk of CVD (HR = 0.31, 95% CI = 0.15–0.65, in the third compared to the first tertile, p for trend = 0.003); similar associations were also observed for dietary intakes of fiber from fruit and vegetable sources. A combination of dietary fiber intake from vegetables, fruits and legumes also had similar impact on the risk of CVD (HR = 0.65, 95% CI = 0.34–1.24, and HR = 0.46, 95% CI = 0.22–0.96, in the second and third tertiles, respectively, p for trend = 0.11).

Table 2. The hazard ratio (95% CI) of coronary heart disease across tertiles of dietary fiber and its categories.

Dietary Fiber Intakes	T1	T2	T3	p for Trend
Total fiber				
Crude	Ref.	0.83 (0.45–1.54)	0.69 (0.36–1.33)	0.56
Model 1	Ref.	0.87 (0.46–1.62)	0.75 (0.38–1.46)	0.69
Model 2	Ref.	0.67 (0.35–1.26)	0.39 (0.18–0.83)	0.05
Soluble fiber				
Crude	Ref.	0.49 (0.26–0.91)	0.39 (0.20–0.76)	0.01
Model 1	Ref.	0.54 (0.29–1.03)	0.41 (0.20–0.82)	0.04
Model 2 [a]	Ref.	0.39 (0.21–0.75)	0.19 (0.09–0.41)	0.001
Insoluble fiber				
Crude	Ref.	0.64 (0.34–1.18)	0.53 (0.28–1.02)	0.15
Model 1	Ref.	0.72 (0.39–1.33)	0.58 (0.29–1.14)	0.25
Model 2 [b]	Ref.	0.54 (0.28–1.03)	0.31 (0.14–0.69)	0.014

Cox proportional hazard regression models were used. Model 1 was adjusted for cardiovascular disease risk score. Model 2 was additionally adjusted for dietary intake of total fats (% of energy), sodium (mg/1000 kcal), and vitamin C (mg/1000 kcal); [a] additionally adjusted for insoluble fiber; and [b] additionally adjusted for soluble fiber.

Table 3. The hazard ratio (95% CI) of coronary heart disease across tertiles of dietary fiber and its categories.

Dietary Fibers	T1	T2	T3	p for Trend
Grain fiber				
Crude	Ref.	0.89 (0.46–1.72)	1.11 (0.59–1.07)	0.79
Model 1	Ref.	0.83 (0.42–1.62)	0.98 (0.52–1.84)	0.84
Model 2	Ref.	0.79 (0.39–1.61)	0.90 (0.44–1.86)	0.82
Legume fiber				
Crude	Ref.	0.61 (0.34–1.11)	0.36 (0.18–0.73)	0.01
Model 1	Ref.	0.59 (0.32–1.09)	0.38 (0.18–0.77)	0.02
Model 2	Ref.	0.47 (0.25–0.89)	0.31 (0.15–0.65)	0.003
Nut fiber				
Crude	Ref.	0.78 (0.43–1.41)	0.47 (0.24–0.94)	0.10
Model 1	Ref.	0.77 (0.43–1.42)	0.54 (0.27–1.07)	0.21
Model 2	Ref.	0.65 (0.33–1.27)	0.49 (0.24–1.02)	0.14
Fruit fiber				
Crude	Ref.	0.74 (0.39–1.39)	0.81 (0.43–1.50)	0.61
Model 1	Ref.	0.74 (0.38–1.41)	0.83 (0.44–1.58)	0.65
Model 2	Ref.	0.56 (0.29–1.09)	0.44 (0.22–0.89)	0.05
Vegetable fiber				
Crude	Ref.	0.83 (0.45–1.52)	0.59 (0.31–1.16)	0.32
Model 1	Ref.	0.82 (0.45–1.51)	0.61 (0.31–1.21)	0.37
Model 2	Ref.	0.64 (0.34–1.20)	0.34 (0.16–0.72)	0.02

Cox proportional hazard regression models were used. Model 1 was adjusted for cardiovascular disease risk score. Model 2 was additionally adjusted for dietary intake of total fats (% of energy), sodium (mg/1000 kcal), and vitamin C (mg/1000 kcal), and other types of dietary fiber (g/day).

4. Discussion

In this prospective cohort study, conducted on a representative Iranian population, a mean 4.7-year follow-up showed that dietary fiber intake especially from legume, fruit, vegetable and nut sources had protective effect against the development of CVD events. Following adjustment of multiple CVD risk factors and dietary variables, most negative trends in the current study remained statistically significant.

Beneficial effects of vegetable fiber in reduced risk of CVD, in our study, could be related to decreased TG and TG to HDL-C ratio during the study follow-up. Lower risk of CVD across increasing intakes of dietary fiber from fruit sources could also be attributed to its inverse association with insulin levels and DBP as well as positive association with HDL-C. Lack of the beneficial effects of grain fiber on the risk of CVD may be explained by its positive relation with CVD risk score at baseline and its association with increased insulin resistance index during the study follow-up. It should be noted that in our study, high intakes of refined grains such as white rice and white breads had major contributions to dietary intakes of grain fiber, whereas the protective effects of grain fiber, reported in some previous studies, were mainly related to whole grains intake [11]. Aside from chance and biases, another explanation is that other characteristics of refined grains such as high-glycemic index nature, rather than fiber per se, may be responsible for the associations observed.

In a 6-year follow-up study among adult men, higher fiber intake (28.9 vs. 12.4 g/day) was inversely related to risk of total myocardial infarction by 0.41 (RR = 0.59, 95% CI = 0.46–0.76); the inverse association was strongest for fatal myocardial infarction (RR = 0.45, 95% CI = 0.28–0.72) [25]. Each 10-g increase in total dietary fiber corresponded to an RR for total myocardial infarction of 0.81 (95% CI, 0.70–0.93); among the three main food contributors to total fiber intake, cereal fiber had a stronger effect on the reduced risk of total myocardial infarction (RR = 0.71, 95% CI = 0.55–0.91 for each 10-g increase in cereal fiber/day) [25]. In another prospective cohort of elderly men, only cereal fiber consumption was associated with lower incident total stroke and ischemic stroke, whereas neither fruit fiber intake nor vegetable fiber intake were associated with incident CVD; compared to cereal fiber from other sources, fiber from dark breads including wheat, rye, and pumpernickel were associated with a lower risk of CVD (HR = 0.76, 95% CI = 0.64–0.90) [26].

Findings of a recent meta-analysis of 22 prospective cohorts showed that total dietary fiber intake was inversely associated with risk of CVD (Risk ratio = 0.91 per 7 g/day, 95% CI = 0.88 to 0.94) and CVD (Risk ratio = 0.91, 95% CI = 0.87–0.94); insoluble fiber and fiber from cereal and vegetable sources were inversely associated with the incident CVD and CVD, whereas fruit fiber intake was only inversely associated with risk of CVD [27]. No clear differences in the effect of dietary fiber intake from various food groups on CVD mortality have been observed in a cohort of adult men, although every additional 10 g/day intake of dietary total fiber reduced CVD mortality by 17% (95% CI = 2%–30%) and all-cause mortality by 9% (95% CI = 0%–18%) [28] (Table 4). The cardioprotective effect of dietary fiber has been found to be stronger for cereal fiber than for fruit or vegetable fiber [29]. In a cross-sectional study conducted on adult men and women, higher intakes of total fiber and insoluble fiber were inversely related to systolic blood pressure [30].

In our previous study, we showed that higher intake of total dietary fiber reduced the risk of metabolic syndrome by 47% (OR = 0.53, 95% CI = 0.39–0.74, p for trend < 0.05); soluble and insoluble fiber intakes were also related to lower risk of metabolic syndrome (OR = 0.60, 95% CI = 0.43–0.84, and OR = 0.51, 95% CI = 0.35–0.72). Similar findings were also observed for dietary fiber from fruits, cereals and legumes sources but not for vegetable and nut fiber [9]. In the National Health and Nutrition Examination Survey, dietary fiber intake was related to a low and intermediate lifetime CVD risk and there was a significant inverse linear association between dietary fiber intake and log-transformed C-reactive protein [31].

Some differences between our findings and those of other cohorts may be related to different dietary habits and dietary patterns; previous studies among Iranians demonstrated some major dietary patterns including traditional dietary pattern with higher load of white rice, traditional breads, vegetables, full-fat dairy products, hydrogenated fats, legumes, dried fruits and nuts; the healthy dietary pattern was related to a higher load of vegetables and fruits, whereas the Western pattern had higher load of fast foods, salty snacks, sweets, mayonnaise, and soft drinks [32,33]. Lack of significant associations between fiber from grains and nuts may be related to types of these food groups consumed among our population. Main grains consumed among the population were refined grains including white rice, and breads with a relatively low-fiber wheat flour; moreover, in our population, nuts were mainly consumed in the form of salty and roasted; these factors may reduce the expected protective effects of fiber from grains and nut sources.

Table 4. The association of dietary fiber intakes and the risk of cardiovascular disease.

Author	Study Population	Findings
Rimm et al. [25]	6-year follow-up study among adult men	Dietary intake of fiber 28.9 vs. 12.4 g/day decreased risk of total myocardial infarction (RR = 0.59, 95% CI = 0.46–0.76) and fatal myocardial infarction RR = 0.45, 95% CI = 0.28–0.72. Cereal fiber reduced risk of total MI (RR = 0.71, 95% CI = 0.55–0.91 for each 10 g/day increase in cereal fiber)
Mozaffarian et al. [26]	8.6-year follow-up of elderly men and women	Highest compared to the lowest quintile of cereal fiber consumption, decreased incident CVD (HR = 0.79; 95% CI = 0.62–0.99) Fruit fiber and vegetable fiber intake were not associated with incident CVD. Higher intake of cereal fiber was associated with lower risk of total stroke, ischemic stroke and ischemic heart disease death.
Streppel et al. [28]	40-year follow-up of adult men	Every additional 10 g/day of dietary fiber intake decreased CVD mortality by 17% (95% CI: 2%, 30%) and all-cause mortality by 9% (0%, 18%).
Threapleton et al. [27]	Meta-analysis of 22 prospective cohorts	Total fiber intake was inversely associated with risk of CVD (RR = 0.91 per 7 g/day, 95% CI = 0.88–0.94) and CVD (RR = 0.91, 95% CI = 0.87–0.94). Each 7 g/day increase in insoluble fiber (RR = 0.82, 95% CI = 0.70–0.96), fiber from cereal (RR = 0.84, 95% CI = 0.76 0.94), and each 4 g/day increase in fiber from vegetable sources (RR = 0.94, 95% CI = 0.89–1.00) decreased risk of CVD and CVD.

MI: Myocardial infarction; CVD: Coronary heart disease; CVD: Cardiovascular disease; HR + Hazard ratio; RR = Relative risk.

Several mechanisms have been proposed to explain beneficial effects of dietary fiber on metabolic pathways; Figure 2 displays some important mechanisms of cardioprotective effects of dietary fiber intakes. Colonic fermentation and subsequent production of short chain fatty acids is another metabolic effect of most types of dietary fiber especially soluble fibers; dietary fiber intake can also regulate gut hormonal responses that may act as satiety factors [34]. The lowering effect of dietary fiber on plasminogen activator inhibitor type 1 and factor VII coagulation activity is also another proposed mechanism for the biological actions of dietary fiber against cardiovascular outcomes [35,36]. Interplay between dietary fiber intakes and the intestinal microbiome has been found to modify the inflammatory responses in the body [37]. Considering the contributory role of gut microbiota in the development of cardiometabolic disorders, such as atherosclerosis, obesity, and type 2 diabetes, and the favorable effects of dietary fiber in modulation of gut microbiota, some cardioprotective properties of dietary fibers may be attributed to this mechanism [38–40].

Some strengths and limitations in the current study should be considered. Among the strength, its prospective population-based design, high participation rate and completeness of the follow-up, and use of a validated comprehensive FFQ to assess regular dietary intakes of the participants provided us an opportunity to investigate the associations of total intakes and different types of dietary fiber with 5-year incidence of CVD, relationship that have not been previously examined among Iranian population. Use of CVD risk score, based on age, total cholesterol, HDL-C, SBP, use of antihypertensive drugs, diabetes, and smoking status, in multivariate models allowed us to account for major CVD confounders without adding many variables that would lead to instability of our models. Of the study limitation, due to potential changes in CVD risk factors during the study follow-up, some degree of misclassification might have occurred which could lead to biased estimated hazard ratios towards the null, as inherent in any prospective study. Furthermore, both the participants' diets and the composition of food may have changed over the follow-up time, leading to errors in assessing dietary exposure of interest. Moreover, the young age of the participants resulted in low incidence of CVD during the study follow-up.

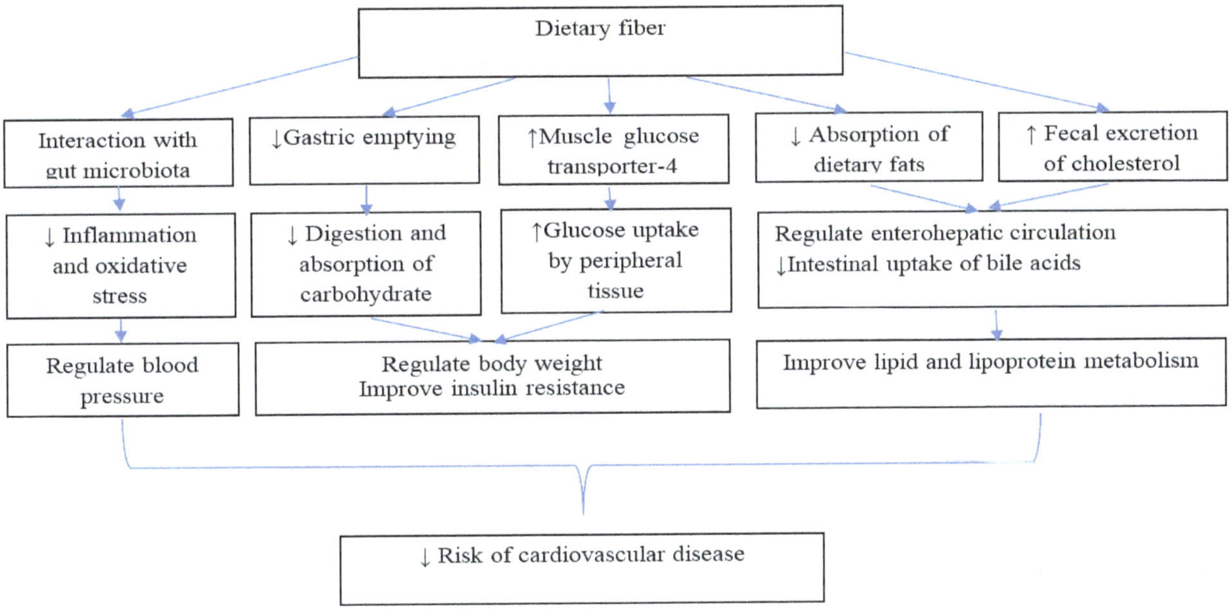

Figure 2. Mechanisms of protective effects of dietary fiber against development of cardiovascular disease. Dietary fiber improved insulin resistance by delaying gastric emptying, reduced absorption and digestion of carbohydrate and increased glucose uptake by peripheral tissue [34]. Dietary fiber also improved lipid and lipoprotein metabolism by decreased absorption of dietary fats, increased fecal excretion of cholesterol and decreased hepatic cholesterol synthesis; dietary fiber especially from cereal sources improved CVD health through multiple mechanisms including lipid reduction, body weight regulation, improved glucose metabolism, blood pressure control, and attenuation of oxidative stress and sub-clinical chronic inflammation [29]. Dietary fiber also modulated gut microbiota and modified cardiometabolic disorders [38–40].

5. Conclusions

In conclusion, our findings provided more evidence to confirm that increased intakes of fiber in a regular diet is an important cardioprotective dietary factor. Both soluble and insoluble dietary fibers have similar beneficial effects against the development of CVD. Dietary fiber intakes from legumes, vegetables and fruits may have stronger impact on cardiovascular outcomes.

Acknowledgments: We thank the TLGS participants and the field investigators of the TLGS for their cooperation and assistance in physical examinations, biochemical and nutritional evaluation and database management. We would like to acknowledge N. Shiva for critical editing of English grammar and syntax of the manuscript. This study was supported by grant No. 121 from the National Research Council of the Islamic Republic of Iran and the Research Institute for Endocrine Sciences of Shahid Beheshti University of Medical Sciences. This study was also supported by the Student Research Committee, Shahid Beheshti University of Medical Sciences (1395/S/47808).

Author Contributions: P.M., Z.B. and F.A. carried out the study design and analysis. P.M., Z.B., S.K.M., A.Z.V. and F.A. prepared the manuscript. All authors read and approved the final manuscript.

References

1. Pereira, M.A.; Liu, S. Types of carbohydrates and risk of cardiovascular disease. *J. Womens Health* **2003**, *12*, 115–122. [CrossRef] [PubMed]

2. Slavin, J.L. Position of the American Dietetic Association: Health implications of dietary fiber. *J. Am. Diet. Assoc.* **2008**, *108*, 1716–1731. [PubMed]
3. Lichtenstein, A.H.; Appel, L.J.; Brands, M.; Carnethon, M.; Daniels, S.; Franch, H.A.; Appel, L.J.; Brands, M.; Carnethon, M.; Daniels, S.; et al. Diet and lifestyle recommendations revision 2006: A scientific statement from the American Heart Association Nutrition Committee. *Circulation* **2006**, *114*, 82–96. [CrossRef] [PubMed]
4. Eilat-Adar, S.; Sinai, T.; Yosefy, C.; Henkin, Y. Nutritional recommendations for cardiovascular disease prevention. *Nutrients* **2013**, *5*, 3646–3683. [CrossRef] [PubMed]
5. Erkkila, A.T.; Lichtenstein, A.H. Fiber and cardiovascular disease risk: How strong is the evidence? *J. Cardiovasc. Nurs.* **2006**, *21*, 3–8. [CrossRef] [PubMed]
6. Eshak, E.S.; Iso, H.; Date, C.; Kikuchi, S.; Watanabe, Y.; Wada, Y.; Wakai, K.; Tamakoshi, A.; JACC Study Group. Dietary fiber intake is associated with reduced risk of mortality from cardiovascular disease among Japanese men and women. *J. Nutr.* **2010**, *140*, 1445–1453. [CrossRef] [PubMed]
7. Kokubo, Y.; Iso, H.; Saito, I.; Yamagishi, K.; Ishihara, J.; Inoue, M.; Tsugane, S.; JPHC Study Group. Dietary fiber intake and risk of cardiovascular disease in the Japanese population: The Japan Public Health Center-based study cohort. *Eur. J. Clin. Nutr.* **2011**, *65*, 1233–1241. [CrossRef] [PubMed]
8. McKeown, N.M.; Meigs, J.B.; Liu, S.; Saltzman, E.; Wilson, P.W.; Jacques, P.F. Carbohydrate nutrition, insulin resistance, and the prevalence of the metabolic syndrome in the Framingham Offspring Cohort. *Diabetes Care* **2004**, *27*, 538–546. [CrossRef] [PubMed]
9. Hosseinpour, S.M.P.; Sohrab, G.; Hosseini-Esfahani, F.; Azizi, F. Inverse association between fruit, legume, and cereal fiber and the risk of metabolic syndrome: Tehran Lipid and Glucose Study. *Diabetes Res. Clin. Pract.* **2011**, *94*, 276–283. [CrossRef] [PubMed]
10. Brown, L.; Rosner, B.; Willett, W.W.; Sacks, F.M. Cholesterol-lowering effects of dietary fiber: A meta-analysis. *Am. J. Clin. Nutr.* **1999**, *69*, 30–42. [PubMed]
11. Liu, S.; Buring, J.E.; Sesso, H.D.; Rimm, E.B.; Willett, W.C.; Manson, J.E. A prospective study of dietary fiber intake and risk of cardiovascular disease among women. *J. Am. Coll. Cardiol.* **2002**, *39*, 49–56. [CrossRef]
12. Azizi, F.; Rahmani, M.; Emami, H.; Mirmiran, P.; Hajipour, R.; Madjid, M.; Ghanbili, J.; Ghanbarian, A.; Mehrabi, Y.; Saadat, N.; et al. Cardiovascular risk factors in an Iranian urban population: Tehran lipid and glucose study (phase 1). *Soz. Praventivmed.* **2002**, *47*, 408–426. [CrossRef] [PubMed]
13. Hosseini-Esfahani, F.; Jessri, M.; Mirmiran, P.; Bastan, S.; Azizi, F. Adherence to dietary recommendations and risk of metabolic syndrome: Tehran Lipid and Glucose Study. *Metab. Clin. Exp.* **2010**, *59*, 1833–1842. [CrossRef] [PubMed]
14. Mirmiran, P.; Esfahani, F.H.; Mehrabi, Y.; Hedayati, M.; Azizi, F. Reliability and relative validity of an FFQ for nutrients in the Tehran lipid and glucose study. *Public Health Nutr.* **2010**, *13*, 654–662. [CrossRef] [PubMed]
15. Panagiotakos, D.B.; Pitsavos, C.; Skoumas, Y.; Stefanadis, C. The Association between Food Patterns and the Metabolic Syndrome Using Principal Components Analysis: The ATTICA Study. *J. Am. Diet. Assoc.* **2007**, *107*, 979–987. [CrossRef] [PubMed]
16. American Diabetes Association. Standards of medical care in diabetes—2014. *Diabetes Care* **2014**, *37*, S14–S80.
17. Chobanian, A.V.; Bakris, G.L.; Black, H.R.; Cushman, W.C.; Green, L.A.; Izzo, J.L., Jr.; Jones, D.W.; Materson, B.J.; Oparil, S.; Wright, J.T., Jr.; et al. The Seventh Report of the Joint National Committee on Prevention, Detection, Evaluation, and Treatment of High Blood Pressure: The JNC 7 report. *JAMA* **2003**, *289*, 2560–2572. [CrossRef] [PubMed]
18. Borai, A.; Livingstone, C.; Kaddam, I.; Ferns, G. Selection of the appropriate method for the assessment of insulin resistance. *BMC Med. Res. Methodol.* **2011**, *11*, 158. [CrossRef] [PubMed]
19. Muniyappa, R.; Lee, S.; Chen, H.; Quon, M.J. Current approaches for assessing insulin sensitivity and resistance in vivo: Advantages, limitations, and appropriate usage. *Am. J. Physiol. Endocrinol. Metab.* **2008**, *94*, E15–E26. [CrossRef] [PubMed]
20. Enzevaei, A.; Salehpour, S.; Tohidi, M.; Saharkhiz, N. Subclinical hypothyroidism and insulin resistance in polycystic ovary syndrome: Is there a relationship? *Iran. J. Reprod. Med.* **2014**, *12*, 481–486. [PubMed]
21. Hadaegh, F.; Harati, H.; Ghanbarian, A.; Azizi, F. Association of total cholesterol versus other serum lipid parameters with the short-term prediction of cardiovascular outcomes: Tehran Lipid and Glucose Study. *Eur. J. Cardiovasc. Prev. Rehabil.* **2006**, *13*, 571–577. [CrossRef] [PubMed]

22. Nejat, A.; Mirbolouk, M.; Mohebi, R.; Hasheminia, M.; Tohidi, M.; Saadat, N.; Azizi, F.; Hadaegh, F. Changes in lipid measures and incident coronary heart disease: Tehran Lipid & Glucose Study. *Clin. Biochem.* **2014**, *47*, 1239–1244. [PubMed]
23. D'Agostino, R.B., Sr.; Vasan, R.S.; Pencina, M.J.; Wolf, P.A.; Cobain, M.; Massaro, J.M.; Kannel, W.B. General cardiovascular risk profile for use in primary care: The Framingham Heart Study. *Circulation* **2008**, *117*, 743–753. [CrossRef] [PubMed]
24. Yilmaz, B.; Sahin, K.; Bilen, H.; Bahcecioglu, I.H.; Bilir, B.; Ashraf, S.; Halazun, K.J.; Kucuk, O. Carotenoids and non-alcoholic fatty liver disease. *Hepatobiliary Surg. Nutr.* **2015**, *4*, 161–171. [PubMed]
25. Rimm, E.B.; Ascherio, A.; Giovannucci, E.; Spiegelman, D.; Stampfer, M.J.; Willett, W.C. Vegetable, fruit, and cereal fiber intake and risk of coronary heart disease among men. *JAMA* **1996**, *275*, 447–451. [CrossRef] [PubMed]
26. Mozaffarian, D.; Kumanyika, S.K.; Lemaitre, R.N.; Olson, J.L.; Burke, G.L.; Siscovick, D.S. Cereal, fruit, and vegetable fiber intake and the risk of cardiovascular disease in elderly individuals. *JAMA* **2003**, *289*, 1659–1666. [CrossRef] [PubMed]
27. Threapleton, D.E.; Greenwood, D.C.; Evans, C.E.; Cleghorn, C.L.; Nykjaer, C.; Woodhead, C.; Cade, J.E.; Gale, C.P.; Burley, V.J. Dietary fibre intake and risk of cardiovascular disease: Systematic review and meta-analysis. *BMJ* **2013**, *347*, f6879. [CrossRef] [PubMed]
28. Streppel, M.T.; Ocké, M.C.; Boshuizen, H.C.; Kok, F.J.; Kromhout, D. Dietary fiber intake in relation to coronary heart disease and all-cause mortality over 40 years: The Zutphen Study. *Am. J. Clin. Nutr.* **2008**, *88*, 1119–1125. [PubMed]
29. Satija, A.; Hu, F.B. Cardiovascular benefits of dietary fiber. *Curr. Atheroscler. Rep.* **2012**, *14*, 505–514. [CrossRef] [PubMed]
30. Aljuraiban, G.S.; Griep, L.M.; Chan, Q.; Daviglus, M.L.; Stamler, J.; Van Horn, L.; Elliott, P.; Frost, G.S. Total, insoluble and soluble dietary fibre intake in relation to blood pressure: The INTERMAP Study. *Br. J. Nutr.* **2015**, *114*, 1480–1486. [CrossRef] [PubMed]
31. Ning, H.; Van Horn, L.; Shay, C.M.; Lloyd-Jones, D.M. Associations of Dietary Fiber Intake with Long-Term Predicted Cardiovascular Disease Risk and C-Reactive Protein Levels (from the National Health and Nutrition Examination Survey Data. *Am. J. Cardiol.* **2014**, *113*, 287–291. [CrossRef] [PubMed]
32. Doostvandi, T.; Bahadoran, Z.; Mozaffari-Khosravi, H.; Mirmiran, P.; Azizi, F. Food intake patterns are associated with the risk of impaired glucose and insulin homeostasis: A prospective approach in the Tehran Lipid and Glucose Study. *Public Health Nutr.* **2016**, *19*, 2467–2474. [CrossRef] [PubMed]
33. Moslehi, N.; Hosseini-Esfahani, F.; Hosseinpanah, F.; Mirmiran, P.; Azizi, F. Patterns of food consumption and risk of type 2 diabetes in an Iranian population: A nested case–control study. *Nutr. Diet.* **2016**, *73*, 169–176. [CrossRef]
34. Weickert, M.O.; Pfeiffer, A.F.H. Metabolic Effects of Dietary Fiber Consumption and Prevention of Diabetes. *J. Nutr.* **2008**, *138*, 439–442. [PubMed]
35. Anderson, J.W.; Tietyen-Clark, J. Dietary fiber: Hyperlipidemia, hypertension, and coronary heart disease. *Am. J. Gastroenterol.* **1986**, *81*, 907–919. [PubMed]
36. Anderson, J.W.; Chen, W.J. Plant fiber. Carbohydrate and lipid metabolism. *Am. J. Clin. Nutr.* **1979**, *32*, 346–363. [PubMed]
37. Kuo, S.M. The interplay between fiber and the intestinal microbiome in the inflammatory response. *Adv. Nutr.* **2013**, *4*, 16–28. [CrossRef] [PubMed]
38. Miele, L.; Giorgio, V.; Alberelli, M.A.; De Candia, E.; Gasbarrini, A.; Grieco, A. Impact of Gut Microbiota on Obesity, Diabetes, and Cardiovascular Disease Risk. *Curr. Cardiol. Rep.* **2015**, *17*, 120. [CrossRef] [PubMed]
39. Hamaker, B.R.; Tuncil, Y.E. A perspective on the complexity of dietary fiber structures and their potential effect on the gut microbiota. *J. Mol. Biol.* **2014**, *426*, 3838–3850. [CrossRef] [PubMed]
40. Parnell, J.A.; Reimer, R.A. Prebiotic fiber modulation of the gut microbiota improves risk factors for obesity and the metabolic syndrome. *Gut Microbes* **2012**, *3*, 29–34. [CrossRef] [PubMed]

16

Validity and Reproducibility of a Habitual Dietary Fibre Intake Short Food Frequency Questionnaire

Genelle Healey [1,2,*], Louise Brough [1], Rinki Murphy [3], Duncan Hedderley [2], Chrissie Butts [2] and Jane Coad [1]

[1] Massey Institute of Food Science and Technology, School of Food and Nutrition, Massey University, Palmerston North 4442, New Zealand; l.brough@massey.ac.nz (L.B.); j.coad@massey.ac.nz (J.C.)

[2] Food, Nutrition and Health, The New Zealand Institute for Plant & Food Research Limited, Palmerston North 4442, New Zealand; duncan.hedderley@plantandfood.co.nz (D.H.); chrissie.butts@plantandfood.co.nz (C.B.)

[3] Faculty of Medical and Health Sciences, The University of Auckland, Auckland 1023, New Zealand; r.murphy@auckland.ac.nz

* Correspondence: genelle.healey@plantandfood.co.nz;

Abstract: Low dietary fibre intake has been associated with poorer health outcomes, therefore having the ability to be able to quickly assess an individual's dietary fibre intake would prove useful in clinical practice and for research purposes. Current dietary assessment methods such as food records and food frequency questionnaires are time-consuming and burdensome, and there are presently no published short dietary fibre intake questionnaires that can quantify an individual's total habitual dietary fibre intake and classify individuals as low, moderate or high habitual dietary fibre consumers. Therefore, we aimed to develop and validate a habitual dietary fibre intake short food frequency questionnaire (DFI-FFQ) which can quickly and accurately classify individuals based on their habitual dietary fibre intake. In this study the DFI-FFQ was validated against the Monash University comprehensive nutrition assessment questionnaire (CNAQ). Fifty-two healthy, normal weight male (n = 17) and female (n = 35) participants, aged between 21 and 61 years, completed the DFI-FFQ twice and the CNAQ once. All eligible participants completed the study, however the data from 46% of the participants were excluded from analysis secondary to misreporting. The DFI-FFQ cannot accurately quantify total habitual dietary fibre intakes, however, it is a quick, valid and reproducible tool in classifying individuals based on their habitual dietary fibre intakes.

Keywords: dietary fibre; short food frequency questionnaire; validation

1. Introduction

Dietary fibre are non-digestible plant polysaccharides found in high amounts in fruits, vegetables, breads and cereals, legumes and nuts and seeds. Dietary fibre has been shown to have important implications on human health, including preventing and alleviating constipation, reducing gastrointestinal cancer incidence and blood glucose levels, lowering blood cholesterol levels and blood pressure, and beneficially modulating gut microbiota [1]. It is also possible that the efficacy of a dietary intervention is altered as a result of the influence habitual dietary fibre intake has on gut microbiota responsiveness and host outcomes. Therefore, being able to quickly assess an individual's habitual dietary fibre intake and classify individuals based on their dietary fibre intakes will prove useful in clinical practice and in nutrition and health research. Dietary assessment methods such as diet records and food frequency questionnaires have inherent limitations such as being difficult to complete accurately, time-consuming and may not accurately assess a person's habitual diet [2]. A small number of dietary fibre assessment questionnaires have been developed, however these questionnaires assess general dietary behaviours, do not estimate total dietary fibre amounts, and/or do not classify individuals based on habitual dietary fibre intakes [3–6]. Therefore, the primary aim of this study was to determine whether a newly developed dietary fibre intake short food frequency questionnaire (DFI-FFQ) can accurately classify individuals based on their habitual dietary fibre intake and the secondary aim of the study was to determine whether the DFI-FFQ can accurately quantify total habitual dietary fibre intakes.

2. Methods

2.1. Subjects

Participants were recruited via email and poster advertisement in multiple locations around Palmerston North, New Zealand. A diverse cross-section of the population was targeted to help ensure a good representation of the New Zealand population was recruited. Sixty-eight individuals provided informed consent to participate in this study, of which fifty-two healthy participants met the inclusion criteria (aged >19 and <65 years, healthy, BMI >18.5 and <30 kg/m^2, no significant weight loss or weight gain within the past year, no significant dietary change within the past year, not pregnant or breastfeeding, no food intolerances which cause gastrointestinal symptoms (i.e., lactose intolerance, gluten sensitivity), no adverse gastrointestinal symptoms, non-smoker and not high alcohol consumers). Participants completed the DFI-FFQ twice, at least 2 weeks apart, and the comprehensive nutrition assessment questionnaire (CNAQ) once. The DFI-FFQ was completed initially, followed by the CNAQ, and lastly the repeated DFI-FFQ was completed. The CNAQ and DFI-FFQ were both completed online. An energy intake: basal metabolic rate (EI:BMR) of <1.1 and >2.19 was used to exclude participants who appeared to have over- or under-reported using the CNAQ [7]. Ethical approval was obtained from the Massey University Human Ethics Committee (Southern A, Application 15/34).

2.2. Development of the DFI-FFQ

The DFI-FFQ (Figure S1) was designed to quickly and accurately classify individuals as low, moderate or high habitual dietary fibre consumers and quantify an individual's habitual dietary fibre intake (g/day). The DFI-FFQ consists of five high dietary fibre containing food groups (vegetables, fruits, breads and cereals, nuts and seeds and legumes) which account for 73.5% of the dietary fibre in a typical New Zealand diet [8]. Examples of what one serve is equivalent to, for each food group, is detailed within the DFI-FFQ. The frequency of consumption for the average number of serves consumed over the past year, was given as follows: Never, <1/month, 1–3/month, 1/week, 2–4/week, 5–6/week, 1/day, 2/day, 3/day, 4/day, 5/day and 6+/day.

2.3. DFI-FFQ Scoring Sheet

A scoring sheet was developed to quantify the amount of dietary fibre consumed and to classify individuals as low, moderate and high dietary fibre consumers. FoodWorks version 7.0.3016 (Xyris Software Pty Ltd., Brisbane, Queensland, Australia) was used to quantify the average amount of dietary fibre provided by the five food groups for each frequency of consumption. An individual's total dietary fibre intake was calculated by adding together the average amount of dietary fibre consumed from each food group in relation to the number of serves consumed.

2.4. Dietary Fibre Classification

The cut-offs used to classify individuals based on their dietary fibre intakes are outlined in Table 1. The high dietary fibre intake cut-offs were selected to reflect the New Zealand Ministry of Health recommended dietary fibre intake guidelines; >25 g/day for females and >30 g/day for males [9]. The low dietary fibre intake cut-offs were selected as the median dietary fibre intake in New Zealand was 17.5 g/day for females and 22.1 g/day for males, which are below recommended amounts [8].

Similar cut-offs have been used previously however the specific cut-offs used in this study were modified to be applicable to a New Zealand population [3].

Table 1. The dietary fibre intake cut-offs used to classify individuals as low, moderate and high dietary fibre consumers.

	Females	Males
Low	<18 g/day	<22 g/day
Moderate	18–24.9 g/day	22–29.9 g/day
High	≥25 g/day	≥30 g/day

2.5. Dietary Assessment Method Used for Comparison

The Monash University online CNAQ was used for comparison with the DFI-FFQ. The 297-item food frequency questionnaire has been shown to be valid in assessing habitual dietary intakes when compared to four 7-day food records, each completed three months apart [10].

2.6. Statistical Analysis

We aimed to recruit enough participants to ensure that correlations over 0.7 would be statistically significant and that the assumptions of *chi-squared* tests would not be over stretched. The relationship between results of the DFI-FFQ when compared to the CNAQ was determined using Spearman correlation, Pearson correlation, Bland-Altman plot, *chi-squared* test and linear weighted kappa score. Test-retest repeatability was assessed using Pearson correlation, Bland-Altman plot and Cronbach's alpha. *T*-tests were used to determine whether there were any differences in dietary fibre intakes between the DFI-FFQ and CNAQ and the repeated DFI-FFQ. A p value of < 0.05 is considered significant. Statistical analysis was carried out using GenStat 17th edition (VSNi Ltd., Hemel Hempstead, UK), Minitab 16th edition (Cronbach's alpha) (Minitab Inc., State College, PA, USA) and the calculator at http://vassarstats.net/kappa.html (kappa score) [11].

3. Results

All eligible participants ($n = 52$) completed the study. The data from 28 participants (54%) were used as the data from 24 participants (46%) were excluded from the analysis secondary to likely misreporting on the CNAQ; with 18 participants (34.5%) having over-reported and six participants (11.5%) having under-reported their energy intakes. The group mean EI:BMR was 2.8 (SD 4.7) prior to exclusion and reduced to 1.6 (SD 0.3) after exclusion. Participant characteristics, total dietary fibre intakes and classifications determined by the DFI-FFQ and CNAQ are summarised in Table 2. The median dietary fibre intake in New Zealand (20.3 g/day) [8] is similar to the average dietary fibre intake of the study cohort, with dietary fibre intakes from both groups being below the New Zealand recommended dietary fibre intake guidelines [9]. The DFI-FFQ took on average 3.5 min to complete in comparison to the estimated completion time of 20–40 min for the CNAQ.

When comparing the DFI-FFQ to the CNAQ for dietary fibre classification, exact agreement occurred 79% of the time and gross misclassification occurred 7% of the time (Table 3). There was a significant difference in dietary fibre intakes between the DFI-FFQ and CNAQ (CNAQ was on average 5 g/day higher than the DFI-FFQ). The two dietary assessment methods were however correlated (Pearson correlation 0.65, Spearman correlation 0.53). A *chi-squared* test indicated an association between the classifications based on the DFI-FFQ and CNAQ ($p = 0.002$) and the linear weighted kappa score showed good agreement [12] (Table 4). The Bland-Altman plot is available within the Supplementary information (Figure S2A).

Table 2. Characteristics, dietary fibre intakes and classifications for the study participants.

Mean (SD)	Male (n = 8)	Female (n = 20)	Total (n = 28)
Participant characteristics			
Age (years)	40 (11.02)	38 (9.37)	39 (9.91)
BMI (kg/m^2)	24 (1.9)	23 (3.1)	24 (2.82)
Ethnicity (No.)			
New Zealand European	4	14	18
Asian	3	0	3
Maori	0	2	2
Other	1	4	5
Dietary fibre intakes and classifications			
DFI-FFQ			
Dietary fibre intake (g/day)	27 (11.77)	23 (10.33)	24 (10.85)
Dietary fibre classification (No.)			
Low	2	5	7
Moderate	2	4	6
High	4	11	15
Monash CNAQ			
Dietary fibre intake (g/day)	31 (11.35)	29 (9.43)	29 (10.09)
Dietary fibre classification (No.)			
Low	1	4	5
Moderate	3	1	4
High	4	15	19

DFI-FFQ: dietary fibre intake short food frequency questionnaire; CNAQ: comprehensive nutrition assessment questionnaire; SD: standard deviation.

Table 3. Comparison in dietary fibre classification between the comprehensive nutrition assessment questionnaire (CNAQ) and the dietary fibre intake food frequency questionnaire (DFI-FFQ).

		CNAQ			Total
		Low	Moderate	High	
DFI-FFQ	Low	5 (18%)	0 (0%)	2 (7%)	7 (25%)
	Moderate	0 (0%)	3 (11%)	3 (11%)	6 (21%)
	High	0 (0%)	1 (3%)	14 (50%)	15 (54%)
Total		5 (18%)	4 (14%)	19 (68%)	28 (100%)

Table 4. Correlation and test-retest repeatability statistical analysis.

Correlation between DFI-FFQ and CNAQ		p Value
Pearson correlation	0.65	<0.001
Spearman correlation	0.53	0.001
Chi-square test	9.6	0.002
Linear weighted kappa *	0.68	
Standard error	0.14	
Magnitude of agreement	Good	
Bland-Altman plot		
Limits of agreement (g/day)	−12.5–22.6	
Standard error	1.7	
Mean difference (g/day)	5	0.007
Test-Retest Repeatability		***p* value**
Pearson correlation	0.94	<0.001
Cronbach's alpha	0.97	
Bland-Altman plot		
Limits of agreement (g/day)	−6.0–9.6	
Standard error	0.72	
Mean difference (g/day)	1.8	0.019

CNAQ: comprehensive nutrition assessment questionnaire; DFI-FFQ: dietary fibre intake short food frequency questionnaire; * One category disagreement had a weight of 3/4 .

Pearson correlation (0.94) and Cronbach's alpha (0.97) showed that the repeated DFI-FFQ correlated. The estimated dietary fibre intake from the second DFI-FFQ was significantly lower than the first DFI-FFQ by 1.8 g/day (Table 4). The Bland-Altman plot is available within the Supplementary information (Figure S2B).

4. Discussion

Presently, there are no known short dietary fibre intake questionnaires that are able to classify individuals based on their habitual dietary fibre intake. Having the ability to be able to quickly and accurately classify an individual based on their dietary fibre intake will prove useful as low dietary fibre intakes have been associated with poorer health outcomes [13]. This study has shown that the DFI-FFQ can accurately classifying individuals based on their habitual dietary fibre intakes.

There was however, a significant difference in habitual dietary fibre intakes between the repeated DFI-FFQs and the DFI-FFQ and CNAQ, which suggests the DFI-FFQ might not accurately quantify total habitual dietary fibre intakes. Research has shown that large food item FFQs overestimate fruit and vegetable consumption, which may help explain the higher dietary fibre intakes determined from the CNAQ [14]. The addition of other dietary fibre contributing food groups, such as cakes and muffins, pies and pastries and biscuits, to the DFI-FFQ may have helped to improve the questionnaire's accuracy in quantifying total habitual dietary fibre intakes as these food groups collectively contribute 6.3% of the dietary fibre in a typical New Zealand diet [8]. Another reason why the DFI-FFQ may not have been able to accurately quantify total habitual dietary fibre intakes may be related to the serving size examples provided. The examples provided did not include all possible foods within a particular food group and relied on participants to use their own judgement regarding the number of serves consumed for foods that were not specifically listed.

There are a handful of short questionnaires that have been developed to assess dietary fibre intakes however these questionnaires assess general dietary behaviours [4–6], do not estimate total dietary fibre amounts [4–6], and/or do not classify individuals based on habitual dietary fibre intakes [3–6]. The DFI-FFQ is novel as it can accurately classify individuals based on habitual dietary fibre intake. Unlike previously developed questionnaires, the DFI-FFQ was validated against an FFQ which assesses dietary intake over the past year, providing a more accurate account of long term rather than current dietary fibre intakes. Additionally, some of the questionnaires were validated using fairly homogenous populations, such as factory workers [3] and patients [5], making these questionnaires less useful in more diverse populations, such as in this study.

When comparing the study cohorts average dietary fibre intake to the Adult Nutrition Survey data [8] it appeared the study cohort has a similar dietary fibre intake to the New Zealand population. Therefore, the DFI-FFQ is a valid tool for classifying individuals based on their habitual dietary fibre intakes in New Zealand. In countries where dietary fibre intakes are distinctly different from New Zealand, the DFI-FFQ may need to be re-validated in these populations.

Forty-six percent of participants were excluded from the study secondary to misreporting on the CNAQ, which reduced the data available for analysis. A known limitation of FFQs is the high rate of misreporting, however the rate of misreporting in this study was much higher than previously reported [15]. It may therefore be useful to compare the DFI-FFQ to another dietary assessment method (i.e., 3- or 7-day diet records, or shorter validated FFQ) to confirm these results. The sample size for this study was small however a sufficient number of participants were recruited based on the sample size calculations, even after exclusion for misreporting. Additionally, other dietary questionnaire validation studies have similarly small participant numbers [16,17]. Despite the limitations discussed, we believe the DFI-FFQ will be a valuable tool in research and clinical practice as it is quick to complete (3.5 min on average), has low respondent burden and is a valid and reproducible method of classifying individuals based on their habitual dietary fibre intakes.

5. Conclusions

The DFI-FFQ has been shown to be a quick, valid and reproducible tool in classifying individuals based on their habitual dietary fibre intakes. The DFI-FFQ cannot however, accurately estimate total habitual dietary fibre intakes.

Author Contributions: G.H. was involved in the conception, study design, recruitment, conducting the study, and writing and editing the manuscript. J.C., C.B., R.M. and L.B. were involved in the conception, study design and editing of the manuscript. D.H. conducted the statistical analysis and was involved in editing the manuscript. All authors read and approved the manuscript.

Acknowledgments: The authors would like to take the opportunity to thank the individuals who participated in this study. The study was supported by the Foods for Health programme (C11X1312). The funds for the Foods for Health programme were provided to a number of collaborating New Zealand organisations, including The New Zealand Institute for Plant & Food Research Limited, by the Ministry of Business, Innovation and Employment, New Zealand Government.

References

1. Fuller, S.; Beck, E.; Salman, H.; Tapsell, L. New horizons for the study of dietary fiber and health: A review. *Plant Foods Hum. Nutr.* **2016**, *71*, 1–12. [CrossRef] [PubMed]
2. Thompson, F.E.; Subar, A.F. Dietary assessment methodology. In *Nutrition in the Prevention and Treatment of Disease*, 2nd ed.; Coulston, A.M., Boushey, C.J., Eds.; Elsevier: London, UK, 2008; pp. 3–39.
3. Roe, L.; Strong, C.; Whiteside, C.; Neil, A.; Mant, D. Dietary intervention in primary care: Validity of the DINE method for diet assessment. *Fam. Pract.* **1994**, *11*, 375–381. [CrossRef] [PubMed]
4. Wright, J.L.; Scott, J.A. The fat and fibre barometer, a short food behaviour questionnaire: Reliability, relative validity and utility. *Aust. J. Nutr. Diet.* **2000**, *57*, 33–39.
5. Shannon, J.; Kristal, A.R.; Curry, S.J.; Beresford, S.A. Application of a behavioral approach to measuring dietary change: The fat- and fiber-related diet behavior questionnaire. *Cancer Epidemiol. Biomark. Prev.* **1997**, *6*, 355–361.
6. Svilaas, A.; Strom, E.C.; Svilaas, T.; Borgejordet, A.; Thoresen, M.; Ose, L. Reproducibility and validity of a short food questionnaire for the assessment of dietary habits. *Nutr. Metab. Cardiovasc. Dis.* **2002**, *12*, 60–70. [PubMed]
7. Black, A.E. Critical evaluation of energy intake using the Goldberg cut-off for energy intake: Basal metabolic rate. A practical guide to its calculation, use and limitations. *Int. J. Obes.* **2000**, *24*, 1119–1130. [CrossRef]
8. Ministry of Health. A Focus on Nutrition Key Findings of the 2008/09 New Zealand Adult Nutrition Survey. Available online: https://www.health.govt.nz/system/files/documents/publications/a-focus-on-nutrition-v2.pdf (accessed on 15 July 2016).
9. Ministry of Health; Department of Health and Ageing. Nutrient Reference Values for Australia and New Zealand. Available online: http://www.health.govt.nz/publication/nutrient-reference-values-australia-and-new-zealand (accessed on 15 July 2016).
10. Barrett, J.S.; Gibson, P.R. Development and validation of a comprehensive semi-quantitative food frequency questionnaire that includes FODMAP intake and glycemic index. *J. Am. Diet. Assoc.* **2010**, *110*, 1469–1476. [CrossRef] [PubMed]
11. Kappa as a Measure of Concordance in Categorical Sorting. Available online: http://vassarstats.net/kappa.html (accessed on 15 July 2016).
12. Masson, L.F.; McNeill, G.; Tomany, J.O.; Simpson, J.A.; Peace, H.S.; Wei, L.; Grubb, D.A.; Bolton-Smith, C. Statistical approaches for assessing the relative validity of a food-frequency questionnaire: Use of correlation coefficients and the kappa statistic. *Public Health Nutr.* **2003**, *6*, 313–321. [CrossRef] [PubMed]
13. Buil-Cosiales, P.; Zazpe, I.; Toledo, E.; Corella, D.; Salas-Salvadó, J.; Diez-Espino, J.; Ros, E.; Navajas, J.F.C.; Santos-Lozano, J.M.; Arós, F.; et al. Fiber intake and all-cause mortality in the Prevención con Dieta Mediterránea (PREDIMED) study. *Am. J. Clin. Nutr.* **2014**, *100*, 1498–1507. [CrossRef] [PubMed]
14. Krebs-Smith, S.M.; Heimendinger, J.; Subar, A.F.; Patterson, B.H.; Pivonka, E. Using food frequency questionnaires to estimate fruit and vegetable intake: Association between the number of questions and total intakes. *J. Nutr. Educ.* **1995**, *27*, 80–85. [CrossRef]

15. Molag, M.L.; De Vries, J.H.; Ocke, M.C.; Dagnelie, P.C.; Van Den Brandt, P.A.; Jansen, M.C.; van Staveren, W.A.; van't Veer, P. Design characteristics of food frequency questionnaires in relation to their validity. *Am. J. Epidemiol.* **2007**, *166*, 1468–1478. [CrossRef] [PubMed]
16. O'Reilly, S.; McCann, L. Development and validation of the Diet Quality Tool for use in cardiovascular disease prevention settings. *Aust. J. Prim. Health* **2012**, *18*, 138–147. [CrossRef] [PubMed]
17. Spoon, M.; Devereux, P.; Benedict, J.; Leontos, C.; Constantino, N.; Christy, D.; Snow, G. Usefulness of the food habits questionnaire in a worksite setting. *J. Nutr. Educ. Behav.* **2002**, *34*, 268–272. [CrossRef]

Permissions

All chapters in this book were first published by MDPI; hereby published with permission under the Creative Commons Attribution License or equivalent. Every chapter published in this book has been scrutinized by our experts. Their significance has been extensively debated. The topics covered herein carry significant findings which will fuel the growth of the discipline. They may even be implemented as practical applications or may be referred to as a beginning point for another development.

The contributors of this book come from diverse backgrounds, making this book a truly international effort. This book will bring forth new frontiers with its revolutionizing research information and detailed analysis of the nascent developments around the world.

We would like to thank all the contributing authors for lending their expertise to make the book truly unique. They have played a crucial role in the development of this book. Without their invaluable contributions this book wouldn't have been possible. They have made vital efforts to compile up to date information on the varied aspects of this subject to make this book a valuable addition to the collection of many professionals and students.

This book was conceptualized with the vision of imparting up-to-date information and advanced data in this field. To ensure the same, a matchless editorial board was set up. Every individual on the board went through rigorous rounds of assessment to prove their worth. After which they invested a large part of their time researching and compiling the most relevant data for our readers.

The editorial board has been involved in producing this book since its inception. They have spent rigorous hours researching and exploring the diverse topics which have resulted in the successful publishing of this book. They have passed on their knowledge of decades through this book. To expedite this challenging task, the publisher supported the team at every step. A small team of assistant editors was also appointed to further simplify the editing procedure and attain best results for the readers.

Apart from the editorial board, the designing team has also invested a significant amount of their time in understanding the subject and creating the most relevant covers. They scrutinized every image to scout for the most suitable representation of the subject and create an appropriate cover for the book.

The publishing team has been an ardent support to the editorial, designing and production team. Their endless efforts to recruit the best for this project, has resulted in the accomplishment of this book. They are a veteran in the field of academics and their pool of knowledge is as vast as their experience in printing. Their expertise and guidance has proved useful at every step. Their uncompromising quality standards have made this book an exceptional effort. Their encouragement from time to time has been an inspiration for everyone.

The publisher and the editorial board hope that this book will prove to be a valuable piece of knowledge for researchers, students, practitioners and scholars across the globe.

List of Contributors

Qi Yang
Center for Marine Drugs, State Key Laboratory of Oncogene and Related Genes, Department of Pharmacy, Renji Hospital, School of Medicine, Shanghai Jiao Tong University, Shanghai 200127, China
Centre for Marine Biopro ducts Development, College of Medicine and Public Health, Flinders University, Adelaide, South Australia 5042, Australia

Qi Liang
Centre for Marine Biopro ducts Development, College of Medicine and Public Health, Flinders University, Adelaide, South Australia 5042, Australia
Shanxi University of Chinese Medicine, Tai Yuan 030619, China

Biju Balakrishnan and Wei Zhang
Centre for Marine Biopro ducts Development, College of Medicine and Public Health, Flinders University, Adelaide, South Australia 5042, Australia

Damien P Belobrajdic
CSIRO Health and Biosecurity, Adelaide South Australia 5000, Australia

Qian-Jin Feng
Shanxi University of Chinese Medicine, Tai Yuan 030619, China

Chengquan Tan, Hongkui Wei, Xichen Zhao, Chuanhui Xu and Yuanfei Zhou
Department of Animal Nutrition and Feed Science, College of Animal Science and Technology, Huazhong Agricultural University, Wuhan 430070, China

Jian Peng
Department of Animal Nutrition and Feed Science, College of Animal Science and Technology, Huazhong Agricultural University, Wuhan 430070, China
The Cooperative Innovation Center for Sustainable Pig Production, Wuhan 430070, China

Sandi L. Navarro and Lesley F. Tinker
Division of Public Health Sciences, Fred Hutchinson Cancer Research Center, Seattle, WA 98109, USA

Marian L. Neuhouser, Shirley A. A. Beresford and Johanna W. Lampe
Division of Public Health Sciences, Fred Hutchinson Cancer Research Center, Seattle, WA 98109, USA
Department of Epidemiology, School of Public Health, University of Washington, Seattle, WA 98105, USA

Ting-Yuan David Cheng
Division of Cancer Prevention and Population Sciences, Roswell Park Cancer Institute, Buffalo, NY 14263, USA

James M. Shikany
Division of Preventive Medicine, University of Alabama at Birmingham, Birmingham, AL 35294, USA

Linda Snetselaar
Department of Epidemiology, University of Iowa, Iowa City, IA 52242, USA

Jessica A. Martinez
Department of Nutritional Sciences, University of Arizona Cancer Center, Tucson, AZ 85724, USA

Ikuko Kato
Department of Oncology and Pathology, Wayne State University, Detroit, MI 48201, USA

Robert S. Chapkin
Program in Integrative Nutrition and Complex Diseases, Texas A&M University, College Station, TX 77843, USA

Pilar Buil-Cosiales and Javier Díez-Espino
Atención Primaria, Servicio Navarro de Salud-Osasunbidea, 08010 Navarra, Spain
Centro de Investigación Biomédica en Red Fisiopatología de la Obesidad y Nutrición (CIBERobn), Instituto de Salud Carlos III, 28029 Madrid, Spain
IdiSNA, Navarra Institute for Health Research, 31008 Pamplona, Navarra, Spain

Miguel Angel Martinez-Gonzalez
Centro de Investigación Biomédica en Red Fisiopatología de la Obesidad y Nutrición (CIBERobn), Instituto de Salud Carlos III, 28029 Madrid, Spain
IdiSNA, Navarra Institute for Health Research, 31008 Pamplona, Navarra, Spain
Department of Preventive Medicine and Public Health, University of Navarra, 31008 Pamplona, Navarra, Spain
Department of Nutrition, Harvard School of Public Health, Boston, MA 02115, USA

Miguel Ruiz-Canela and Estefania Toledo
Centro de Investigación Biomédica en Red Fisiopatología de la Obesidad y Nutrición (CIBERobn), Instituto de Salud Carlos III, 28029 Madrid, Spain
IdiSNA, Navarra Institute for Health Research, 31008 Pamplona, Navarra, Spain
Department of Preventive Medicine and Public Health, University of Navarra, 31008 Pamplona, Navarra, Spain

Ana García-Arellano
Department of Emergency, Complejo Hospitalario de Navarra Servicio Navarro de Salud-Osasunbidea, 31008 Pamplona, Navarra, Spain

Moul Dey
Department of Health and Nutritional Sciences, South Dakota State University, Brookings, SD 57007, USA

Bret Rust and Nancy L. Keim
Department of Nutrition, University of California at Davis, 1 Shields Ave, Davis, CA 95616, USA
Western Human Nutrition Research Center, USDA-ARS, 430West Health Sciences Drive, Davis, CA 95616, USA

Danielle N. Cooper, Angela De Leon and Julita E. Baker
Department of Nutrition, University of California at Davis, 1 Shields Ave, Davis, CA 95616, USA

Mary E. Kable, William Horn and Dustin Burnett
Western Human Nutrition Research Center, USDA-ARS, 430West Health Sciences Drive, Davis, CA 95616, USA

Maria L. Marco
Food Science and Technology, University of California at Davis, 1 Shields Ave, Davis, CA 95616, USA

Samsu U. Nurdin
School of Biological Sciences, Flinders University, Adelaide, SA 5042, Australia
Department of Agricultural Product Technology, Lampung University, Bandar Lampung 35145, Indonesia
Flinders Centre for Innovation in Cancer, Adelaide, SA 5042, Australia

James C. R. Stangoulis
School of Biological Sciences, Flinders University, Adelaide, SA 5042, Australia

Catherine A. Abbott
School of Biological Sciences, Flinders University, Adelaide, SA 5042, Australia
Flinders Centre for Innovation in Cancer, Adelaide, SA 5042, Australia

Graeme P. Young
Flinders Centre for Innovation in Cancer, Adelaide, SA 5042, Australia

Richard K. Le Leu
Flinders Centre for Innovation in Cancer, Adelaide, SA 5042, Australia
CSIRO Food and Nutrition, Adelaide, SA 5000, Australia

Claus T. Christophersen
CSIRO Food and Nutrition, Adelaide, SA 5000, Australia
School of Medical and Health Sciences, Edith Cowan University, Joondalup, WA 6027, Australia

Robert E. Steinert and Daniel Raederstorff
DSM Nutritional Products Ltd., R & D Human Nutrition and Health, Basel 4057, Switzerland

Thomas M. S. Wolever
Glycemic Index Laboratories, Inc., Toronto, ON M5C 2N8, Canada

Rafaëlle M. A. van Gijssel
The Department of Epidemiology, Erasmus MC, University Medical Center, Office Na-2909, Rotterdam 3000 CA, The Netherlands
The Generation R Study Group, Erasmus MC, University Medical Center, Rotterdam 3000 CA, The Netherlands

Kim V. E. Braun, Oscar H. Franco and Trudy Voortman
The Department of Epidemiology, Erasmus MC, University Medical Center, Office Na-2909, Rotterdam 3000 CA, The Netherlands

Jessica C. Kiefte-de Jong
Department of Global Public Health, Leiden University, The Hague 3595 DG, The Netherlands
The Department of Epidemiology, Erasmus MC, University Medical Center, Office Na-2909, Rotterdam 3000 CA, The Netherlands

Vincent W. V. Jaddoe
The Department of Epidemiology, Erasmus MC, University Medical Center, Office Na-2909, Rotterdam 3000 CA, The Netherlands
The Generation R Study Group, Erasmus MC, University Medical Center, Rotterdam 3000 CA, The Netherlands
The Department of Pediatrics, Erasmus MC, University Medical Center, Rotterdam 3000 CA, The Netherlands

Tahir Rasool Qamar, Fatima Syed, Muhammad Nasir and Sanaullah Iqbal
Department of Food Science and Human Nutrition, University of Veterinary & Animal Sciences, Lahore 54000, Punjab, Pakistan

Habib Rehman
Department of Physiology, University of Veterinary & Animal Sciences, Lahore 54000, Punjab, Pakistan

Muhammad Nauman Zahid
Department of Population Medicine and Diagnostic Sciences, Cornell University, Ithaca, NY 14850, USA

Rui Hai Liu
Department of Food Science, Cornell University, Ithaca, NY 14850, USA

Sibylle Kranz
Department of Kinesiology, University of Virginia, Charlottesville, VA 22904, USA

Kevin W. Dodd
National Cancer Institute, Bethesda, MD 20892, USA

Wen Yen Juan
Nutrition Assessment and Evaluation, Office of Nutrition and Food Labeling, Center for Food and Applied Nutrition, United States Food and Drug Administration, College Park, MD 20740, USA

LuAnn K. Johnson and Lisa Jahns
United States Department of Agriculture, Agricultural Research Service, Grand Forks Human Nutrition Research Center, Grand Forks, ND 58203, USA

Maria L. Stewart and J. Paul Zimmer
Global Nutrition R & D, Ingredion Incorporated, 10 Finderne Ave, Bridgewater, NJ 08807, USA

Vicky A. Solah, Deborah A. Kerr, Wendy J. Hunt, Haelee K. Fenton and Stuart K. Johnson
School of Public Health, Faculty of Health Sciences, Curtin University, Perth WA 6845, Australia

Carol J. Boushey
Epidemiology Program, University of Hawaii Cancer Center, Honolulu, HI 96813, USA

Edward J. Delp
Video and Image Processing Laboratory, School of Electrical and Computer Engineering, Purdue University, West Lafayette, IN 47907, USA

Xingqiong Meng
Flinders Centre for Innovation in Cancer, School of Medicine, Flinders University, Adelaide 5001, Australia

Roland J. Gahler
Factors Group R & D, Burnaby, BC V3N4S9, Canada

Anthony P. James
School of Public Health, Faculty of Health Sciences, Curtin University, Perth WA 6845, Australia
Curtin Health Innovation Research Institute, Faculty of Health Sciences, Curtin University, Perth WA 6845, Australia

Aqif S. Mukhtar
School of Public Health, Faculty of Health Sciences, Curtin University, Perth WA 6845, Australia
Centre for Population Health Research, Faculty of Health Sciences, Curtin University, Perth WA 6845, Australia

Simon Wood
School of Public Health, Faculty of Health Sciences, Curtin University, Perth WA 6845, Australia
InovoBiologic Inc., Calgary, AB Y2N4Y7, Canada
Food, Nutrition and Health Program, University of British Columbia, Vancouver, BC V6T1Z4, Canada

Athanasios Koutsos
Hugh Sinclair Unit of Human Nutrition and the Institute for Cardiovascular and Metabolic Research (ICMR), Department of Food and Nutritional Sciences, University of Reading, Whiteknights, Reading RG6 6AP, UK
Nutrition & Nutrigenomics Unit, Department of Food Quality and Nutrition, Research and Innovation Centre, Fondazione Edmund Mach (FEM), Via Mach 1, 38010 San Michele all'Adige, TN, Italy

Julie A. Lovegrove
Hugh Sinclair Unit of Human Nutrition and the Institute for Cardiovascular and Metabolic Research (ICMR), Department of Food and Nutritional Sciences, University of Reading, Whiteknights, Reading RG6 6AP, UK

Maria Lima, Lorenza Conterno, Martina Bianchi, Francesca Fava and Kieran M. Tuohy
Nutrition & Nutrigenomics Unit, Department of Food Quality and Nutrition, Research and Innovation Centre, Fondazione Edmund Mach (FEM), Via Mach 1, 38010 San Michele all'Adige, TN, Italy

Mattia Gasperotti and Urska Vrhovsek
Metabolomics Unit, Department of Food Quality and Nutrition, Research and Innovation Centre, Fondazione Edmund Mach (FEM), Via Mach 1, 38010 San Michele all'Adige, TN, Italy

Parvin Mirmiran, Zahra Bahadoran and Sajad Khalili Moghadam
Nutrition and Endocrine Research Center, Student Research Committee, Research Institute for Endocrine Sciences, Shahid Beheshti University of Medical Sciences, No. 24, Shahid-Erabi St., Yeman St., Velenjak, Tehran 19395-4763, Iran

Azita Zadeh Vakili
Cellular and Molecular Endocrine Research Center, Obesity Research Center, Research Institute for Endocrine Sciences, Shahid Beheshti University of Medical Sciences, No. 24, Shahid-Erabi St., Yeman St., Velenjak, Tehran 19395-4763, Iran

Fereidoun Azizi
Endocrine Research Center, Research Institute for Endocrine Sciences, Shahid Beheshti University of Medical Sciences, No. 24, Shahid-Erabi St., Yeman St., Velenjak, Tehran 19395-4763, Iran

Genelle Healey
Massey Institute of Food Science and Technology, School of Food and Nutrition, Massey University, Palmerston North 4442, New Zealand
Food, Nutrition and Health, The New Zealand Institute for Plant & Food Research Limited, Palmerston North 4442, New Zealand

Duncan Hedderley and Chrissie Butts
Food, Nutrition and Health, The New Zealand Institute for Plant & Food Research Limited, Palmerston North 4442, New Zealand

Louise Brough and Jane Coad
Massey Institute of Food Science and Technology, School of Food and Nutrition, Massey University, Palmerston North 4442, New Zealand

Rinki Murphy
Faculty of Medical and Health Sciences, The University of Auckland, Auckland 1023, New Zealand

Index

www.ingramcontent.com/pod-product-compliance
Lightning Source LLC
LaVergne TN
LVHW080928210926
848485LV00004B/754
9781646465651